BILINGUAL SPEECH-LANGUAGE PATHOLOGY

AN HISPANIC FOCUS

CULTURE, REHABILITATION, AND EDUCATION SERIES
SERIES EDITOR
Orlando L. Taylor, Ph.D.

Bilingual Speech-Language Pathology: An
Hispanic Focus
Edited by Hortencia Kayser, Ph.D.

Integrating Language and Learning for
Inclusion: An Asian/Pacific Focus
Edited by Li-Rong Lilly Cheng, Ph.D.

BILINGUAL
SPEECH-LANGUAGE
PATHOLOGY

AN HISPANIC FOCUS

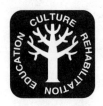

EDITED BY

HORTENCIA KAYSER, PH.D.
UNIVERSITY OF ARIZONA
TUCSON, ARIZONA

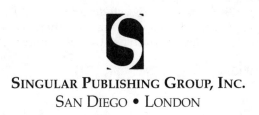

SINGULAR PUBLISHING GROUP, INC.
SAN DIEGO • LONDON

Singular Publishing Group, Inc.
4284 41st Street
San Diego, California 92105-1197

19 Compton Terrace
London, England N1 20N

© 1995 by Singular Publishing Group, Inc.

Typeset in 10/12 Palatino by So Cal Graphics
Printed in the United States of America by McNaughton & Gunn

Library of Congress Cataloging-in-Publication Data

Bilingual speech-language pathology: an Hispanic focus / edited
 by Hortencia Kayser
      p.   cm. — (Culture, rehabilitation, and education series)
   Includes bibliographical references and index.
   ISBN 1-56593-205-6   (pb)
   1. Language disorders.   2. Speech disorders.   3. Hispanic
Americans—Language.   4. Hispanic American handicapped—
Rehabilitation.   I. Kayser, Hortense Garcia Ramirez, 1947–
II. Series
RC429.856 1995
616.85'5—dc20   95-9820
                                                           CIP

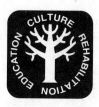

CONTENTS

Foreword by Orlando L. Taylor, Ph.D.   **IX**

Preface   **XIII**

Contributors   **XVII**

Acknowledgments   **XIX**

1   An Emerging Specialist: **1**
The Bilingual Speech-Language Pathologist
Hortencia Kayser, Ph.D.

PART I
SPEECH AND LANGUAGE DEVELOPMENT,
DISORDERS, ASSESSMENT,
AND INTERVENTION   15

2   Spanish Phonological Development   **17**
Brian A. Goldstein, Ph.D.

3   Spanish Morphological and Syntactic Development   **41**
Raquel T. Anderson, Ph.D.

4   "Early Intervention? Qué Quiere Decir Éso?" / . . .   **75**
What Does That Mean?
Rosemary Quinn, Ph.D.

5   Narrative Development and Disorders in Spanish-speaking   **97**
Children: Implications for the Bilingual Interventionist
Vera F. Gutierrez-Clellen, Ph.D.

6 Language Assessment and Instructional Programming **129**
for Linguistically Different Learners: Proactive
Classroom Processes
Elizabeth D. Peña, Ph.D., and
Luciano Valles, Jr., M.S.

7 Considerations in the Assessment and Treatment of **153**
Neurogenic Communication Disorders in Bilingual Adults
Belinda A. Reyes, Ph.D.

PART II
ASSESSMENT ISSUES AND CONSIDERATIONS **183**

8 Bilingualism, Myths, and Language Impairments **185**
Hortencia Kayser, Ph.D.

9 Interpreters **207**
Hortencia Kayser, Ph.D.

10 Intelligence Testing of Hispanic Students **223**
Jozi DeLéon, Ph.D.

11 Assessment of Speech and Language Impairments **243**
in Bilingual Children
Hortencia Kayser, Ph.D.

12 Language Samples: Elicitation and Analysis **265**
Hortencia Kayser, Ph.D., and
María Adeliada Restrepo, M.A.

PART III
CONCLUSIONS **289**

13 Research Needs and Conclusions **291**
Hortencia Kayser, Ph.D.

APPENDIXES

A English and Spanish Professional Terminology **307**

B   Spanish Case History Form   **313**

C   English and Spanish Parent Letter   **321**

Index   **329**

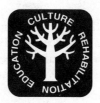

FOREWORD

This book is first in a series of books on "Culture, Rehabilitation, and Education in Culturally and Linguistically Diverse Populations." The series represents the first major effort to present, in a comprehensive, interdisciplinary manner, the state of the literature on culture and its impact on rehabilitation in a variety of fields, especially the field of communication disorder.

The series focuses on this rather broad array of disciplines in response to the changing environment in which health care, rehabilitation, and education are offered, particularly in the United States. It is increasingly the rule that speech-language clinicians, teachers, social workers, psychologists, nurses, physical therapists, and others work in collaboration to provide services for the **whole** person. For school-age individuals, one cannot readily divorce the services provided to individuals who are disabled in clinics and hospitals from those provided in schools. Thus, the eclectic approach of this series will enable readers to see how culture affects the full range of services offered to individuals who are disabled in a variety of settings and from a variety of disciplines.

At the dawn of the 21st century, the topic of cultural diversity has permeated virtually all disciplines within the social, behavioral, and rehabilitation sciences, as well as the field of education. Beginning in the late 1960s and continuing to the present, research, theory, and clinical practice have increasingly considered topics pertaining to culture as they relate to the nature and acquisition of "normal" behavior and function, and to issues pertaining to the nature, assessment, and management of various disorders and disabilities.

Scholars and practitioners have advanced several reasons for increased interest in cultural considerations in understanding normal behavior and disabilities. Some of these reasons have focused on the rapid demographic changes that have occurred in the United States.

Others have focused on the establishment of increased ethical and legal requirements for gender, race, and disability equity. Still others have focused on theoretical requirements for considering cultural issues in addressing topics of development (acquisition), assessment, and intervention.

The demographic issue cannot be overemphasized. According to the 1990 census, for example, people of color (African Americans, Hispanics, Asian Americans, Native Americans, Aleuts, Eskimos, Pacific Islanders, and others) comprised almost 28% of the American population. Moreover, they comprised more than 35% of the school-age children and were the majority of the population in most of America's urban centers. If current birth rates and immigration patterns continue, they will comprise a majority of the American population by the middle of the 21st century. This is true already in the state of California, and will become so in Texas by the turn of the century. More importantly, these rapidly growing populations will continue to comprise a substantial portion of the pool of individuals seeking services from professionals in the rehabilitation and educational fields.

To assure that these professionals are prepared to provide such services, it is important—indeed imperative—that they are well informed on the nature of culture and its effect on normal behavior and disability. In the field of communication disorders, for example, clinicians must be fully informed on the nature of the family and community environments in which speech and language behavior are acquired. They must know how to infuse notions pertaining to cultural diversity into assessment, diagnostic, and intervention strategies.

A good case also can be made to use legal issues and legislative mandates to validate the notion of cultural considerations in the rehabilitation fields and education. In addition to the presence of such laws as the Americans with Disabilities Act, federal law, for example, requires nondiscrimination in the assessment, diagnosis, educational placement, and provision of rehabilitation services to children with communicative disorders and other special needs in public school settings. Clearly, the intention and substance of these laws and mandates cannot be achieved unless the professional workforce is well informed on the nature of culture and its effect on education and rehabilitation.

More important than demographic and legal issues, for purely theoretical reasons the topic of culture and cultural diversity should permeate every aspect of the disciplines that provide services to the disabled. Even without the legal, ethical, or demographic factors, we are required to address the nature of culture if we are to have valid notions about the nature of normal and disabled behavior and function. The reasons for such a claim is obvious.

First, all behavior—and especially communicative behavior—is acquired within a family/community context. With respect to communication, for example, culture determines everything from the language/dialect to be acquired, and their cognitive underpinnings, to how communication is used as a function of purpose, audience, and meaning.

Second, the determination of what is and is not "normal"—and what to do about "abnormal" behavior and function—is culturally determined. Also, certain culturally based genetic, social, physical, and nutritional issues can result in differences in prevalence and etiology considerations for some disorders in different groups (e.g., sickle cell anemia in African Americans).

Finally, intervention issues in all disciplines should be culturally driven if they are to be effective. Everything from the instruments employed to assess behavior and the interactions with the client and family members to the underlying intervention strategies and the materials used in intervention settings should all be culturally driven.

The focus on bilingual populations for the first book in this series is not accidental. Increasingly, the population of the United States consists of individuals who speak a language other than English, or live in homes where more than one language is spoken, or personally speak two or more languages, with English **perhaps** being one of them. In those cases where the person speaks more than one language, the level of proficiency in any one of them may vary. Indeed, the individual may not be proficient in **any** of the languages that he or she speaks, even the dominant language.

No matter what the circumstances are, the number of languages spoken, or the matter of proficiency or dominance, the rehabilitation specialist or educator will increasingly encounter bilingual—or even multilingual—persons seeking services. For example, close to 10% of the American people are Hispanic—many of whom are bilingual— and this population increased by approximately 50% between the period 1980–1990. At its current rate of growth, this population is expected to overcome African Americans to become the nation's largest minority by the year 2000.

In this book, Kayser and her collaborators present a thorough analysis of the theories, issues, and myths pertaining to language and cognitive assessment, education, and intervention with bilingual children and adults. Relying on the wealth of research that has emerged over the past 25 or so years, the book provides a source book for clinicians, educators, academicians, researchers, and students to understand the nature and acquisition of normal language and acquisition in bilingual populations, with a focus on Spanish and Spanish-English bilingual persons.

Focusing heavily on the Hispanic population, the book presents culturally and linguistically valid ways for assessing language and communication in bilingual children and adults and how to appropriately provide educational and clinical management services to bilingual individuals. Contrary to most books in communication disorders which focus almost exclusively on children, Kayser and her co-authors consider the full age range of individuals within the bilingual population from the very young child through aged adults.

A new America—a multicultural America—is just over the horizon. As a result, rehabilitation workers, communication disorders specialists, and educators will face new challenges—and opportunities—in the years ahead. However, the emergence of new basic and applied data and theory pertaining to culture, behavior, disability, and intervention will permit us to meet these challenges and opportunities with unprecedented success.

Orlando L. Taylor, Ph.D.

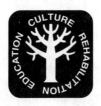

PREFACE

Over the years I have developed outlines on topics for presentations I thought were important for speech-language pathologists who provide services to Hispanic children to understand and know. Over the years these topics have become areas of expertise for some outstanding new doctorates in the field of bilingual speech-language pathology. This book is a presentation of these authors' work and my own thoughts and research on bilingualism, assessment, and research methodology. Much of what is presented in this book is a combination of literature review, case studies, original unpublished research, and the authors' perspectives and experiences with Hispanic children and adults. I have also included material from interviews with clinicians who work with Hispanic students.

This book was written for speech-language pathologists who work with Spanish-English speaking children and adults with communicative impairments. The clinician may be bilingual, English speaking only, or desire to become bilingual. The information may be introductory for some clinicians, but hopefully it will be new and advanced information for the majority of speech-language pathologists who read this book. This book does not cover every possible topic that affects Hispanic populations; but it focuses on the areas that most frequently confront clinicians in practice, such as phonological and language disorders, early intervention, narrative development, school-age populations, and adults. The purpose of this book is to present clinicians with information that combines research and application so that it can serve as a resource in the management of Hispanic children and adults with communicative impairments.

This book is divided into three parts with an introductory and concluding chapter concerning research. In Chapter 1, I review the standards defined by the American Speech-Language-Hearing Association for academic and language proficiency for bilingual speech-language pathologists and then provide suggestions for developing these competencies.

Part I has six chapters devoted to the topics of speech and language development, disorders, and intervention with Hispanic children and adults. Each of the authors has developed an expertise concerning Spanish speaking individuals at different age levels and language skills. In Chapter 2, Brian Goldstein provides a review of the Spanish phonological system, dialects, normative data, assessment, and intervention with children with phonological disorders. In Chapter 3, Raquel Anderson discusses the morphosyntactic patterns of Spanish, development of these features in children, and the use of this information in assessment and intervention. In Chapter 4, Rosemary Quinn reviews the traditional understanding of early language socialization practices and relates them to literature and research on Hispanics. She then discusses how this information can be used to adapt early intervention services for Hispanic populations. Vera Gutierrez-Clellen presents a thorough review of the development of narratives in children in Chapter 5 and discusses samples of her research with Spanish-speaking children. Elizabeth Peña and Luciano Valles then discuss, in Chapter 6, the instructional needs and adaptations necessary for Hispanic students in the classroom and the changing roles of the speech-language pathologist. In Chapter 7, Belinda Reyes discusses the many issues related to language in adult bilinguals and the different needs of the Hispanic adult neurogenic patient.

Part II has five chapters devoted to issues related to the assessment of Spanish-speaking children. In Chapter 8, the development of bilingualism and myths that exist among speech-language pathologists about bilingualism and communicative impairments are discussed. These myths are prevalent among practicing clinicians who do not understand the dynamics of learning two languages. In Chapter 9, I discuss the issues related to the selection, training, and use of interpreters in the assessment process. Jozi DeLéon, a bilingual special educator and educational diagnostician, then presents a review of the practices and her own experiences in intelligence testing of Hispanic students in Chapter 10. Recommended procedures for speech and language assessment are presented in Chapter 11. Maria Adelaida Restrepo and I present the elicitation and analysis of language samples in Chapter 12. This chapter is of special significance because it details analysis procedures for Spanish speakers.

Chapter 13 is on research and my concluding remarks. I present an argument that researchers and research methodology must change and adapt to the culture and population that is being studied. The chapter includes a review of a working group on minority research and training needs held by the National Institute on Deafness and Other Communication Disorders. This chapter is a call for clinicians to become field researchers to expand the knowledge concerning Hispanic children and adults. Suggestions are made concerning the first steps toward research mentorship and collaboration with university researchers.

Speech-language pathologists face a formidable task in providing appropriate services to Hispanic populations. This book is an attempt to gather information that will help clinicians in their daily decisions in assessment and intervention with Hispanic children and adults.

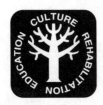

CONTRIBUTORS

Raquel T. Anderson, Ph.D.
Indiana University
Bloomington, Indiana

Jozi DeLéon, Ph.D.
New Mexico State University
Las Cruces, New Mexico

Brian A. Goldstein, Ph.D.
St. Louis University
St. Louis, Missouri

Vera F. Gutierrez-Clellan, Ph.D.
San Diego State University
San Diego, California

Hortencia Kayser, Ph.D.
University of Arizona
Tucson, Arizona

Elizabeth Peña, Ph.D.
University of Texas at Austin
Austin, Texas

Rosemary Quinn, Ph.D.
University of Texas—
    Pan American
Edinburg, Texas

Maria Adelaida Restrepo, M.A.
University of Arizona
Tucson, Arizona

Belinda Reyes, Ph.D.
University of Texas at El Paso
El Paso, Texas

Luciano Valles, Jr., M.S.
University of Massachusetts
Amherst, Massachusetts

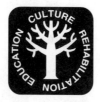

ACKNOWLEDGMENTS

I want to thank the Department of Speech and Hearing Sciences and the National Center for Neurogenic Communication Disorders, University of Arizona, who helped support part of the writing of this book (Research and Training Center Grant No. 1P60 DC-01409, National Institute on Deafness and Other Communication Disorders). Also, I am grateful to the many bilingual graduate students whom I have had the honor of teaching and mentoring over the years. They worked many long hours in transcribing, typing, and giving me feedback on my thoughts, manuscripts, and lectures. Their dedication to the field of speech-language pathology and the Hispanic population they serve has always encouraged me about the future of this profession.

DEDICATION

Some wonderful women helped mold me as a person, educator, and researcher. This book is dedicated to:

Guadalupe Garcia Ramirez (1907–1961),
a Godly woman and my mother;

Frances Ramos, Cecilia Rodriguez, and Eugenia Gomez,
my sisters and spiritual mothers;

Guadalupe Valdes, Ph.D., and Rosalinda Barrera, Ph.D.,
my first Hispanic professors and role models;

Marylee Norris, M.S., and Jennifer Watson, Ph.D.,
friends who understood and supported my work with Hispanic students;

Daisy Tomassini-Gancitano, Ph.D.
a friend who taught me the value of rest;

Audrey Holland, Ph.D., and Tanya Gallagher, Ph.D.,
friends and research mentors who have helped me to focus my research goals and career.

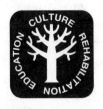

CHAPTER 1

AN EMERGING SPECIALIST: THE BILINGUAL SPEECH-LANGUAGE PATHOLOGIST

HORTENCIA KAYSER, Ph.D.

My career began in May of 1975 when I obtained a B.S. degree in Speech Pathology from a university in North Texas. Having received little professional guidance in my training program I quickly bid farewell to my university life and in September embarked on my first career experience as a public school speech-language pathologist in South Texas. I soon found myself providing therapy to predominately Mexican American and African-American children whose cultural and linguistic differences, unfortunately, made them prime candidates for

(continued)

special education services. I can still remember how I felt during those 4 years (working) when I would have conversations with fellow colleagues who were monolingual clinicians, and it was assumed that I would know the answers to all the language and academic woes of bilingual children. The emotions ranged from inadequacy to anger to intense moral obligation and responsibility to find the answers. Many people assumed that by nature of my Mexican American background and being bilingual I would have the answers.

Upon completion of my masters degree from the bilingual speech-language pathology program at Texas Christian University, I headed West . . . to Tucson, Arizona and entered the world of hospital rehabilitation services as a bilingual speech-language pathologist for my CFY. During my 18 months at the rehabilitation hospital, I found my job description growing by the day. I became a counselor, interpreter, family advocate, social worker, translator, and spokesperson for concerns expressed by my clients and their families. Any interest on my part to specialize in an area was met with, "oh, but you're bilingual; you don't have the luxury to specialize. You need to know about all disorders because you're needed in all areas." Feeling a need to return to public school work, I obtained a position with a local school district. During my 9 years in the Tucson schools, I worked primarily as a member of a bilingual diagnostic team. Those years as a public school clinician were some of the most important learning experiences I have had. The wealth of knowledge I received and accumulated from the children I evaluated, the parents I conferenced with, and my fellow colleagues has enriched me professionally in a way I am unable to express adequately in words.

Graciela Garcia, M.S., CCC-SLP
Clinical Instructor
University of Texas at Pan American
Edinburg, Texas

ASHA-certified bilingual speech-language pathologists are rare in the profession. In this elite group of clinicians, the number who have been educated and trained as bilingual specialists is even smaller. Those who have practiced as bilingual clinicians without specific training recognize that there are limitations to their clinical competencies because of this omission in their graduate education. Once these individuals face the multifaceted situations that arise in assessment and intervention with bilingual, bicultural clients, continuing education in multicultural topics becomes a priority. Bilingual clinicians across the country are concerned about the quality of the services they provide. They are also concerned about issues that distinguish them as a group, such as speciality recognition, second language competency, academic competencies, and, to the non-native speaker of Spanish, cultural sensitivity. Speciality recognition with standards and guidelines may be part of the future for these clinicians. What many speech-language pathologists do not know is that standards concerning academic, clinical, and language proficiency have been developed by the American Speech-Language-Hearing Association (ASHA). The purpose of this chapter is to discuss ASHA's role in defining competencies and language proficiency of bilingual specialists and how these competencies can be developed.

⊔

POSITION STATEMENTS

Although ASHA has attempted to address the issues surrounding competencies for bilingual clinicians, the specific knowledge base and linguistic competencies are generally defined by a small number of academicians, as well as individual bilingual clinicians. ASHA initially recommended academic competencies through a position statement concerning the "Clinical Management of Communicatively Handicapped Minority Language Populations" (ASHA, 1985). The purpose of this position statement was to "recommend competencies for assessment and remediation of communicative disorders of minority language speakers and to describe alternative strategies that can be utilized when those competencies are not met" (p. 29). Five competencies for bilingual clinicians were identified as necessary for the assessment and remediation in the minority language. These included: (1) language proficiency: native or near native fluency in both the minority language and the English language; (2) normative processes: the ability to describe the process of normal speech and language acquisition for both bilingual and monolingual individuals and how those processes are manifested in oral and written language; (3) assessment: the ability to administer and interpret formal and informal assessment procedures to distinguish between communication difference and communication disorders; (4) intervention: the ability to apply intervention strategies for treatment of communicative disorders in the minority language; and (5) cultural sensitivity: the ability to recognize cultural factors that affect the delivery of speech-language pathology and audiology services to the minority language speaking community. This position statement was of particular importance because it served as the basis for curriculum development for many minority emphasis programs. The actual content for these courses depended on the individual universities. Some programs in speech-language pathology had only one course that was seminar and discussion based, whereas other universities offered two or three courses that emphasized sociolinguistics, second language acquisition, and assessment and intervention. Therefore, the specific content that a bilingual clinician should know has not been determined by any group or organization.

Within ASHA, two groups have attempted to assist clinicians with the academic competencies to serve bilingual, bicultural populations. The Multicultural Issues Board (ASHA, 1995) has developed current reading lists that can be used by clinicians as well as graduate students for independent study. The ASHA Hispanic Caucus has attempted to network clinicians for independent study. There are resources, but clinicians must seek out these individuals, agencies, and organizations to obtain the information.

One attempt by ASHA to outline linguistic competency was through the development of a definition for a bilingual speech-language pathologist and audiologist. The primary purpose for the ASHA definition of "bilingual" was to protect the public from clinicians who claim to have bilingual abilities when in fact they may not speak the second language fluently (ASHA, 1989). This definition offered guidelines for bilingual professionals as well as professionals who aspired to become bilingual. The definition (ASHA, 1989) states:

> Speech-language pathologists or audiologists who present themselves as bilingual for the purposes of providing clinical services must be able to speak their primary language and to speak (or sign) at least one other language with native or near-native proficiency in lexicon (vocabulary), semantics (meaning), phonology (pronunciation), morphology/syntax (grammar), and pragmatics (uses) during clinical management. (p. 93)

This definition was a compromise between two extremes of the association membership. There are bilingual clinicians who adhere to a strict definition of bilingualism, that is, the clinician must be balanced and have equal abilities in both languages. The other extreme is defended by clinicians and agencies who recognize that there are not enough native speakers of Spanish who can qualify under the strict definition. Once a compromise definition was presented to the Executive Board of ASHA, the definition was slightly revised. After presentation to the Legislative Council for vote as a position statement of the association, the definition was once again revised. The definition was debated, but it was passed by the Legislative Council.

What does this definition mean to practicing ASHA-certified clinicians? It sets a standard for bilingualism in the professions of speech-language pathology and audiology. ASHA-certified clinicians who identify themselves as bilingual are now bound by the ASHA Code of Ethics for practice. Clinicians who are not near native-like in the second language can be brought before the Board of Code of Ethics (ASHA, 1994) for practicing in the minority language when their linguistic skills are not adequate. But what happens to clinicians who want to become bilingual or the assimilated Hispanic who understands Spanish and desires to become actively proficient in Spanish? This will be discussed in the next section on language proficiency.

I consider myself an "academic bilingual." Being of Scandinavian descent and having grown up in northern Minnesota, I grew up in an English only home. In ninth grade, I took my first of three high school Spanish courses. During my third year, I was fortunate to be able to spend 15 days in Spain with my Spanish class. After that trip to Spain, I made it a personal goal to become fluent in Spanish. My parents were very supportive of this goal. Having participated in eye care missions to Mexico, Guatemala, and Colombia, my mother and step-father instilled within me an interest in and appreciation for other cultures. In addition, they introduced me to two women, one from Colombia and one from Argentina, and I was able to practice my classroom Spanish in a very meaningful way. I spent one semester of my college years at the Universidad de las Americas in Puebla, Puebla, Mexico. I looked for ways I could use my Spanish within the field of speech-language pathology and enrolled into the bilingual program in speech-language pathology at Texas Christian University. Currently, I am a staff speech-language pathologist in the outpatient speech clinic. Approximately 50 percent of my personal caseload is made up of children from Spanish-speaking or bilingual homes. I evaluate two to three new patients per week,

(continued)

most of whom are Spanish-speaking. In addition, I have a small private practice. Within this private practice, I see one child individually, and I also provide evaluations for a Head Start center. The majority of my Spanish-speaking clients are of Mexican or Puerto Rican descent. Many are from inner city neighborhoods and would be considered low socio-economic status.

Deanine Paulson, M.S., CCC-SLP
Children's Memorial Hospital
Chicago, Illinois

⊥┐

COMPETENCIES OF BILINGUAL SPEECH-LANGUAGE PATHOLOGISTS

LANGUAGE COMPETENCIES

In the last 20 years, the American Speech-Language-Hearing Association has seen a growth in the number of Hispanic (ASHA, 1993) clinicians. The ASHA census reported that in 1975 there were 50 Hispanic ASHA-certified clinicians. In 1993 there were 705 Hispanic speech-language pathologists certified by ASHA (ASHA, 1993). Although the number of bilingual, bicultural clinicians (certified and uncertified) in the United States is not known, it is possible that many of these individuals are not linguistically prepared to address the needs of the Hispanic communicatively impaired. An area of concern for many faculty and agencies is the **English** language proficiency of Hispanic clinicians. The level of proficiency in the **Spanish** language does not often receive the attention and importance that it deserves. Hispanic clinicians who are primarily Spanish speaking must "prove" their English competency, but primarily English-speaking clinicians do not have to develop or demonstrate competency in Spanish. An agency and faculty of a speech-language pathology program should be concerned about bilingual clinical competencies.

Certification of bilingual competencies has been recommended for clinicians, especially for those who are not certain about their linguistic level in English or Spanish. Certification of language proficiency can be obtained through language testing services or through testing services in university language programs or by State Education Agencies that certify bilingual education teachers. Whichever mechanism is chosen by the clinician, testing of language proficiency ensure native, nonnative, and near-native bilingual clinicians and their clients that the level of English or Spanish ability is appropriate for "clinical management"(ASHA, 1989. p. 93).

HETEROGENEITY OF BILINGUAL CLINICIANS

Bilingual individuals are a heterogeneous group who have differing levels of proficiency in the two languages. Westby (1991) describes the language use of bilinguals as a continuum. Traditional individuals will prefer to use the native language in the home and community. Neo-traditionalists generally prefer using the native language at home but have adopted the second language for other domains, such as school and work. Transitional persons prefer the native language in the home and intimate social relationships, but use English for community and external relationships. Bicultural individuals use English as the preferred language and the parents prefer the home language. Acculturated persons use English in the home and community and have lost use of the native language. Pan-Renaissance individuals, who are not bilingual, use English as their primary and only language. No two persons are similar in their abilities to speak the same two languages.

Many bilingual clinicians are concerned about their own bilingualism. Some individuals expect perfection from themselves and those they serve. But frequently, clinicians may have excellent abilities in English and average abilities in Spanish or vice versa. Very few bilingual persons have equal abilities in the two languages. Additionally, many individuals may believe that once bilingual always bilingual, this is not the case (Baetens-Beardsmore, 1986). Bilingual speakers do quickly lose the ability to speak a language that is not actively used with other speakers of that language. For example, Hispanic clinicians may lose some ability to speak their home language during undergraduate and graduate training. The same is true for students who are gaining proficiency in English. Bilingualism is dynamic, and fluency does change without practice.

LANGUAGE AND CULTURE

Linguistic competency in English and Spanish is important, but we often forget that the clinician's culture also is brought into the use of these languages. Saville-Troike (1986) defines culture as the knowledge individuals need to be functional members of a community. This includes the rules for interactions, appropriate behaviors, and the regulation of interactions with individuals from different cultural backgrounds. When there is contact with another culture, the individual members of the community may either assimilate and acculturate the new group's view of the world. *Acculturation* is acceptance of selected rules for interactions and different values of the second culture, while still adhering to the rules of the home culture. *Assimilation* is the acceptance of various values, ideas, and so on of the new culture and rejection of differing cultural values and expectations from the home culture (Peñalosa, 1980). Bilingual-bicultural clinicians have differing levels of acculturation and assimilation. They bring with them individual life experiences that will make them appear either more traditional or very "Americanized," and many fall between these two extremes.

NATIVE AND NONNATIVE BILINGUALS

Hispanic clinicians from Latin American countries do not have the same experiences as Hispanic clinicians born in the United States who were reared in communities where two languages were spoken. Latin Americans face formidable tasks in learning a new culture and language that are different from their own backgrounds. Their tasks are to develop an awareness of a new culture and to learn as much as possible about the people they will serve. The same is true for the Anglo bilingual student who must learn about the Hispanic cultures and population. Latin American and Anglo bilingual students may become bilingual and culturally sensitive to the second culture, but may never become bicultural (Kayser, 1993).

BICULTURALISM IN NATIVE BILINGUALS

Bicultural sensitivity and awareness is an important aspect of becoming a bilingual speech-language pathologist. Clinicians must be sensitive to their own biculturalism. There may be behaviors or roles between speakers that are acceptable in one culture but are considered inappropriate in the second culture. As an example, a young Anglo clinician may feel that it is acceptable to counsel an Hispanic mother on language development or behavior management of children. But, for some young Hispanic women, this situation may be difficult or awkward because their traditional cultural rule would state that an older woman with children would know more about child rearing than a young woman with no children. There must be an awareness of what "feels uncomfortable," and clinicians must identify measures that are effective in that culture.

Bilingual-bicultural clinicians must also become metaculturally aware of their verbal and nonverbal interactions. Each clinician brings her or his own cultural expectations into the clinical situation. Taylor (1986) describes cultural assumptions, verbal and nonverbal behaviors, and rules of interaction that clinicians bring to the clinical event. He states that clients also bring their own assumptions about behaviors that are appropriate for interactions. When bilingual-bicultural clinicians enter the clinician-client exchange with monolingual speakers of either language, they face the possibility of miscommunication that springs from their bilingualism and biculturalism. Clinician interactions with Hispanic clients may have transference of elements from the mainstream Anglo culture, and interactions with mainstream Anglo clients may have elements from the Hispanic culture. These elements may be phonological, morphological, semantic, syntactic, and/or pragmatic. For example, Spanish uses context in combination with nonspecific markers such as this, that, and those to refer to objects. The Spanish speaker learns to combine observation, context, and the nonspecific referents to communicate. Hispanic clinicians may use this style of speaking and use nonspecific pronouns while speaking in English. This element from Spanish has transfered to English. Clinicians should learn to recognize these features in their own speech, language, and nonverbal behaviors.

Recognition and identification of these features in communication can be facilitated through discussions with supervisors, other minority and majority clinicians, and continual self-monitoring. Monitoring of speech and language behaviors can be achieved through videotaping sessions and open discussion about what behaviors appeared to be awkward and what style of speech is more appropriate. These types of discussions with colleagues provide opportunities to recognize the effectiveness of and differences in styles of communication. The Hispanic and mainstream cultures cannot be underestimated in their effects on the clinical interactions during assessment and intervention.

CLINICAL PRACTICUM IN ENGLISH AND SPANISH

Ethically, to practice as a bilingual speech-language pathologist or audiologist, clinicians must have the clinical training to be able to provide services in both languages. The ability to speak two languages is not enough. Practice in the use of professional language in specific situations such as interviewing, assessing, and providing intervention for children and adults, as well as counseling, is needed for main-stream English-speaking students; the same clinical skills are needed in the Spanish language. Bilingualism can be developed with time and encouragement, but the individual must have more than an occasional encounter with an Hispanic client to become competent as a bilingual speech-language pathologist.

There are a number of suggestions for clinicians who desire to increase their bilingualism. These include: video libraries of a variety of evaluations, intervention, and conference sessions and clinical observations with a bilingual clinician in the area, a neighboring state, or in a Spanish-speaking country. It may also be feasible to arrange clinical sabbaticals at a university that trains bilingual clinicians. This would allow the speech-language pathologist an opportunity to observe, participate, and receive feedback from bilingual clinical supervisors who regularly train bilingual student clinicians.

DEVELOPING BILINGUALISM

Individuals can become balanced bilinguals through a number of exercises and experiences. Practice in pronunciation or accent reduction is only a small part of the goal. There must be role playing of specific situations and clinical events. Videotaping the clinician's conference sessions, assessment, and intervention sessions are helpful in identifying areas for practice. Group sessions with other bilingual professionals are especially helpful.

Clinicians who begin the process of bilingualism with minimal second language speaking ability (e.g., rudimentary syntax) may need additional experiences to develop near-native proficiency in the second language as required by ASHA's bilingual definition. If a clinician is experiencing great difficulty in expression in the second language, practice with native monolingual speakers (e.g., church, Latin or mainstream organizations, etc.) is recommended. A summer Spanish or English language immersion program may also be helpful for some individuals.

I was born in Hollis, New York, the product of Puerto Rican parents. While in elementary school, my parents decided it was time to return to the homeland, Puerto Rico. This is where I was raised and spent my later elementary and adolescent years. After high school graduation, I moved to New York to pursue a college education: the first in my immediate family. I arrived in New York in 1979, and thanks to a full scholarship, obtained a bachelor's degree in Speech Communication from Long Island University, Brooklyn Campus. In 1984 I was accepted into the master's program in Speech-Language Pathology at Teachers College, Columbia University. By the time I started my Clinical Fellowship Year I knew that working with the adult neurologically impaired population was my interest area, as well as the assessment and treatment of dysphagia. Although I have been well able to pursue this route, I also felt a "pull" toward pediatric issues in bilingualism. This was fueled, in part, by my increasing awareness of widespread misdiagnoses of bilingual children and the lack of appropriate speech-language services available to the Hispanic community. At present, I am in private practice in Brooklyn, New York. My associate and I provide speech-language and dysphagia services to acute care and long-term care settings; teach undergraduate courses in anatomy and physiology of the head and neck; and serve a primarily bilingual pediatric population in our office.

Luis F. Riquelme, M.S., CCC-SLP
Riquelme & Santo
Speech-Language Pathology
Brooklyn, New York

ACADEMIC COMPETENCIES

The academic competencies for bilingual clinicians, as stated in the position statement on Clinical Management of Communicatively Handicapped Minority-Language Populations (ASHA, 1985), focus on three areas: normal processes, assessment, and intervention. The question for most clinicians is how to attain these competencies. Continuing education is the most obvious answer, but convention sessions often provide either basic information or technical research, or assume considerable background knowledge on the topic.

For a clinician who lives near a university with an Hispanic emphasis program, the solution would be to enroll in a course(s). If this is not possible an alternative would be to write the faculty member and ask if the course could be taken by correspondence or independent study. Another possibility would be to ask the instructor for the syllabus and follow the course outline and readings independently. There are clinicians who do not reside near a university and do not have access to libraries. For these clinicians, independent study may involve teleconferences, videoconferences, computer networking, and audiotapes.

Documentation of all coursework taken on specific topics is necessary only for the clinician's own benefit and as a resource for other staff clinicians and professionals. Independent reading and documentation of academic competencies for bilingual clinicians are not required, yet clinicians know that knowledge in these areas does increase their credibility with other professionals who may not understand the needs of Hispanic children and adults. Clinicians can document their attendence in coursework, workshops, and inservices into notebooks identified as normal processes, assessment, and intervention. A clinician's ability to refer to research, books, articles, charts, and tables concerning second language acquisition, Spanish language development, nonbiased assessment, and best practices in intervention during school and clinical staffings will increase other professionals' confidence in the clinician's recommendations and also ensure better services for clients.

⌐┐

CONCLUSIONS

The purpose of this chapter was to discuss the clinical and academic competencies recommended for bilingual speech-language pathologists. ASHA's position statement on the Clinical Management of Communicatively Handicapped Minority Language Populations (ASHA, 1985) and the Definition for Bilingual Speech Language Pathologists and Audiologists (ASHA, 1989) served as the basis for this discussion. Language proficiency and academic competencies are both important issues in effective assessment and intervention by bilingual clinicians with Hispanic populations. Strategies to attain these competencies were suggested.

Bilingual speech-language pathologists are an emerging group of specialists. Their success in clinical practice will depend on their continuing education and the application of this knowledge.

⌐

REFERENCES

American Speech-Language-Hearing Association. (1985). Clinical management of communicatively handicapped minority language populations. *Asha 27*(6), 29–32.

American Speech-Language-Hearing Association. (1989). Definition: Bilingual speech-language pathologists and audiologists. *Asha, 31*(3), 93.

American Speech-Language-Hearing Association. (1993). *Demographic profile of the ASHA membership and affiliation.* Rockville, MD: Author.

American Speech-Language-Hearing Association. (1994). Code of Ethics. *Asha, 36*(Suppl. 13), 1–2.

American Speech-Language-Hearing Association. (1995). Reading lists on multicultural populations for independent study. Rockville, MD: Author.

Baetens-Beardsmore, H. (1986). *Bilingualism: Basic principles* (2nd ed.). San Diego, CA: College-Hill Press.

Kayser, H. (1993). Supervision of the Hispanic graduate student. *Supervisor's Forum, 1*(1), 12–23.

Peñalosa, F. (1980). *Chicano sociolinguistics: A brief introduction.* Rowley, MA: Newbury House.

Saville-Troike, M. (1986). Anthropological considerations in the study of communication. In O. Taylor (Ed.), *Nature of communication disorders in culturally and linguistically diverse populations* (pp. 47–72). San Diego, CA: College-Hill Press.

Taylor, O. (1986). Historical perspectives and conceptual framework. In O. Taylor (Ed.), *Nature of communication disorders in culturally and linguistically diverse populations* (pp. 1–18). San Diego, CA: College-Hill Press.

Westby, C. (1991, April). *Culture, families, language and learning: Appreciating the differences.* Paper presented at the Texas Speech-Language-Hearing Association, Houston.

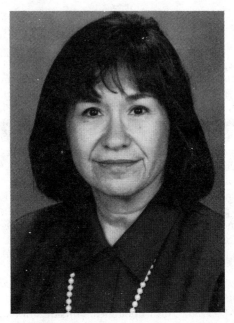

HORTENCIA KAYSER, Ph.D.

Dr. Kayser is an instructor in the Department of Speech and Hearing Sciences at the University of Arizona. She received her master's degree in 1975 from the University of Arizona and her doctorate in 1985 from New Mexico State University. Dr. Kayser's primary interest in speech-language pathology is in child language, with research in the socialization and conversational language use of bilingual preschool and school-age Hispanic children. Her previous position was the Coordinator of the Bilingual Speech-Language Pathology program at Texas Christian University, Fort Worth, Texas.

PART I

SPEECH AND LANGUAGE DEVELOPMENT, DISORDERS, ASSESSMENT, AND INTERVENTION

The chapters in Part I review the literature on Spanish speech and language development and disorders, assessment, and intervention from infancy through adulthood. Each chapter also includes the authors' experiences, clinical observations, and unpublished research notes concerning these topics. Of particular interest are the case studies that are presented to exemplify the use of the developmental information available to clinicians.

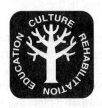

CHAPTER 2

SPANISH PHONOLOGICAL DEVELOPMENT

BRIAN A. GOLDSTEIN, PH.D., CCC-SLP

Researchers in speech-language pathology have a long history of describing the phonological acquisition process in English-speaking children. The characterization of phonological patterns in large numbers of normally developing children began in the 1930s (e.g., Wellman, Case, Mengert, & Bradbury, 1931) and has continued into the 1990s (e.g., Smit, Hand, Freilinger, Bernthal, & Bird, 1990). Simultaneous with the exploration of the speech characteristics in normally developing children was a trend to describe the phonological patterns in English-speaking children with phonological disorders (e.g., Hawk, 1936). The pursuit of this path is, of course, preeminent in speech-language pathology whose main mission is to remediate speech and language disorders. Although there is a large and diverse body of research identifying phonological patterns in English-speaking children, both normally developing and children with phonological disorders, that is not the case for children who speak Spanish.

Due to a lack of information on phonological acquisition in the Latino population in general and across the various Spanish dialects in particular, speech-language pathologists face a difficult task in providing appropriate diagnostic and intervention services to Spanish-speaking children. For Spanish-speaking children, consequences of the general lack of developmental phonological data and the specific lack of phonological data from more than one dialect group include (a) the delay or absence of diagnostic and intervention services, (b) the inappropriate labeling of phonological skills in both normally developing children and children with phonological disorders, (c) the misdiagnosis of a phonological disorder by using data collected from other Spanish dialect groups, and (d) the misdiagnosis of a phonological disorder by using data collected from English speakers. By providing speech-language pathologists with current information on Spanish phonological development, the risk of these effects can be reduced. The description of Spanish phonology and its dialects, phonological patterns in normally developing children and children with phonological disorders, and appropriate assessment and intervention techniques will allow clinicians to possess the requisite knowledge to gauge phonological development in Spanish-speaking children.

The purpose of this chapter is to present an overview of the issues related to phonological development and disorders in Spanish-speaking children. The chapter is divided into the following sections: (1) Spanish consonant and vowel system; (2) Spanish dialects; (3) normative data (including cross-dialectal information on both normally developing children and children with phonological disorders); (4) assessment; and (5) intervention. The last section presents case studies designed to highlight a number of the issues discussed throughout the chapter.

⊔

SPANISH CONSONANT AND VOWEL SYSTEM

In this section, a brief overview of the Spanish consonant and vowel system is presented. (For a more complete analysis, see Iglesias and Anderson, 1993.) This survey includes information on the consonants and vowels found in "standard" Spanish, including their allophonic variations. Subsequently, details will be provided on the primary Spanish dialects spoken in the United States, the Cuban, Mexican, and Puerto Rican dialects.

"STANDARD" SPANISH

For ease of discussion, a version of Spanish which does not exist, "standard" Spanish, will be examined. Although a standard version of Spanish is not actually spoken by anyone, describing this system lays the groundwork for and helps in understanding the numerous Spanish dialects. The phonemes and allophones of Spanish are listed in Table 2–1.

There are five primary vowels in Spanish, the two front vowels are /i/ and /e/, and the three back vowels are /u/, /o/, and /a/.

TABLE 2–1
Phonemes and allophones of standard Spanish (based on Iglesias & Anderson, 1993).

Phonemes	Allophone(s)
i	i
e	e
u	u
o	o
a	a
p	p
b	b, β
t	t
d	d, ð
k	k
g	g, ɣ
f	f, ɸ
x	x, h
s	s
w	w, u, gw
j	j, i, dʒ
tʃ	tʃ
l	l
ɾ	r, l
r	r, R
m	m
n	n
ɲ	ɲ

There are 18 phonemes in "standard" Spanish: the voiceless unaspirated stops, /p/, /t/, and /k/; the voiced stops, /b/, /d/, and /g/; the voiceless fricatives, /f/, /x/, and /s/; the affricate, /tʃ/; the glides, /w/ and /j/; the lateral, /l/; the tap /ɾ/ and trill /r/; and the nasals, /m/, /n/, and /ɲ/.

SPANISH DIALECTS

The existence of differences between Spanish dialects further complicates the process of characterizing phonological patterns in Spanish-speaking children. Unlike English, in which dialectal variations are generally defined by variations in vowels, Spanish dialectal differences primarily affect consonant sound classes rather than vowels or a few specific phonemes. The two most prevalent dialect groups of Spanish in the United States are Southwestern United States and Caribbean resulting from the "large number of Mexican immigrants, the migration of large numbers of Puerto Ricans, and the immigration of political refugees from Cuba, El Salvador, and Nicaragua" (Iglesias & Anderson, 1993, p. 151). Because speech-language pathologists may not be aware of important phonological and/or phonetic differences among the predominant dialects of Spanish spoken in the United States, information on the phonological features of these principle Spanish dialects will be presented.

The primary dialect features of the Mexican, Cuban, and Puerto Rican dialects of Spanish which *differ* from "standard" Spanish are listed in Table 2–2. Although there may be other dialect features not described here, these seem to characterize the majority of features exhibited by the speakers in these three dialect groups. By delineating specific features, there is no implication that (a) every feature is always evidenced in the same manner or (b) every speaker of a particular dialect utilizes each and every dialect feature listed below.

The dialect differences primarily affect certain sound classes over others. Fricatives and liquids (in particular /s/, /ɾ/, and /r/) tend to show more variation than either stops, glides, or the affricate. The differences between Spanish dialects make it paramount that speech-language pathologists be aware of the dialect the children are speaking. Otherwise, there may be the likelihood of misdiagnosis. This issue will be discussed in more detail in the section on phonological development in preschool children with phonological disorders.

TABLE 2–2
Description of Mexican, Cuban, and Puerto Rican Spanish.

	Allophone			
Phone	**Mexican**	**Cuban**	**Puerto Rican**	**Environment**
b	v	–	–	Free variation
d	–	Ø	–	Word final
k,g	Ø	–	–	Abutting consonants
f	–	–	ɸ	I
s	Ø	Ø	Ø	F
	h	h	h	F
	–	–	Ø, C#C	F [lob braso]
ð	–	Ø	Ø	V_V
x	h	h	h	I, F
	ʃ	–	–	I
tʃ	–	ʃ(women)	ʃ	I
n	–	ŋ	ŋ	Before pause or V
ɾ(tap)	–	Ø, CC	–	Abutting CC [kweppo]
	–	I(rare)	I	_[+anterior] ([t,d)]
	–	–	I	F
	–	–	i	Abutting CC (rural)
r(trill)	R(rare)	–	R	I
	–	–	x	I
l	–	–	r(rural)	F

Key: "–" = not typically exhibited in that dialect; Ø = deleted; I = syllable–initial;
F = syllable–final
Sources: Canfield, 1981; Cotten & Sharp, 1988; Lombardi & de Peters, 1981; Navar-
ro–Tomás, 1966.

⌐ㄱ

NORMATIVE DATA

When attempting to assess phonological patterns in English-speaking
children, speech-language pathologists can compare a child's performance against a reliable referent (collected from both normally developing children and children with phonological disorders) and thus

determine if the child exhibits a phonological disorder. This allows for appropriate diagnostic classification and intervention services. This process is not as simple for Spanish-speaking children. Currently, identification of phonological disorders in Spanish-speaking children is considerably more difficult for a number of reasons. First, the relevant data do not exist in great numbers. Although some data on the phonological patterns in normally developing Spanish-speakers are available (e.g., Goldstein, 1988; Jimenez, 1987; Stepanof, 1990), little data have been gathered from Spanish-speaking children with phonological disorders. Second, it is inappropriate to use normative phonological data gathered from English-speaking children to assess Spanish-speaking children. Although in the past clinicians have attempted to generalize normative phonological data collected from English-speaking children to diagnose Spanish-speaking children, this comparison is not valid. Finally, developmental phonological data cannot necessarily be generalized from one dialect group to another. The existing data on both normally developing children and children with phonological disorders typically have been collected from Mexican (e.g., Gonzalez, 1978) or Mexican-American children (e.g., Acevedo, 1991; Meza, 1983).

In the sections that follow, the data available on phonological acquisition in normally developing children and children with phonological disorders are presented for Spanish-speaking children (a) less than 3-years-old, (b) in preschool, and (c) in elementary school. Although these data are presented as monolithic, there are differences among studies in sample size, type of assessment, age range of the subjects, and so on.

PHONOLOGICAL DEVELOPMENT IN NORMALLY DEVELOPING CHILDREN YOUNGER THAN 3 YEARS OLD

The phonological development of normally developing children younger than 3 years of age has been studied primarily in three areas: (a) babbling, (b) vowel development, and (c) phonological development in 2-year-olds. First, because babbling has been shown to be connected to later phonological development, the characteristics of babbling are described from a cross-linguistic perspective with specific reference to Spanish-speaking children. Second, information on the accuracy of vowel productions is provided. During an assessment, speech-language pathologists usually do not typically consider the production of vowels, assuming that they are always accurate. That is not always the case, however, especially for very young normally developing children and children with phonological disorders. Finally, phonological skills in 2-year-olds will be presented because clinicians continue to provide diagnostic and intervention services to younger children.

BABBLING

There has been much discussion in recent years concerning the link between babbling and later phonological development. (See Locke, 1983 for a detailed discussion along with more recent work by Bleile, Stark, and McGowan, 1993.) The data appear to show a relationship between early segmental production and subsequent phonological development, indicating that speech-language pathologists must attend to the child's productions before 2 years of age.

Cross-linguistically, infants seem to exhibit common patterns of production (e.g., Boysson-Bardies & Vihman, 1991; Vihman, Velleman, & McCune, 1994). For example, children primarily will produce consonant-vowel (CV) canonical shapes (e.g., [mama]) with consonant segments more likely to be produced in syllable-initial position. They are less likely to produce consonants in syllable-final position. Place of articulation for consonants will likely be labial and dental as opposed to palatal and velar, and the manner of articulation will tend to be represented by oral and nasal stops over fricatives and liquids. Moreover, the children's phonetic repertoires will contain few rare or nonuniversal consonants. That is, it is unusual for infants to produce sounds that are not common across the world's languages (e.g., clicks or pharyngeal fricatives).

Consistent with the data presented above, Oller and Eilers (1982) found a predominance of CV syllables in Spanish-speaking children with consonants tending to be singleton, unaspirated stops. They also noted that these children produced more syllable-initial than syllable-final consonants. In syllable-final position, fricatives or affricates were more common than stops; in fact, it was rare for the children to produce syllable-final stops at all.

VOWELS

The acquisition and development of vowels in children have also received increased attention recently (e.g., Clement & Wijnen, 1994;

Oller & Eilers, 1982; Otomo & Stoel-Gammon, 1992; Pollock & Keiser, 1990) although few studies have examined the production of vowels in Spanish-speaking children. Oller and Eilers (1982) found that the mean proportion occurrence of vowel-like productions in 12- to 14-month-old English- and Spanish-speaking children was remarkably similar. In general, they noted that the children were likely to produce more anterior-like vowels than posterior-like ones. The rank order of the first 10 vowels in Spanish-speaking infants were: (1) [ɛ]; (2) [æ]; (3) [e]; (4) [i]; (5) [a]; (6) [ʌ]; (7) [ʊ]; (8) [u]; (9) [ɪ]; (10) [o] (p. 573). Maez (1981) indicated that by 18 months, the three subjects in her study had mastered (i.e., produced correctly at least 90% of the time) the five basic Spanish vowels, [i], [e], [u], [o], and [a]. Her study, however, focused on consonant development, and she did not indicate if any vowel errors occurred.

2-YEAR-OLDS

The few studies that have examined phonological acquisition and development in normally developing Spanish-speaking 2-year-olds generally fall into two categories: (1) those examining primarily segmental production and (2) those examining primarily the evidence of phonological process. Of the five studies which will be summarized here, one used subjects of Chilean descent (Pandolfi & Herrera, 1990), two used subjects of Puerto Rican descent (Anderson & Smith, 1987; Vivaldi, 1990), and three used subjects of Mexican-American descent (Gonzalez, 1983; Maez, 1981; Mann, Kayser, Watson, & Hodson, 1992). Mann et al. (1992) also examined phonological development in 3- and 4-year-olds in their study. Those data are presented in a later section.

The results of the segmental studies (Anderson & Smith, 1987; Gonzalez, 1983; Maez, 1981) indicated that, in general, normally developing Spanish-speaking children had developed most of the phonetic system by 2 years, 6 months. Specifically, they showed good production of oral and nasal stops and glides; fair production of voiceless fricatives; and poor production of the affricate, voiced spirants, and liquids. The results of the phonological process studies (Anderson & Smith, 1987; Mann, et al., 1992; Pandolfi & Herrera, 1990; Vivaldi, 1990) demonstrated that processes occurring over 50% of the time tended to be syllable structure processes, typically, cluster reduction and weak syllable deletion. Processes occurring 25–50% of the time included initial, medial, and final consonant deletion, with velar fronting and assimilation occurring less than 25% of the time.

PHONOLOGICAL DEVELOPMENT IN NORMALLY DEVELOPING PRESCHOOL CHILDREN

Studies examining phonological development in Spanish-speaking children have concentrated on development in preschool children (i.e., 3- to 5-year-olds). These studies have focused on the acquisition of phonetic inventories (Acevedo, 1991; De la Fuente, 1985; Eblen, 1982; Jimenez, 1987; Summers, 1982), although there have been some studies describing sound classes (e.g., Macken, 1975, 1978; Macken & Barton, 1980) and phonological processes (Cabello, 1986; Goldstein, 1988; Stepanof, 1990). Moreover, the majority of both segment- and phonological process-based studies have used Mexican (Gonzalez, 1978; Summers, 1982) or Mexican-American (Acevedo, 1991; Eblen, 1982; Jimenez, 1987) children as subjects although there have been studies examining children acquiring Bolivian Spanish (Fantini, 1985), Dominican Spanish (De la Fuente, 1985), and Puerto Rican Spanish (Anderson & Smith, 1987; Goldstein, 1988; Goldstein & Iglesias, in press; Gonzalez, 1981).

The data from segment-based studies suggested that normally developing Spanish-speaking children accurately produced most segments at a relatively early age (Maez, 1981). More specifically, by 5 years of age, the following phonemes were found *not* to be mastered: /g/, /f/, /s/, /ɲ/, /ɾ/, /r/ (Acevedo, 1991; De la Fuente, 1985; Fantini, 1985; Gonzalez, 1978; Mason, Smith, & Hinshaw, 1976; Summers, 1982). Studies examining more general patterns of phonological development are more recent compared with phonetic studies.

In general, it seems that Spanish-speaking children have suppressed (i.e., are no longer productively using) the majority of phonological processes by the time they reach 3½ years of age (Becker, 1982; Diamond, 1983; Goldstein, 1988; Gonzalez, 1981; Mann et al., 1992; Stepanof, 1990). The results of these studies indicated that commonly occurring processes (evidenced more than 10% of the time) were postvocalic singleton omission, stridency deletion, tap/trill /r/, consonant sequence reduction, and final consonant deletion. Less commonly occurring processes (exhibited less than 10% of the time) tended to be fronting (both velar and palatal), prevocalic singleton omission, assimilation, and stopping.

PHONOLOGICAL DEVELOPMENT IN PRESCHOOL CHILDREN WITH PHONOLOGICAL DISORDERS

Although there have been quite a number of studies characterizing phonological patterns in normally developing children, this information remains sparse for Spanish-speaking children with phonological disorders. Two studies which have examined the phonological characteristics in Spanish-speaking preschool children with phonological disorders are Goldstein (1993) and Meza (1983). Goldstein (1993) used the *Assessment of Phonological Disabilities—Spanish* (APD-S) (Iglesias, 1978) to examine 54 Spanish-speaking children of Puerto Rican descent with phonological disorders, ranging in age from 3;1 to 4;8. Of the 54 children, 20 were 3-year-olds (10 males and 10 females) and 34 were 4-year-olds (24 males and 10 females). Meza (1983) examined the occurrence of phonological processes in 20 highly unintelligible preschool Mexican-American children using the *Assessment of Phonological Processes—Spanish* (APP-S) (Hodson, 1986).

Despite differences between Meza's and Goldstein's study in assessment instrument, sample size, and dialect group, a comparison between the two studies provides useful information concerning the percentage of children (as opposed to mean percentage-of-occurrence for individual phonological processes) exhibiting phonological processes.

The results shown in Table 2–3 indicate that the percentage of Spanish-speaking children with phonological disorders who exhibit specific processes is similar. However, there are two exceptions, cluster reduction and weak (unstressed) syllable deletion. It is possible to account for the discrepancy in cluster reduction by the manner in which that process was defined in the two studies. According to Meza's definition, the reduction of any two contiguous segments was termed "consonant sequence reduction" (p. 55); this definition applied to both abutting consonants and word-initial clusters. In Goldstein (1993), cluster reduction was defined as the elimination of

TABLE 2–3

Percentage of children exhibiting phonological processes.

Process*	Meza (1983)	Goldstein (1993)
Cluster reduction	100	83
Unstressed syllable deletion	100	81
Stopping	80	93
Palatal fronting	40	20
Liquid simplification	95	94
Assimilation	95	87

*Only processes targeted in both studies are listed.

any element of a two-member, word-initial consonant pair. In the case of weak (unstressed) syllable deletion, 100% of the children exhibited this process in Meza's study compared with 81% in Goldstein's study. This variance can be accounted for by a dialect difference between the forms of Mexican and Puerto Rican Spanish. In Puerto Rican Spanish, there is a propensity to delete unstressed syllables which does not occur in the Mexican dialect. For example, the word *escoba* (broom) is typically produced as [eskoβa] in the Mexican dialect but as [koβa] in the Puerto Rican dialect. Thus, the deletion of an unstressed syllable would count as an error for children speaking the Mexican dialect but not for children speaking the Puerto Rican dialect.

Given that the phonological processes exhibited by children with phonological disorders who speak two distinct Spanish dialects are similar, these results seem to suggest that collecting phonological data from various dialect groups is unnecessary. That is, it might be assumed, *incorrectly*, that, as long as dialect is taken into account, acquisition data collected from one dialect group can be generalized to another dialect group. This is true, however, only in terms of the types of phonological processes evident in these children. As indicated above, the percentage of children exhibiting cluster reduction and weak syllable deletion differed across dialect groups. These differences may not be paramount in terms of differentially diagnosing a normally developing child from one with a phonological disorder. Dialect differences, however, may need to be taken into account in the course of intervention, for example, in determining the order in which processes should be remediated. Furthermore, this similarity of results across dialect groups must be viewed with caution because (1) different assessment tools were used and (2) the phonological patterns in only two dialect groups of children with phonological disorders have been examined.

PHONOLOGICAL DEVELOPMENT IN NORMALLY DEVELOPING SCHOOL-AGE CHILDREN

We have seen that by the time Spanish-speaking children reach the age of 5, most phonological processes are suppressed, and the majority of consonants are mastered. However, Spanish-speaking children will continue to make some errors, typically substitutions and distortions as opposed to omissions, at least until the age of 7. Beyond the age of 7, they may continue to exhibit some residual errors, particularly on consonant clusters (Mason et al., 1976).

The studies that have examined phonological patterns in Spanish-speaking children older than 5 years of age have focused on segmental production as opposed to more general patterns (i.e., phonological processes) and have used children speaking the Mexican/Mexican-American dialect of Spanish (Bailey, 1982; Evans, 1974; Gonzalez, 1978; Macy, 1979; Mason et al., 1976) to the exclusion of any other dialect group. Because children at this age should be accurately producing the vast majority of consonant segments, phonological development in school-age children will be described by indicating phones that are *not* mastered.

By the time Spanish-speaking children reach first grade, only a few specific phones are likely to show any errors at all. These phones are contained in four sound classes: fricatives, liquids, the affricate, and clusters. Fricatives which may continue to show inconsistent production include [x], [s], and [ð] (Gonzalez, 1978; Mason et al., 1976). The affricate [tʃ] may be in error as well (Evans, 1974). Not surprisingly, the liquids [ɾ], [r], and [l], and some consonant clusters will also exhibit errors (Bailey, 1982). Macy (1979) indicates further that the majority of cluster errors in this age group will involve /s/-clusters.

PHONOLOGICAL DEVELOPMENT IN SCHOOL-AGE CHILDREN WITH PHONOLOGICAL DISORDERS

Very few studies have examined phonological patterns in Spanish-speaking school-age children with phonological disorders. Bichotte, Dunn, Gonzalez, Orpi, and Nye (1993) examined (a) normal English dominant, (b) normal Spanish dominant, and (c) disordered Spanish dominant children. For the purposes of this discussion, the focus will be on the results from the last category, disordered Spanish dominant children. Subjects consisted of 10 Spanish dominant males ranging in age from 6;3 to 8;0. Each child was assessed using the *Assessment of Phonological Processes—Spanish* (APP-S) (Hodson, 1986). The results suggested that, in general, these children with phonological disorders showed significantly more errors for consonant sequence reduction, stridents, and velars than their normally developing peers. In addition, processes exhibiting percentages-of-occurrence greater than 20% included stridents, tap/trill /r/, and glides. These data are mostly consistent with the types of errors (i.e., difficulty with tap/trill /r/, stridents, and velars) made by normally developing school-age children (e.g., Bailey,

1982; Mason et al., 1976) and younger Spanish-speaking children who are phonologically disordered (Goldstein, 1993; Meza, 1983).

SUMMARY OF NORMATIVE DATA

In summary, the normative data show that normally developing Spanish-speaking infants will tend to produce CV syllables containing oral and nasal stops with front vowels. It is likely that, by the time normally developing Spanish-speaking children reach 3 years of age, they will use the dialect features of the community and will have mastered the vowel system and most of the consonant system. By the end of preschool, normally developing children will exhibit some difficulty with consonant clusters and a few phones, specifically, [ð], [x], [s], [n], [tʃ], [ɾ], [r], and [l]. To one degree or another, these children will still occasionally exhibit the following phonological processes: cluster reduction, unstressed syllable deletion, stridency deletion, and tap/trill /r/ deviation, but will likely have suppressed velar and palatal fronting, prevocalic singleton omission, stopping, and assimilation. For some Spanish-speaking children, phonetic mastery will continue into the early elementary school years when they continue to show some, although infrequent, errors on the fricatives [x] and [s], the affricate [tʃ], the liquids [ɾ, r, l], and consonant clusters.

CASE STUDIES

Stoel-Gammon and Dunn (1985) have suggested that the highest (although not the only) priorities for treatment occur on segments and phonological patterns that most affect intelligibility, on patterns that cut across sound classes, and on patterns that disappear at the earliest age from the speech of normally developing children. (See Table 2–4 for considerations in the assessment and treatment of Spanish-speaking children.)

There are a number of issues to address concerning the treatment of phonological disorders in Spanish-speaking children. First, the effectiveness of specific treatment techniques has not been addressed. Speech-language pathologists have used treatment techniques with Spanish-speaking children that were designed for English-speaking children. There is no reason to believe that these techniques will not be effective for Spanish-speakers, but there are no data to judge either

TABLE 2–4

Considerations in the assessment and treatment of Spanish-speaking children.

I. Considerations for Phonological Assessment (after Bernthal & Bankson, 1993, pp. 222–223)
   A. Use an assessment tool designed specifically to assess Spanish-speaking children
   B. Take the child's dialect into account
   C. Describe the phonological status of an individual
   D. Determine if the child's phonological system is sufficiently different from normal development to warrant intervention
   E. Determine treatment direction
   F. Make predictive and prognostic statements relative to phonological change with or without intervention
   G. Monitor change in phonological performance
   H. Identify factors that may be related to the presence or maintenance of a phonological disability

II. Phonological Assessment Tools for Spanish-speaking Children
   A. *Austin Spanish Articulation Test* (Carrow, 1974)
   B. *Assessment of Phonological Processes—Spanish* (Hodson, 1986)
   C. *Assessment of Phonological Disabilities* (Iglesias, 1978)
   D. *Southwest Spanish Articulation Test* (Toronto, 1977)

III. General Considerations in the Treatment of Phonological Disorders (after Stoel-Gammon & Dunn, 1985, pp. 166–167)
   A. Developing a treatment plan based on underlying factors that contribute to etiology of the disorder (e.g., auditory status, structural adequacy, and motoric abilities
   B. Consider each child as an individual
   C. Use normal acquisition data as a guide to planning treatment goals
   D. Have a philosophical framework (e.g., phone mastery vs. phonological processes)
   E. Teach the child to monitor responses
   F. Measuring progress with an initial baseline, intermittent testing to determine progress, and testing for generalization.
   G. Factors to consider when selecting targets
      1. The phones in the child's repertoire
      2. The frequency of occurrence of the phone in the language
      3. Age of acquisition and ease of production of the phone
      5. Stimulability
      6. Age of client

---

way. Second, there are no studies to indicate when it is appropriate to conduct treatment for phonological disorders in Spanish and when treatment should be administered in English. The decision to intervene in English or Spanish begins with an appropriate and thorough assessment. During this process, Mann and Hodson (1994) caution that clinicians should not judge the child's language proficiency on short interactions but should attempt to complete phonological analyses in both languages. The assessment then will determine in which language intervention should take place. Finally, the acquisition of phonological skills by Spanish-speaking children during the course of treatment is one area in which there is an acute lack of data. Although some longitudinal data have been obtained from English-speaking children (e.g., Vihman & Greenlee, 1987), currently no longitudinal data are available on the treatment of phonological disorders in Spanish-speaking children.

In summary, there are little, if any, data addressing treatment efficacy, language of instruction, and phonological development in Spanish-speaking children. To illustrate the concepts in goal planning presented above and to discuss other issues specific to the treatment of phonological disorders in Spanish-speaking children, two case studies will be presented.

CASE 1: E.E.

E.E. is a 3 year 10-month-old female who speaks the Puerto Rican dialect of Spanish. E.E. has attended a bilingual (Spanish-English) Head Start for 2 months. Prior to her enrollment, E.E. was exposed to little or no English. The *Assessment of Phonological Disabilities—Spanish* (APD-S) (Iglesias, 1978) was used to assess E.E. Because E.E. uses the Puerto Rican dialect of Spanish, her results are calculated and analyzed taking into account the features of Puerto Rican Spanish. To account for dialect features in her particular speech community, the clinician consulted available information on the dialect features of Puerto Rican Spanish (e.g., Terrell, 1981) and sampled the adult speakers in the child's linguistic community to seek out any other dialect features not commonly noted in descriptions of this dialect of Spanish. This sampling revealed one dialect feature employed by adult speakers in the community but not widely reported in discussions of Puerto Rican Spanish. Adults in E.E.'s linguistic community produced /doktoɾ/ ("doctor") as [dostol] (Goldstein, 1993). Thus, her production of /doktoɾ/ as [dostol] was not counted as an error. If this specific dialect feature had not been taken into account, E.E. would have been penalized for making an "error" that was, in fact, a dialect feature. "Errors" can only be counted as such when they are in conflict with the child's dialect. In another example from the Puerto Rican dialect of Spanish, word-final /s/ is deleted. For example, /dos/ (two) is produced as [doː] (the vowel is generally lengthened). E.E.'s production of [doː] should *not* be and was not counted as an instance of final consonant deletion. However, if she had produced /floɾ/ (flower) as [flo], the production would be scored as an instance of final consonant deletion because the deletion of word-final /ɾ/ is not a feature of the dialect.

The failure of speech-language pathologists to account for dialectal features in the phonological systems of Spanish-speaking children may result in misdiagnosing these children as phonologically disordered. If speech-language pathologists are not aware of or unsure about the particular features of a child's dialect, they can locate this information from adult informants, interpreters/support personnel (following ASHA's guidelines), and published books and articles on Spanish dialects (e.g., Cotten & Sharp, 1988; Terrell, 1981).

The results shown in Figure 2–1 indicate that E.E. presents with a moderate-severe phonological disorder and is 25% intelligible in spontaneous conversation. E.E. exhibits six processes with percentages of occurrence over 10%: liquid simplification, weak syllable deletion, cluster reduction, initial consonant deletion, velar fronting, and stopping. E.E. utilizes cluster reduction and initial consonant deletion at high percentages-of-occurrence, 91% and 60%, respectively, with weak syllable deletion being exhibited moderately, 43%. Liquid simplification, velar fronting, and stopping occur at 17%, 13%, and 13%, respectively.

To remediate E.E.'s phonological disorder, the speech-language pathologist would likely use a phonological approach because she exhibits such unusually high percentages-of-occurrence on two of the processes. Using this type of approach requires the speech-language pathologist to target certain processes over others and then to decide which specific process (or processes) to target initially.

In E.E.'s case, three processes, cluster reduction, initial consonant deletion, and weak syllable deletion, are highly evident in her speech and would be considered appropriate initial targets for remediation. Based on the guidelines provided previously (see Table 2–4), the speech-language pathologist would likely begin therapy with E.E. targeting initial consonant deletion and weak syllable deletion. Initial consonant deletion should be targeted because her use of that process shows a very

Name: E.E.
Date of Birth: 12/8/87
Date of Assessment: 10/28/91   Age: 3;10
Examiner: B.G.
Intelligibility: 25%

Processes	Percentage-of-Occurrence
Cluster Reduction	91
Initial Consonant Deletion	60
Weak Syllable Deletion	43
Liquid Simplification	17
Velar Fronting	13
Stopping	13
Final Consonant Deletion	9
Assimilation	2
Palatal Fronting	0

FIGURE 2-1
Results of E.E. on the *Assessment of Phonological Disabilities.*

high percentage of occurrence, impacts greatly on intelligibility, and is rarely, if ever, evident in the speech of normally developing Spanish-speaking preschool children. Weak syllable deletion would also be a target for remediation. Because syllabicity is such an important aspect in Spanish phonological development, and there are few monosyllabic words in Spanish, clinicians would probably target weak/unstressed syllable deletion in children who were deleting unstressed syllables in two syllable words (Mann & Hodson, 1994). It is equally important that speech-language pathologists decide which phonological processes *not* to target initially. Mann and Hodson (1994) note that the clinician would likely not initiate treatment by targeting a phonological process such as final consonant deletion because there are so few final consonants in Spanish and the use of this process is unlikely to greatly affect intelligibility. Although E.E. exhibits cluster reduction at a higher percentage of occurrence than initial consonant deletion, it probably would not be one of the processes initially targeted because the use of that process does not affect intelligibility as much as the use of initial consonant deletion. Moreover, as indicated in the section on normative data, errors on clusters are commonly noted in normally developing Spanish-speaking preschool children, whereas initial consonant deletion is not.

CASE 2: M.F.

M.F. is a 6-year-old male who speaks the Mexican dialect of Spanish. M.F. attended a bilingual (Spanish-English) Head Start for 2 years, a bilingual kindergarten for 1 year, and is currently enrolled in a bilingual first grade classroom. The *Assessment of Phonological Processes—Spanish* (APP-S) (Hodson, 1986) was used to assess M.F. Based on the results of the evaluation, he presents with a mild phonological disorder and is 90 to 95% intelligible in spontaneous conversation. Because M.F. uses the Mexican dialect of Spanish, his results are calculated taking into account the features of Mexican Spanish.

Given that M.F. in particular and Spanish-speaking children in general in the United States typically are exposed to English to some degree, speech-language pathologists must decide in which language or languages to assess these children. Clinicians can assess the child in Spanish-only, English-only, or in both English and Spanish. Even if the child seems to be either a dominant English speaker or a dominant Spanish speaker, it is common practice to assess phonological skills in both languages (Mann & Hodson, 1994).

As can be seen in Figure 2–2, M.F. exhibits only one process with a percentage of occurrence over 10%, 44% for liquid /r/. The remaining processes that are evident in his speech (consonant sequence reduction, syllable reduction, stridents, and liquid /l/) occur less than 10% of the time. As noted in the section on normative data, some errors on the tap/trill /r/ are typically evident in Spanish-speaking 6-year-olds. However, based on the guidelines of the APP-S, "liquid /r/" would be targeted for treatment because it shows a percentage of occurrence greater than 40%. Unlike E.E., in which a phonological technique would be warranted, a more phonetic approach might be more appropriate in this case because the child's errors are concentrated on one phoneme.

⼬

CONCLUSION

The amount of research examining phonological development and disorders in Spanish-speaking children has increased, albeit slowly, over the past 10 to 15 years. Speech-language pathologists must be mindful of the gaps in our knowledge base to ensure that they are not basing diagnostic decisions and intervention services on limited normative information. There are a number of specific areas in which more

Name: M.F.
Date of Birth: 8/21/85
Date of Assessment: 8/11/91　　　　　　　**Age:** 6;0
Examiner: B.G.
Intelligibility: 90–95%

Processes*	**Percentage-of-Occurrence**
Phonological Omissions	
Consonant Sequence Reduction	8
Syllable Reduction	2
Class Deficiencies	
Stridents	9
Liquid /r/	44
Liquid /l/	2

*Only processes with percentages greater than 0% are listed

FIGURE 2-2
Results of M.F. on the *Assessment of Phonological Processes—Spanish.*

data need to be acquired. First, the majority of studies on phonological development in Spanish-speakers have focused on preschool children (i.e., those aged 3;0–5;0). Very few studies have examined the acquisition and development of both vowels and consonants in both normally developing children and children with phonological disorders, especially those aged 2;0–3;0 and children over 5. Furthermore, speech-language pathologists treating phonological disorders in Spanish-speaking children have no information on the patterns of phonological change during treatment. Second, the description of phonological patterns in both normally developing children and children with phonological disorders has not typically been examined in exacting detail either through the specific description of substitution and vowel errors or by the consideration of recent advances in phonological theory such as nonlinear phonology (see Bernhardt & Stoel-Gammon, 1994, for a description of this theory). Finally, a full accounting of the features of Spanish dialects commonly spoken in the United States is needed to accurately assess and treat Spanish-speaking children. This would include the examination of phonological patterns in normally developing children and children with phonological disorders speaking a variety of Spanish dialects and the completion of comprehensive adult dialect feature studies. These examinations will aid speech-language pathologists in making appropriate diagnostic decisions so that they can accurately distinguish phonological differences from disorders and plan for the treatment of phonological disorders.

⊓

REFERENCES

Acevedo, M. (1991, November). *Spanish consonants among two groups of Head Start children*. Paper presented at the annual convention of the American Speech-Language-Hearing Association, Atlanta, GA.

Anderson, R., & Smith, B. (1987). Phonological development of two-year-old monolingual Puerto Rican Spanish-speaking children. *Journal of Child Language, 14*, 57–78.

Bailey, S. (1982). *Normative data for Spanish articulatory skills of Mexican children between the ages of six and seven*. Unpublished master's thesis, San Diego State University, San Diego, CA.

Becker, M. (1982). *Phonological analysis of speech samples of monolingual Spanish-speaking intelligible four-year-olds*. Unpublished master's thesis, San Diego State University, San Diego, CA.

Bernhardt, B., & Stoel-Gammon, C. (1994). Nonlinear phonology: Introduction and clinical application. *Journal of Speech and Hearing Research, 37*, 123–143.

Bernthal, J. & Bankson, N. (1993). *Articulation and phonological disorders* (3rd ed.). Englewood Cliffs, NJ: Prentice-Hall.

Bichotte, M., Dunn, B., Gonzalez, L., Orpi, J., & Nye, C. (1993, November). *Assessing phonological performance of bilingual school-age Puerto Rican children*. Paper presented at the annual convention of the American Speech-Language-Hearing Association, Anaheim, CA.

Bleile, K., Stark, R., & McGowan, J. (1993). Speech development in a child after decannulation: Further evidence that babbling facilitates later speech development. *Clinical Linguistics and Phonetics, 7*(4), 319–337.

Boysson-Bardies, B., & Vihman, M. (1991). Adaptation to language: Evidence from babbling and first words in four languages. *Language, 67*(2), 299–319.

Cabello, A. (1986). *A comparison of phonological processes evidenced by intelligible and unintelligible Spanish-speaking Mexican-American children*. Unpublished manuscript, San Diego State University, San Diego, CA.

Canfield, D. L. (1981). *Spanish pronunciation in the Americas*. Chicago: University of Chicago Press.

Carrow, E. (1974). *Austin Spanish Articulation Test*. Austin, TX: Learning Concepts.

Clement, C., & Wijnen, F. (1994). Acquisition of vowel contrasts in Dutch. *Journal of Speech and Hearing Research, 37*, 83–89.

Cotton, E., & Sharp, J. (1988). *Spanish in the Americas.* Washington, DC: Georgetown University Press.

De la Fuente, M. T. (1985). *The order of acquisition of Spanish consonant phonemes by monolingual Spanish speaking children between the ages of 2.0 and 6.5.* Unpublished doctoral dissertation, Georgetown University, Washington, DC.

Diamond, F. (1983). *Phonological analysis of Spanish utterances of normally-developing bilingual Mexican-American children.* Unpublished master's thesis, San Diego State University, San Diego, CA.

Eblen, R. (1982). A study of the acquisition of fricatives by three-year-old children learning Mexican Spanish. *Language and Speech, 25*, 201–220.

Evans, J. S. (1974). Word pair discrimination and imitation abilities of preschool Spanish-speaking children. *Journal of Learning Disabilities, 7*, 573–580.

Fantini, A. (1985). *Language acquisition of a bilingual child: A sociolinguisitc perspective (to age 10).* San Diego, CA: College-Hill Press.

Goldstein, B. (1988). *The evidence of phonological processes of 3- and 4-year old Spanish-speakers.* Unpublished master's thesis, Temple University, Philadelphia.

Goldstein, B. (1993). *Phonological patterns in speech-disordered Puerto Rican Spanish-speaking children.* Unpublished doctoral dissertation, Temple University, Philadelphia.

Goldstein, B., & Iglesias, A. (in press). Phonological patterns in normally developing 4-year-old Spanish-speaking preschoolers of Puerto Rican descent. *Language, Speech, and Hearing Services in the Schools.*

Gonzalez, A. (1981). *A descriptive study of phonological development in normal speaking Puerto Rican preschoolers.* Unpublished doctoral dissertation, Pennsylvania State University, State College, PA.

Gonzalez, G. (1983). The acquisition of Spanish sounds in the speech of two-year-old Chicano children. In R. Padilla (Ed.), *Theory technology and public policy on bilingual education* (pp. 73–87). Rosslyn, VA: National Clearinghouse for Bilingual Education.

Gonzalez, M. M. (1978). Cómo detectar al niño con problemas del habla (Identifying speech disorders in children). México: Editorial Trillas.

Hawk, S. (1936). Speech defects in handicapped children. *Journal of Speech Disorders, 1*, 101–106.

Hodson, B. (1986). *Assessment of Phonological Processes—Spanish.* San Diego, CA: Los Amigos Association.

Iglesias, A. (1978). *Assessment of phonological disabilities.* Unpublished assessment tool, Ohio State University, Columbus.

Iglesias, A., & Anderson, N. (1993). Dialectal variations. In J. Bernthal & N. Bankson (Eds.), *Articulation and phonological disorders* (3rd ed., pp. 147–161). New York: Prentice-Hall.

Jimenez, B. C. (1987). Acquisition of Spanish consonants in children aged 3–5 years, 7 months. *Language Speech and Hearing Services in the Schools, 18*(4), 357–363.

Locke, J. (1983). *Phonological acquisition and change.* New York: Academic Press.

Lombardi, R. P., & de Peters, A. B. (1981). *Modern spoken Spanish: An interdisciplinary perspective.* Washington, DC: University Press of America.

Macken, M. (1975). The acquisition of intervocalic consonants in Mexican Spanish: A cross sectional study based on imitation data. *Papers and Reports on Child Language Development, 9,* 29–42.

Macken, M. (1978). Permitted complexity in phonological development: One child's acquisition of Spanish consonants. *Lingua, 44,* 219–253.

Macken, M., & Barton, D. (1980). The acquisition of the voicing contrast in Spanish: A phonetic and phonological study of word-initial stop consonants. *Journal of Child Language, 7,* 433–458.

Macy, A. (1979). *Normative data for Spanish articulatory skills of Mexican children between the ages of five and six.* Unpublished master's thesis. San Diego State University, San Diego, CA.

Maez, L. (1981). *Spanish as a first language.* Unpublished doctoral dissertation, University of California, Santa Barbara.

Mann, D., & Hodson, B. (1994). Spanish-speaking children's phonologies: Assessment and remediation of disorders. *Seminars in Speech and Language, 15*(2), 137–147.

Mann, D. P., Kayser, H., Watson, J., & Hodson, B. (1992, November). *Phonological systems of Spanish-speaking Texas preschoolers.* Paper presented at the annual convention of the American Speech-Language-Hearing Association, San Antonio, TX.

Mason, M., Smith, M., & Hinshaw, M. (1976). *Medida Española de articulación* (Measurement of Spanish Articulation). San Ysidro, CA: San Ysidro School District.

Meza, P. (1983). *Phonological analysis of Spanish utterances of highly unintelligible Mexican-American children.* Unpublished master's thesis, San Diego State University, San Diego, CA.

Navarro-Tomás, T. (1966). *El Español en Puerto Rico* (Spanish in Puerto Rico). Río Piedras, Puerto Rico: Editorial Universitaria Universidad de Puerto Rico.

Oller, D. K., & Eilers, R. (1982). Similarity of babbling in Spanish- and English-learning babies. *Child Language, 9,* 565–577.

Otomo, K., & Stoel-Gammon, C. (1992). The acquisition of unrounded vowels in English. *Journal of Speech and Hearing Research, 35,* 604–616.

Pandolfi, A. M., & Herrera, M. O. (1990). Producción fonológica diastratica de niños menores de tres años (Phonological production in children less than three-years old). *Revista Teorica y Aplicada, 28,* 101–122.

Pollock, K., & Keiser, N. (1990). An examination of vowel errors in phonologically disordered children. *Clinical Linguistics and Phonetics, 4*(2), 161–178.

Smit, A., Hand, L., Freilinger, J., Bernthal, J., & Bird, A. (1990). The Iowa articulation norms project and its Nebraska replication. *Journal of Speech and Hearing Disorders, 55,* 779–798.

Stepanof, E. R. (1990). Procesos phonologicos de niños Puertorriqueños de 3 y 4 años evidenciado en la prueba APP-Spanish (Phonological processes evidenced on the APP-Spanish by 3- and 4-year-old Puerto Rican children). *Opphla, 8*(2),15–20.

Stoel-Gammon, C., & Dunn, C. (1985). *Normal and disordered phonology.* Baltimore: University Park Press.

Summers, J. A. (1982). *Normative data for Spanish articulation skills of Mexican children between the ages of four and five.* Unpublished master's thesis, San Diego State University, San Diego, CA.

Terrell, T. (1981). Current trends in the investigation of Cuban and Puerto Rican phonology. In J. Amastae & L. Elías-Olivares (Eds.), *Spanish in the United States: Sociolinguistic aspects* (pp. 47–70). Cambridge: Cambridge University Press.

Toronto, A. (1977). *Southwestern Spanish Articulation Test.* Austin, TX: National Education Laboratory Publishers.

Vihman, M., & Greenlee, M. (1987). Individual differences in phonological development: Ages one and three years. *Journal of Speech and Hearing Research, 30,* 503–521.

Vihman, M., Velleman, S., & McCune, L. (1994). How abstract is child phonology? Toward an integration of linguistic and psychological approaches. In M. Yavas (Ed.), *First and second language phonology* (pp. 9–44). San Diego: Singular Publishing Group.

Vivaldi, A. (1990). *Phonological process use and dissolution in the acquisition of Puerto Rican Spanish.* Unpublished doctoral dissertation, New York University, New York.

Wellman, B., Case, I., Mengert, I., & Bradbury, D. (1931). Speech sounds of young children. *University of Iowa Studies in Child Welfare* (No. 5). Iowa City: University of Iowa Press.

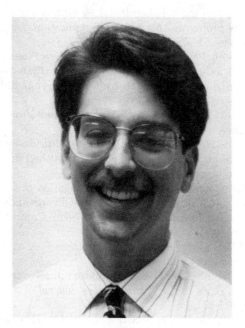

BRIAN GOLDSTEIN, Ph.D.

Dr. Goldstein is an Assistant Professor in the Department of Communication Disorders at Saint Louis University in St. Louis, Missouri. He received a masters degree in 1988 and a doctorate in 1993 from Temple University. Dr. Goldstein has worked extensively with Latino children and their families. His research has focused on both language and phonological development and disorders in Spanish-speaking children. His previous employment positions include speech-language pathologist at the Rainbow Community Head Start in Philadelphia and at the Massachusetts General Hospital in Boston.

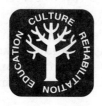

CHAPTER 3

SPANISH MORPHOLOGICAL AND SYNTACTIC DEVELOPMENT

RAQUEL T. ANDERSON, PH.D., CCC-SLP

Morphosyntactic development has been an area of active research in the fields of language development and disorders (Bowerman, 1985; Connell, 1986; Cziko, 1989; Gleitman, 1990). A significant amount of data have been obtained describing typical patterns of grammatical development in monolingual speakers. Most of the data have been obtained on English-speaking children. Although less data are available on other languages, there is sufficient information to aid clinicians working with children from a variety of linguistic backgrounds (Leonard, Sabbadini , & Leonard, 1987; Leonard, Sabbadini, Volterra, & Leonard, 1988; Pizzuto & Caselli, 1992; Slobin, 1995). Spanish is an excellent example. The last two decades have seen an increase in the number of investigations that have particularly addressed Spanish morphosyntactic development (González, 1983; Máez, 1983; Merino,

1992; Merino, 1992; Pérez-Pereira, 1989; Romero, 1985). The data collected in these investigations provide clinicians who are working with Spanish-speaking children with criteria for determining whether a language impairment exists and for planning and implementing an intervention plan.

In addition to this information, the Spanish-speaking clinician who has had experience working with Spanish-speaking children has experiential knowledge of typical and atypical development. Through interactions with language-impaired children, as well as typical language learners, the clinician may gain knowledge about Spanish and its typical developmental course. The clinician may also learn procedures that aid in effectively evaluating morphosyntactic skills, as well as for providing intervention in this area. As a clinician who is particularly interested in morphology and syntax and who has had more than a decade of experience working with language-impaired Spanish-speaking children, I will present in this chapter both data gathered from research and information gathered from clinical experience.

The purpose of this chapter is to provide speech-language pathologists with information that will assist them in the assessment and treatment of Spanish-speaking children with morphosyntactic deficits. The chapter is divided into three major areas, beginning with a discussion of salient morphosyntactic patterns of Spanish which will aid the clinician in understanding important characteristics of the language. Second, relevant developmental data are presented both from published research and from my experience with Spanish-speaking children. Finally, two case studies of children who evidence atypical morphosyntactic development are presented along with a discussion of the assessment and intervention procedures that have been effective.

The importance of morphology and syntax in assessment of language-impaired children needs to be emphasized. Most research in the area of language disorders has stated that children with language impairment, especially children who have been diagnosed as specific language impaired and/or language-learning disabled, have particular difficulty in the areas of syntax and morphology (Connell & Stone, 1992; Leonard et al., 1987; Paul & Alforde, 1993). This suggests that language form needs to be addressed in the assessment and intervention processes. Although other areas need to be addressed as well, speech-language pathologists should not lose sight of structural components of language when assessing language skills in Spanish-speaking children.

ᄓ

BASIC CHARACTERISTICS: SPANISH MORPHOLOGY AND SYNTAX

Before discussing morphosyntactic aspects of Spanish, it is important to stress that any clinician working with a Spanish-speaking population needs to consider the Spanish variant used by the community, as well as the amount of contact that exists with English. Although most of the research conducted on dialectal differences in Spanish has focused on phonology and vocabulary, the limited data that are available on morphosyntactic development suggest that cross-dialectal morphosyntactic differences exist (López-Ornat, 1988). In addition, phonological differences across Spanish variants affect the surface representation of morphosyntactic structures. Spanish dialects in which the /s/ phoneme has as allophonic variants /h/ and/or omission in postvocalic position are excellent examples of this effect. A study conducted by Terrell (1978) on monolingual Puerto Rican Spanish-speakers, where this pattern is part of the variant's phonology, suggests that speakers of this dialect mark plurality only once in the noun phrase (e.g., /las casa grande/). This pattern would suggest a difficulty with noun phrase agreement, while in reality, this is the production pattern of the speakers of that Spanish variant.

Contact with English can also affect the form of Spanish. As has been observed in the linguistics literature, as languages come in contact, the languages involved tend to adopt each other's features (Silva-Corvalán, 1986). In the United States, where Spanish and English are in contact, the clinician needs to be aware of the possible effects that English form may have on Spanish form. This linguistic phenomenon stresses the importance of clinicians obtaining information concerning the child's linguistic community and the structure of the Spanish variant used in that community.

INFLECTIONAL MORPHOLOGY

VERB MORPHOLOGY

Spanish, in contrast to English, is a highly inflected language. This is especially apparent in its verb system. Spanish verbs are inflected for tense, person, number, mood and aspect. There are three types of stem classes: a– (e.g., *hablar*/to speak-talk, *cantar*/to sing, *llorar*/to cry), e– (e.g., *tener*/to have, *comer*/to eat, *beber*/to drink), and i– (e.g., *dormir*/to sleep, *reir*/to laugh, *seguir*/to follow). Of these stem classes, the a– stem is considered the unmarked form, as it is the most frequent and the earliest acquired stem class (Schnitzer, 1993). The inflectional morphology will vary according to the verb stem class. Table 3–1 presents an example of a Spanish verb form, *hablar* (to talk/speak) and its inflection for the simple tenses. As can be noted, there are different inflections for person, number, mood (subjunctive-indicative) and aspect (imperfect-perfect). Examples of inflectional morphology for e– and i– stems are presented in Appendix 3-A.

As in English, the Spanish verb system is inflected for tense. The three major tenses—present, future, and past are differentially inflected in Spanish. Whereas English only has one inflectional form for person— the third person singular present /s/, Spanish has various inflectional

TABLE 3–1

Verb conjugation for simple tenses and person for the verb *hablar* (to talk/speak).

	Singular			Plural		
Tense	**1st**	**2nd**[a]	**3rd**	**1st**	**2nd**[b]	**3rd**
Present indicative	hablo	hablas	habla	hablamos	hablan	hablan
Imperfect indicative	hablaba	hablabas	hablaba	hablábamos	hablaban	hablaban
Preterit	hablé	hablaste	habló	hablamos	hablaron	hablaron
Future	hablaré	hablarás	hablará	hablaremos	hablarán	hablarán
Conditional	hablaría	hablarías	hablaría	hablaríamos	hablarían	hablarían
Present subjunctive	hable	hables	hable	hablemos	hablen	hablen
Imperfect subjunctive	hablara/ hablase	hablaras/ hablases	hablara/ hablase	habláramos/ hablásemos	hablaran/ hablasen	hablaran hablasen

[a]2nd person singular *usted* follows the conjugation for third person singular (*el/ella*).

[b]Conjugation for *vosotros* is not included, as many Spanish variants spoken in the United States and Latin America do not include this form. The plural form *ustedes* is used, following conjugation for third person plural *ellos/ellas* .

forms for indicating person (see Table 3–1). Note that the person inflection in Spanish also differentiates between singular and plural forms.

The Spanish verb system permits differences in tense aspect. The two aspects coded within the verb morphology are perfect and imperfect. Aspect permits the speaker to indicate differences in duration of the action (Solé & Solé, 1977). For example, perfect aspect signals that the action expressed in the verb form was completed (e.g., *Yo hablé ayer*/I talked yesterday—action of talking was completed). The preterit tense, as well as all conjugations with an auxiliary verb (e.g., *Yo he hablado*/I have talked) signal the perfect aspect. On the other hand, imperfect aspect signals that the action has not been completed (e.g., *Yo hablaba con mi madre cuando oí el disparo*/I was talking to my mother when I heard the shot.). All simple tenses, with the exception of the preterit, express the imperfect aspect.

In addition to aspect, Spanish verb morphology permits the speaker to express differences in mood and the speaker's perception of the action. In Spanish, three verb moods are distinguished: the indicative, the imperative, and the subjunctive (Solé & Solé, 1977) (see Table 3–1). When the speaker uses a verb form inflected in the indicative mood, he is perceiving the action coded in the verb as one that has or will occur. In other words, the speaker is certain that the action did occur, is occurring, or will occur. The imperative mood is used when the speaker is presenting the action as a command or as a suggestion (*Habla*/[You] talk). In instances where the speaker considers that the action coded in the verb as probable, but not certain, the subjunctive mood is used (*Ojalá hable mucho*/Let's hope he talks a lot).

Spanish, as English, has an auxiliary verb system. Three verb forms that occur as main verbs are also used as auxiliary verbs. These are *estar* (to be), *haber* (to have), and *andar* (to walk). The latter verb is used most frequently in some Spanish variants. When used, its meaning is equivalent to the auxiliary verb estar (e.g., *Yo estaba hablando—Yo andaba hablando*/I was talking). This pattern of use for the verb *andar* as an auxiliary is evidenced in some Mexican Spanish variants (González, 1983). Table 3–2 presents examples of compound verb tenses with their person and number inflection.

Spanish verb morphology also has irregular forms that do not follow the usual conjugation pattern. Spanish irregular verb forms modify the verb stem. Not all person and tense inflections will be irregular. For example, the first person present indicative form of the verb *caber* (to fit) is *quepo*, whereas the second person inflection for this tense is *cabe*. The first person form is irregular for this tense, but the second person

TABLE 3–2
Verb conjugation for compound tenses for the verb *hablar* (to talk/speak).

	Singular			Plural		
Tense	**1st**	**2nd**[a]	**3rd**	**1st**	**2nd**[b]	**3rd**
Present progressive	estoy hablando	estás hablando	está hablando	estamos hablando	están hablando	están hablando
Present perfect indicative	he hablado	has hablado	ha hablado	hemos hablado	han hablado	han hablado
Past perfect indicative	había hablado	habías hablado	había hablado	habíamos hablado	habían hablado	habían hablado
Preterit perfect	hube hablado	hubiste hablado	hubo hablado	hubimos hablado	hubieron hablado	hubieron hablado
Future perfect	habré hablado	habrás hablado	habrá hablado	habremos hablado	habrán hablado	habrán hablado
Conditional perfect	habría hablado	habrías hablado	habría hablado	habríamos hablado	habrían hablado	habrían hablado
Present perfect	haya hablado	hayas hablado	haya hablado	hayamos hablado	hayan hablado	hayan hablado
Past perfect subjunctive	hubiera/ hubiese hablado	hubieras/ hubieses hablado	hubiera/ hubiese hablado	hubiéramos/ hubiésemos hablado	hubieran/ hubiesen hablado	hubieran/ hubiesen hablado

form is not. Other examples of irregular verb conjugations are presented in Table 3–3.

An important contrast between Spanish and English verb morphology is present in the verb forms known as copulas. These are the linking verbs (Lund & Duchan, 1993). In English, one verb form is used mainly to link or join the subject of the sentence with a description. This is the verb "to be." In Spanish, two verb forms are distinguished: *ser* and *estar*. These two verbs are not interchangeable. They have distinct syntactic and semantic functions. Solé and Solé (1977) state that both *ser* and *estar* occur in the following contexts: (1) with adverbs of place to express origin (e.g., *El es de Puerto Rico*/He is from Puerto Rico; *El está en Puerto Rico*/He is in Puerto Rico) and (2) with

TABLE 3–3

Examples of irregular verb forms.

Verb	Conjugation	Person	Tense
caber (to fit)	cupo	3rd singular	preterit
dormir (to sleep)	duermo	1st singular	present indicative
saber (to know)	se	1st singular	present indicative
poner (to put)	pusieron	3rd plural	preterit
aprobar (to approve)	apruebas	2nd singular	present indicative

adjectivals (e.g., *Ramón es muy guapo*/Ramón is very handsome; *Ramón está muy guapo*/Ramón is very handsome). The difference between the two forms lies mainly on the meaning conveyed. *Estar* refers to a state of being, not a quality. It denotes an attribute or aspect that is not constant. *Ser*, on the other hand, refers to a quality of the subject and it thus relates to a more constant and stable attribute. For example, the sentence *Es de Puerto Rico* is interpreted as the individual being of that country. The sentence *Está en Puerto Rico* is interpreted as the individual visiting the country, but not necessarily being of Puerto Rican origin. The same can be said about attributes. A sentence such as *Es guapo* indicates that the subject of the sentence is indeed handsome. If, instead of using *ser*, *estar* is used (i.e., *Está guapo*), the subject is at that moment handsome, but this attribute is not necessarily a quality of that individual. Syntactically, *ser* can co-occur with past participles, forming a passive construction (e.g., *El niño es perseguido por el perro*/The boy is chased by the dog). *Estar* takes present participles, forming present progressive constructions (e.g., *El niño está jugando*/The boy is playing) (Solé & Solé, 1977).

PRONOUN CASE

The Spanish pronominal system differs considerably from the English pronominal system in its surface representation. A summary of the pronouns present in Spanish by grammatical case is presented in Table 3–4. Included are subject pronouns, object pronouns (reflexive and nonreflexive), and possessive pronouns. Although not presented in this table, two other subject pronouns occur in certain Spanish variants. These are for second person singular and plural forms (*vos* and *vosotros*, respectively) and take the place of the pronouns *tú* and *ustedes*.

TABLE 3–4

Spanish pronoun forms.

Person	Subject	Object Nonreflexive	Object Reflexive	Possessive[a]
1st singular	yo	me	me	mío(a)
2nd singular informal	tú	te	te	tuyo(a)
2nd singular formal	usted	le/lo/la[a]	se	suyo(a)
3rd singular	él /ella[a]	lo/le/la[a]	se	suyo(a)
1st plural	nosotros(as)[a]	nos	nos	nuestro(a)
2nd plural	ustedes	les/los/las[a]	se	suyo(a)
3rd plural	ellos/ellas[a]	les/los/las[a]	se	suyo(a)

[a]Gender is expressed in these pronouns. Possessives also incorporate plural morphemes (e.g., *La canasta es mía*/The basket is mine; *Las canastas son mías*/The baskets are mine).

Spanish is a pro-drop language (Hyams, 1986, 1992). As a result, subject pronouns are frequently deleted. Information concerning who the subject of the sentence is (i.e., person) is coded in the verb. When subject pronouns are used, these are most frequently produced for pragmatic reasons, mainly to stress who the subject of the sentence is (*Yo me lo comí*/I [and nobody else] ate it). In addition, in variants where phonological patterns affect the use of morphological markers for expressing person, subject pronouns are used more frequently, especially with the person forms that lose this contrast (Hochberg, 1986).

Object pronouns are markedly different from English object pronouns. In Spanish, object pronouns are clitic; thus, they always occur adjacent to a verb (e.g., *Te busqué*/I looked for you). They can be positioned before (preclitic) or after (enclitic) the verb. If two or more object pronouns co-occur with the verb, they must all be positioned before or after the verb. The specific position will depend on the configuration of the verb that relates to them. Solé and Solé (1977) indicate that, if the verb is in the indicative or subjunctive mood or if the verb occurs within a negative imperative sentence, the pronouns are placed before the verb phrase. Object pronoun postposition occurs with affirmative commands, infinitives, and present participles. Table 3–5 presents examples of preclitic and enclitic pronominal constructions.

English and Spanish differ with respect to reflexive constructions. Unlike English, most of the pronominal forms used to code nonreflex-

TABLE 3–5
Examples of preclitic and enclitic pronominal constructions.

Verb Form/Mood	Preclitic Construction	Enclitic Construction
Indicative mood	Lo pinté ayer. (I painted it yesterday.)	
Subjunctive mood	Espero que te guste. (I hope you like it.)	
Imperative within negative construction	No te atrevas. (Don't you dare.)	
Imperative in affirmative construction		Búscalo. (Look for it.)
Infinitive constructions		Quiero ayudarte. (I want to help you.)
Present participles		Hablándole la calmarás. (By speaking to her, you will calm her.)

ive relationships are used for coding reflexive relationships (e.g., *Me pinté*/I painted myself; *Me pintaste*/You painted me). The only exception is the pronoun *se*, which is used as the reflexive pronoun for second person formal *usted*, and the third person singular and plural referents (e.g., *La pinté*/I painted her; *Se pintó*/She painted herself). Unlike English, where the use of a reflexive pronoun can be optional (e.g., I bathed/I bathed myself), in Spanish, when the reflexive is a direct object, it is obligatory. This is because their elision would cause ambiguity as to whom the recipient of the action is (e.g., *El bañó*/He bathed someone; *El se bañó*/He bathed himself). This characteristic of the Spanish language renders reflexive constructions a more frequent occurrence than in English.

Reflexive pronouns can also occur in utterances where the verb has traditionally been categorized as intransitive (i.e., a verb that does not take a direct or indirect object). García (1975) named these "Romance reflexives." Examples of these are presented in Table 3–6. Spanish also uses the third person reflexive pronoun *se* in sentence constructions where the subject is not specified (García, 1975; Gili

TABLE 3–6
Examples of romance reflexive constructions.

Romance Reflexive Constructions	English Equivalent
El vaso se cayó de la mesa.	The glass fell from the table.
La máquina de coser se rompió.	The sewing machine broke.
El muchacho se va a bajar del carro.	The young man is going to get out of the car.
Yo me salí de la fila.	I left the line.
Tú te viniste temprano.	You came back early.

Gaya, 1943; Langacker, 1970; Otero, 1973; Schroten, 1972). This use of the pronoun has been termed by Spanish linguists as the impersonal *se* (e.g., *Se venden libros*/Books are sold here). These patterns of use of reflexive pronouns stress the saliency of these forms in the language and the various functions they serve.

NOUN PHRASE MORPHOLOGY

Spanish, in contrast to English, assigns grammatical gender to nouns, Thus, nouns are either assigned the feminine or the masculine gender. As in English, Spanish marks nouns for number. In general, feminine gender is ascribed to nouns ending in /a/ and to nouns that relate specifically to this gender (e.g., girl, lady, mother). Masculine gender is given to nouns ending in /o/ and those that refer to a male entity (e.g., boy, mailman, male teacher). For nouns ending in a consonant or with another vowel, specific rules apply. Two grammatical morphemes are used for establishing plurality. The bound morpheme /s/ is used with nouns that end in a vowel, and the bound morpheme /es/ is used for nouns ending in a consonant. The reader is referred to Spanish grammar books for more precise rules for establishing gender and number (e.g., Solé & Solé, 1977).

Within a noun phrase, all constituents must agree with the noun in both gender and number. In addition to the noun, determinants and adjectives, in general, are marked for number and gender. All Spanish determinants, with the exception of possessives and numerals, must agree with the noun for gender and must encode the same number distinction as the noun. Most adjectives follow this pattern. Table 3–7 presents examples of noun phrase agreements for gender and number.

Spanish has a variety of determinant forms, and they vary according to gender and number. In addition, there is the use of a neuter definite article *lo* . This form does not occur before concrete nouns. Its purpose is to nominalize an attribute that describes some aspect of an event, an idea, or a noun (Solé & Solé, 1977). It also occurs in instances where the gender or number is unspecified. Table 3–8 presents a summary of these determinants with examples.

TABLE 3–7
Examples of noun phrase agreement.

Spanish Noun Phrase	English Equivalent
la muchacha alta	the tall young woman
el bebé bonito	the pretty baby
la comida caliente	the hot food
el muchacho alto	the tall young man
las canastas llenas	the filled baskets
los abrigos largos	the long coats
loa calcetines rotos	the torn socks

TABLE 3-8
Spanish determinants.

Spanish Form	Indefinite Articles	Definite Articles	Demonstratives
Singular			
Feminine	una (una flor, una amiga, una casa)	la (la flor, la amiga, la casa)	esta (esta flor, esta amiga, esta casa)
Masculine	un (un vaso, un avión, un amigo)	el (el vaso, el avión, el amigo)	este (este vaso, este avión, este amigo)
Neuter	uno (uno bonito, uno alegre)	lo (lo bonito, lo alegre)	esto (esto bonito, esto alegre)
Plural			
Feminine	unas (unas flores, unas amigas, unas casas)	las (las flores, las amigas, las casas)	estas (estas flores, estas amigas, estas casas)
Masculine	unos (unos vasos, unos aviones, unos amigos)	los (los vasos, los aviones, los amigos)	estos (estos vasos, estos aviones, estos amigos)

BASIC CHARACTERISTICS OF SPANISH SYNTACTIC STRUCTURE

The following discussion centers on general characteristics of clause word order (sentence), noun phrase word order, formation of negative sentences, formation of wh- and yes/no questions, and use of complex sentences. A comprehensive discussion of Spanish syntax is beyond the scope of this chapter and the reader is encouraged to review basic Spanish syntax.

CLAUSAL WORD ORDER

In general, Spanish is more flexible than English with respect to ordering the phrases within an utterance. Although it is mainly a subject-verb-object language, variations to this pattern are acceptable. Because Spanish is a more morphologically rich language than English, it provides for more flexibility in phrase order within the sentence. Thus, the ordering of noun phrases and verb phrases within the sentence may be variable. Examples of this variability are presented in Table 3–9. In addition to this variability, subject omission is acceptable in Spanish. As mentioned previously, verb inflection provides the listener with information concerning person reference.

TABLE 3-9
Examples of word order variations in Spanish clauses.

Spanish Construction	English Translation
La luna se ve linda.	The moon looks pretty.
Se ve linda la luna.	Looks pretty the moon.
El hombre caminaba en la montaña.	The man walked in the mountains.
Caminaba en la montaña el hombre.	Walked in the mountains the man.
Caminaba el hombre en la montaña.	Walked the man in the mountains.
Nosotras fuimos al parque.	We went to the park.
Fuimos al parque.	(We) went to the park.
Las gallinas corrieron muy rápido.	The chickens ran very fast.
Corrieron muy rápido.	(The chickens) ran very fast.
Yo sabía que no era cierto.	I knew it wasn't true.
Sabía que no era cierto.	(I) knew it wasn't true.

NOUN PHRASE WORD ORDER

The basic word order in Spanish noun phrases is NP (DET) + NOUN + (ADJECTIVE). This contrasts with English, in which the noun phrase constituents are ordered so that all modifiers precede the noun. Examples of noun phrase constructions were presented in Table 3–7. As with other grammatical aspects, there are some Spanish noun phrase constructions in which the adjective precedes the noun. Some examples are the use of a numeral (*dos libros*/two books), the use of the comparative terms *gran, buen* (e.g., *gran maestro*/great teacher; *un buen muchacho*/a good young man), and the use of ordinal numbers or adjectives (e.g., *el primer hombre*/the first man; *el último varón*/the last male).

NEGATIVE SENTENCE FORMATION

Spanish negative sentence formation is structurally simpler than English negative sentence formation. Negative sentences in Spanish are formed by inserting a negative adverb before the verb phrase. Examples of these adverbs are *nunca* (never) and *no* (no, not). In addition, Spanish permits double negative constructions. Table 3–10 provides the reader with examples of negative sentence transformations in Spanish.

TABLE 3–10
Spanish negative transformations.

Affirmative Form	Negative Form
Yo lo vi ayer. (I saw him yesterday.)	Yo no lo vi ayer. (I didn't see him yesterday.)
Quizo hacerte sentir mal. (He wanted to make you feel bad.)	No quizo hacerte sentir mal. (He didn't want to make you feel bad.)
Manuel siempre venía temprano. (Manuel was always early.)	Manuel no venía temprano. (Manuel was never early.) Manuel no venía temprano nunca. (Manuel wasn't early never.)[a]

[a]Incorrect sentence form.

QUESTION FORMATION

Question forms in Spanish, unlike English, do not require the use of the auxiliary verb system. In addition, when the Spanish verb within the question is a compound form (i.e., aux + verb), there is no auxiliary verb inversion. Furthermore, subject-verb inversion is not always necessary. In general, then, Spanish yes/no questions are marked by rising intonation. Wh- questions are formed by adding a question pronoun in the initial sentence slot followed by the verb phrase and an optional noun phrase. Examples of yes/no and wh- questions in Spanish are presented in Table 3–11.

COMPLEX SENTENCES

As in English, Spanish complex sentences include coordination and subordination. Coordinated sentences are joined by the use of conjoiners like "and" (*y*), "but" (*pero*), "nor" (*ni*), and "or" (*o*). Coordination can occur at the sentence level (e.g., *El fue al cine y ella le habló*/He

TABLE 3–11
Question forms in Spanish.

Question Form	English	Spanish
Yes/no	Are you sleepy?	¿Tienes sueño?
	Do you want some?	¿Quieres un poco?
	Is the boy walking?	¿El niño está caminando? ¿Está caminando el niño?
Wh-		
What/qué	What do you want?	¿Qué quieres?
Who/quién	Who is talking?	¿Quién está hablando?
Where/dónde	Where is the basket?	¿Dónde está la canasta?
When/cuándo	When are you coming back?	¿Cuándo regresas?
Which/cuál	Which is the one?	¿Cuál es?
How/cómo	How do you do that?	¿Cómo haces eso?
Why/por qué	Why did he leave?	¿Por qué se fue?

went to the movies and she talked to him), in the predicate (e.g., *El fue al cine y a la tienda*/He went to the movies and to the store), and in the subject (e.g., *María y José fueron al parque*/Mary and Joseph went to the park). Subordinated sentences are formed by the use of a relative pronoun, such as "that" (*que*), "what" (*que*), "how" (*cuan, como*), and "because" (*porque*). They can also occur within the predicate (e.g., *El hace cuanto quiere*/He does what he pleases), and within the subject (e.g., *El hombre que estaba sentado habló*/The man that was seated spoke). Embedded sentences function as complex verb phrases, adverbial clauses, subject clauses, and relative clauses. Table 3–12 provides some examples of complex sentences in Spanish.

⊔

GRAMMATICAL DEVELOPMENT IN SPANISH-SPEAKING CHILDREN

Prior to presenting the developmental data that have been recorded for Spanish-speaking children, several cautionary statements must be made. The investigations in the area of morphosyntactic development

TABLE 3–12
Examples of Spanish embedded sentences.

Type of Complex Sentence	Spanish Construction	English Construction
Complex verb phrases	Ramón espera que le escribas.	Ramón hopes that you will write to him.
	El muchacho quiere irse temprano.	The young man wants to leave early.
Adverbial clauses	Ya que está muy lejos, no podremos llegar hoy.	Since it is so far away, we will not be able to get there today.
Subject clauses	El niño se haya ido no es extraño.	That he has left is not odd.
Relative clauses	La perra que se escapó es de los vecinos.	The dog that ran away is our neighbor's.

have varied in design. Some have been longitudinal (e.g., Máez, 1983), but most have been cross-sectional (e.g., Anderson, 1987; González, 1983). In addition, most research paradigms have relied on data collection through spontaneous speech samples (e.g., Linares-Orama & Sanders, 1977; Máez, 1983). Therefore, developmental patterns are inferred. This may not be the most appropriate means for assessing the development of specific forms, because the frequency of occurrence of morphosyntactic structures is dependent on the context for communication. Thus, frequency of occurrence may not be the best indicator for establishing order of acquisition of specific grammatical morphemes.

Two other methodological differences relate directly to the subjects used in these studies. Investigations on Spanish language development have included subjects from various Spanish-speaking countries (e.g., Puerto Rico: Anderson, 1987; Morales, 1986a; Romero, 1985; Chile: Peronard, 1985; Mexico: Kernan & Blount, 1966) in addition to Spanish-speaking children living in the United States. Dialectal differences and exposure to English may differentially affect morphosyntactic development in Spanish-speaking children (López-Ornat, 1988). Another difference pertaining to the population sampled is the age range chosen for study. Most studies include 3-year-old children as the youngest subjects. Studies are now including 2-year-old children, but many of the developmental data do not encompass this important age range.

In the present discussion, pertinent data on morphosyntactic development will be summarized in terms of age range and development of specific structures. This information is presented in Table 3–13. As can be seen in the table, age ranges have been used for describing developmental patterns across noun phrase morphology, verb morphology, and sentence structure. Although some studies have used mean length of utterance (MLU) ranges for describing developmental trends, I will not do so for two reasons. First, studies that have presented MLU scores for Spanish-speaking children have varied considerably in their procedures for counting morphemes (Kvaal, Shipstead-Cox, Nevitt, Hodson, & Launer, 1988; Linares-Orama & Sanders, 1977; Máez, 1983). As a result, it is difficult to compare results. Second, MLU was developed for English (Brown, 1973), and not for Spanish. Both languages vary considerably with respect to inflection. Thus, it has not been established that MLU is an adequate measure of language development in Spanish. The information provided in the literature on morphosyntactic development will be sup-

TABLE 3–13

Summary of developmental data for morphosyntactic development in Spanish-speaking children.

Age Range	Verb Morphology	Noun Phrase Elaboration	Prepositional Phrases	Syntactic Structure

2;0–3;0	Present indicative
	Simple preterit
	Imperative
	Periphrastic
	   future
	Copulas ser/estar
		Indefinite and definite
		   articles
		Article gender
		   Plural /s/
		   Plural /es/
			en
			con
			para
			a
			de
				Sentences with
				   copula verbs
				Use of clitic
				   direct object
				Reflexive
				   constructions
				(S)VO
				   sentences
				Yes/no
				   questions
				Negative with
				   no before verb
				   phrase
				Imperative
				   sentences
				Wh- questions
				   qué
				   quién
				   dónde
				   para qué
				   cuándo
				   por qué
				   cómo
				   de quién
				   con quién
				Embedded
				   sentences
				Embedded
				   direct object

3;0–4;0	Imperfect preterit
	Past progressive
	Ir progressive
	   past/present
	Compound preterit
	Present subjunctive
		Grammatical
		   gender in nouns
		   and adjectives
		Use of quantifiers
			hasta
			entre
			desde
			sobre
				Wh- questions
				   established
				Use of full set
				   of negatives
				Subjunctive
				   clauses
				Embedding

4;0–5;0	Past subjunctive
	Present perfect
	   indicative
		Gender in clitic
		   3rd person
		   pronouns		

Sources: González (1978, 1983); Kvaal et al. (1988); Máez (1983); Merino (1992); Morales (1986a, 1986b); Pérez-Pereira (1989); Peronard (1985); Romero (1985).

plemented by clinical observations made by the author during her experience with Spanish-speaking language impaired children.

DEVELOPMENT OF VERB MORPHOLOGY

Most of the data collected for verb morphology have been in the area of tense, with some mention of mood and aspect. The age range of acquisition of verb tense are presented in Table 3–14. The patterns observed suggest that the first form to develop are simple tenses, specifically the present indicative (*Yo hablo*/I speak) and simple preterit (*Yo hablé*/I spoke). The first compound form to be evidenced

TABLE 3–14
Age ranges for the development of verb inflection in Spanish-speaking children.

Tense	Age Range (years;months)								
	2;0	2;6	3;0	3;6	4;0	4;6	5;0	5;6	6;0
Present indicative	——	——							
Simple preterit	——	——							
Imperative	——	——							
Copulas	——	——							
Present progressive	——	——							
Compound preterit			——	——	——				
Periphrastic future				——	——	——			
Imperfect preterit				——					
Present subjunctive					——	——	——	——	——
Past progressive					——				
Past subjunctive						——	——		

Note: Beginning of line indicates initial age when appearance of the specific tense was noted. Line demarcates ranges in the acquisition of the forms.

Sources: González (1983); Máez (1983); Morales (1986a, 1986b); Pérez-Pereira (1989); Romero (1985).

is the present progressive (*Yo estoy hablando*/I am speaking). In addition, the periphrastic future (*Yo voy a hablar*/I am going to speak), which implies a complex sentence structure, is also an early acquired form. All these tenses are acquired by 3 years of age. In fact, some investigators indicate appropriate use of these tenses by the first half of the third year (2;6 years) (González, 1983; Morales, 1986a, 1986b). At this age, both indicative and imperative mood forms are observed (*Mira*/Look; *Hablo*/I talk).

The imperfect forms begin to be observed more consistently at 3 years of age (*Yo hablaba*/I was speaking). past progressive forms also begin to emerge at this time, as well as some compound tenses, such as the compound preterit (*Yo había hablado*/I had spoken). It is during the 3-year-old period that verbs inflected in the subjunctive mood emerge. These, nevertheless, are produced inconsistently, especially since the subjunctive mood occurs in complex sentences (e.g., *Yo quiero que te vayas*/I want you to leave). From 4 to 5 years of age, other subjunctive forms, specifically the past tense, emerge (e.g., *Yo creía que tú habías ido*/I thought you had gone). In my clinical experience, subjunctive mood is an aspect of verb inflection that is particularly difficult for language-impaired children to acquire. In typical language learners, I have observed stable use of the subjunctive inflection by 5 years of age.

Some data have been collected on person inflection. Nevertheless, these have been difficult to interpret. During spontaneous speech production, person distinctions made depend on conversational context. Lack of use of a specific person form does not necessarily mean that children do not have this form in their expressive repertoire. Error data would aid in studying the development of person distinctions (i.e., error patterns in the use of person inflection). Regrettably, studies have not analyzed these. From the data presented in the various studies on verb inflection, it can be inferred that by 2 years of age, correct inflection for singular forms for all persons is evidenced (González, 1983; Máez, 1983). Production of plural inflection is acquired later, but still early (by approximately 3 years of age) (González, 1983). My experience with both typical and atypical language learners suggests that the acquisition of person distinctions occurs very early in the development of verb inflection and is not usually significantly impaired in children with language disabilities.

Other patterns of morphological development have been reported in the literature. With respect to verb stem inflection, Schnitzer (1993) indicates that a– stems are acquired earlier than the other stem forms. In addition, the pattern of regularizing irregular verb forms is also evidenced in Spanish-speaking children (e.g., *Sabo/se*; *poniste/pusiste*). This can be observed in children throughout their preschool years. Furthermore, it is quite possible that, in some dialects, these forms are in fact used. In working with children where one of the parents is English dominant, I have observed this parent over-regularize irregular forms; thus, it is essential to obtain information concerning language input, not only frequency, but type.

The copulative verbs *ser* and *estar* are present very early. These have been observed in children as young as 20 months of age (Máez, 1983). González (1983) indicates that the copula verbs were the most frequently occurring verbs in the language samples of 2;0-year-old Mexican-American children. In a study by Sera (1992), the pattern of contrastive use of both copula verbs was assessed in Spanish-speaking Cuban-American children between the ages of 3;6 and 11;1. Her results suggest that children first learn to contrast between these forms in a context by context basis, and that the first cues for establishing the contrast between *ser* and *estar* are syntactic. Children were able to assign *ser* and *estar* following adult rules to adjectives (e.g., *Es bonita*/She is pretty, versus, *Está bonita*/She is, at this moment, pretty). Nevertheless, they tended to use *estar* more frequently when using a locative adverb, thus not establishing a difference in meaning through the contrastive use of the two copula verbs.

DEVELOPMENT OF NOUN PHRASE INFLECTION

A summary of developmental patterns observed in the development of noun phrase morphology is presented in Table 3–13. By 2 years of age, both definite and indefinite articles are present in Spanish-speaking children's noun phrases (Máez, 1983). Plural forms also emerge during the third year of life (2;0–2;11 years) (Kvaal, et al., 1988). Of the two plurals, the /s/ plural is used before the /es/ plural. In terms of noun phrase agreement morphemes, correct use of gender appears early in the use of both female and male gender definite and indefinite articles (Máez, 1983). By 3 years of age, the correct gender in the adjective is acquired (Merino, 1992). By 4 years of age, correct gender in the use of third person pronouns appears (Merino, 1992). Clinical experience suggests that grammatical gender is generally not impaired in monolingual Spanish-speaking language-disordered children. The errors produced occur mainly in instances where the child overgeneralizes the regular rule to all forms (e.g., *la azúcar/el azúcar; el mano/la mano; la agua/el agua*). Error productions for article-noun gender agreement have been observed in children exposed to English. This has been especially apparent in instances where one of the primary caretakers is English-dominant and tends to make the same types of errors. As mentioned previously, it is essential to study the child's Spanish language input when assessing morphosyntactic skills.

Data on noun phrase agreement for plural are scarce. The data presented in the developmental literature suggest that this is acquired, at least for article-noun plural agreement, by 2;6 years. The reader is cautioned on dialectal differences and plural agreement, as studies have shown differential patterns for marking plurality in noun phrases across Spanish-speakers (Terrell, 1978).

THE DEVELOPMENT OF PERSONAL PRONOUNS

The developmental literature available on personal pronoun development suggests that these forms are acquired by monolingual Spanish-speaking children by 3 years of age (Anderson, 1987; Schum, Conde & Díaz, 1992). Developmental data on personal pronoun development are presented in Table 3–15. As can be observed, the first person

TABLE 3–15

Spanish personal pronoun development.

Pronoun	Age Range (years;months)			
	2;0	2;6	3;0	3;6
Yo	——————————			
Tú	——————————			
El/ella	———————————————————			
Me	———————————————————			
Te	———————————————————			
La/lo	———————————————————			
Se	———————————————————			

Note: Clitic pronouns include both reflexive and nonreflexive uses. Plural forms were evidenced in Schum et al. (1992) at approximately 2;6 years for subject pronoun forms.

Sources: Anderson (1987); Schum et al. (1992).

forms to develop are first and second person (*yo, tú, me, te*). Third person forms develop later. Children evidence the use of *yo* and *tú* by 2 years of age (Anderson., 1987; Schum et al., 1992). By approximately 2;6, the use of third person subject pronouns is observed. Although Spanish permits the elision of subject pronouns, these are the first forms to be acquired by Spanish-speaking children. This has been observed in both spontaneous speech data (Schum et al., 1992), as well as the data obtained from structured activities (Anderson, 1987). Correct use of object pronouns, in both reflexive and nonreflexive constructions can be observed as early as 2 years of age. All singular object pronouns are acquired by 3 years of age. Plural clitic pronouns *los/las/les* are seen to emerge approximately at 2;9 years of age.

The most frequent error pattern reported in the production of pronouns, specifically the clitic pronouns, is the omission of the pronominal form (*Yo ví; Yo te ví*/I saw; I saw you) (Anderson, 1987; Schum et al., 1992). This pattern has also been observed in other languages that have clitic pronouns, such as Italian (Pizzuto & Caselli, 1992). The omission of the clitic pronouns is a salient characteristic of the expressive language of language-impaired Italian-speaking children (Leonard et al., 1988). In my experience with Spanish-speaking language-impaired children, this pattern is also present in their oral language.

DEVELOPMENT OF SYNTACTIC STRUCTURE

The majority of the studies of syntactical development have been conducted by González (1978) with Mexican-American children. The reader is again advised to consider dialectal differences across Spanish-speaking countries and communities.

A vast array of clause structures have been noted in Spanish-speaking children. General patterns of development are summarized in Table 3–13. González (1978) indicates that at 2 years of age, children use sentences with both copula verbs. This includes clauses with the omission of the subject, as well as with the production of the subject (e.g., *Está ahí/La pelota está ahí*, [The ball] is there). These include the use of a noun phrase for the copula *ser* or an adverb for the copula *estar*. Included in the clause structure at this time are the clitic pronouns, but these are not consistent in the children's speech. By 2;6, the use of clitic pronoun forms within the sentence is more frequent. In addition, children evidence use of direct objects within the clause (e.g., *Agarré la pelota*/[I] grabbed the ball). By 3 years of age, the Spanish-speaking children studied by González (1978) had a variety of sentence forms, including forms with variations in the usual word order (i.e., SVO). González (1978) indicates that in sentences where the SVO order is not followed, instances of lack of subject-verb agreement may be seen as late as 5 years of age. This is a pattern that has also been observed in older children, as well as adults, albeit infrequently. Thus, if lack of subject-verb agreement occurs sporadically in sentences that do not follow the SVO order, it does not indicate a deficiency in morphosyntactic skills.

The development of prepositions in Spanish was studied by Peronard (1985). She followed three monolingual Spanish-speaking Chilean children for approximately 2 years to 4 years of age. The first prepositions to emerge were those expressing place, company, and instrument. These were the following: *en, con, para, a, de*. All three children were producing these prepositions at 2 years of age. The last prepositions to emerge in the children's spontaneous speech were *hasta, entre, desde*, and *sobre*. These were observed most frequently between 3 and 4 years of age.

Certain types of sentences are established quite early in Spanish-speaking children. Various sentence transformations are seen in the speech of children by 2;6. These include the negative transformation, the question formation, imperative sentences, and embedded sentences. According to González (1978), the use (Subject) + no + verb phrase can be seen at this age. By 3;6, the Mexican-American children he studied demonstrated the correct use of the full set of negatives in Spanish.

Use of rising intonation is the basic pattern in Spanish for the production of yes/no questions. This can be observed in children as young as 2;0. Wh- questions are also present at this time and include *qué* (what), *quién* (who), and *dónde* (where) (González, 1978). At 2;6, questions with *para qué* (for what), *cuándo* (when), *por qué* (why), and *cómo* (how), emerge. By 2;9, González (1978) states that children utilize *de quién* (whose) and *con quién* (with whom). He adds that by 3 years of age, the children studied used a wide variety of wh- questions. Because Spanish question formation does not include auxiliary verb inversion, children master yes/no and wh- question transformations early.

During the early stages of language development, imperatives consist mainly of one-word utterances or verb + direct object (González, 1978). By 2;6, the use of imperative sentences is established and correlates with the development of aspect for verb inflection. The first embedded sentences to emerge in Spanish are those with the periphrastic future. These are observed at 2;6 (Morales, 1986a). Other embedded sentences that begin to emerge at this age are those in which the embedded clause functions as a direct object. This clause tends to occur at the end of the sentence and thus follows the general operating principle in language development presented by Slobin (1985) "pay attention to the ends of utterances." With the appearance of the subjunctive mood, embedded clauses with the subjunctive begin to emerge at approximately 3 years of age. Nevertheless, the child will initially begin using the indicative mood for the subjunctive mood (e.g., *Quería que me des/Quería que me dieras*—I wanted you to give me).

ㄣ

CASE STUDIES

The following two case studies are from Spanish-speaking Mexican-American children. Although exposed to English, both children are Spanish dominant. The first child to be presented is completing her second semester of treatment. The second child has received treatment for approximately 4 years. For both children, therapy has been provided in Spanish. Their primary language deficits were morphology and syntax, but they differed with respect to the specific areas of difficulty. Specifically, one child appeared to be at an earlier stage of morphosyntactic development (Case 1), whereas the other was more advanced in both the use of inflectional morphology and syntax (phrase and clause structure) (Case 2). Furthermore, morphology was targeted for both children, and syntax (word order) was targeted for one child. These case studies illustrate possible morphosyntactic deficits in Spanish-speaking children. The rationale for choosing specific targets for intervention, as well as the procedures used will be discussed.

CASE 1: F.N.

F.N. is a 5-year-old child. She is the oldest of three children. Spanish is the only language spoken at home. English and Spanish are spoken at the preschool. She has been receiving therapy in our clinic for one-and-a-half semesters. Initial evaluation results indicated that F.N. presented a moderate phonological impairment, as assessed by the *Assessment of Phonological Processes—Spanish* (APP-S) (Hodson, 1986). Phonological error patterns included consonant sequence reductions (e.g., [ne ɣ o]/[ne ɣr o]), unstressed syllable deletions in multisyllabic words (e.g., [tena]/[estampa]), and class deficiencies for the flap /ɾ/ and the trill /r/ (e.g., [nalis]/[na ɾ is]; [jajo]/[ra ð jo]). Language samples obtained during child-mother and child-clinician interaction revealed a significant delay in expressive language, with morphosyntactic skills being a major area of deficiency. F.N.'s productions consisted primarily of one-word utterances. Noun phrases included primarily an article and a noun. Verb inflection was significantly delayed. F.N. used verbs in the infinitive form (e.g., *ahorita poner eso*/*ahorita pones eso*). Omission of copulas in obligated instances was also apparent (e.g., *esa linda*/*esa es linda*). Results from the *Spanish Structured Photographic Expressive Language Test—Preschool* (Werner & Kresheck, 1989) paralleled these findings.

Therapy addressed both articulation and expressive language. Language goals were established to develop verb inflection. These goals have considered the interaction between phonological errors and morphological skills. The morphological forms targeted are not affected by the child's phonological errors. These are person and tense inflection. For both targets, the use of the flap /ɾ/, and the trill /r/ are not needed. In addition, final /s/ is produced by the child and syllable omissions are present only in the initial weak syllables of multisyllabic words. Correct production of consonant clusters is not necessary for the production of verb tense and inflection. It is also important to state that the literature that suggests that morphology should not be targeted in phonologically disordered children pertains to English-speaking children (Lund & Duchan, 1993). Spanish is a morphologically rich language that relies much more on inflection for meaning. It is possible that what is suggested for English may not be applicable to Spanish.

Three person inflection forms have been targeted simultaneously: first, second informal, and third person singular. Two tenses have been used: present indicative (e.g., *hablo*/*hablas*/*habla*) and simple preterit (e.g., *hablé*/*hablaste*/*habló*). The choice for person and tense relates directly to order of acquisition (see Table 3–13). Due to the fact that –a stem inflection is the most frequently occurring and earlier acquired form (Schnitzer, 1993), these verbs were used as initial targets. A contrastive approach to the treatment of verb morphology was used. Through structured play activities, the clinician, child, and "other" (i.e., doll) performed a variety of actions. The clinician began with first and second person contrast (*Yo pinto/Tú pintas*), and when the child evidenced correct use of these forms, she incorporated the third person form (*Ella pinta*). The order for person followed what was established for personal pronoun distinctions, as these pronouns were introduced in the activities (see Table 3–15). After first and second person inflection was established for present indicative, the simple preterit was introduced. Here, the contrast was in terms of the time when the action took place. Thus, the same person referent was used in the contrasting utterance pair (*Yo pinto/Yo pinté*). Through actual performance of the action, the different inflections of time/tense were made more apparent to the child. At present, F.N. consistently uses both tenses, as well as first and second person inflection in her spontaneous speech. In addition, she adequately uses copula verbs. Following the developmental patterns presented in Table 3–13, future goals should include noun phrase elaboration, use of prepositional phrases, and use of other verb tenses, as well as aspect (imperfect/perfect distinction). Noun phrase elaboration should incorporate the use of adjectives with correct use of gender and placement within the phrase. The periphrastic future and the present progressive should follow for verb tense. Once these have been acquired, the use of the imperfect preterit tense as it contrasts with the simple preterit needs to be introduced. Prepositions initially targeted should be *en* (in), *a* (to), followed by *de* (of), *con* (with), and *para* (for), as these are acquired earlier.

CASE 2: I.B.

I.B. is a 9-year-old Spanish-speaking male. He was diagnosed by a team of professionals at a local Child Study Center as presenting moderate mental retardation, microcephaly, and cerebral palsy. A speech-language evaluation revealed a significant delay in phonological development, as well as in expressive and receptive language. Therapy was recommended and focused on both articulation and language skills. Language therapy had focused on the development of simple complete sentences, use of locative adverbs, and verb inflection for tense.

During the first year of intervention at our center, several errors were noted in his expressive language. Although extremely verbal, I.B. had difficulty with phrase order within the sentence. This affected subject-verb agreement for person (e.g., *La casa limpió yo/Yo limpié la casa*). He also demonstrated difficulty with the correct use of possessive pronouns, as these contrasted with possessive adjectives. I.B. consistently used the possessive pronoun for the possessive adjective (*mía casa/mi casa*). Treatment goals were developed to address word order and use of possessive adjectives.

Procedures for working with correct word order relied mainly on modeling and imitation within a role- and structured play interaction in the clinical setting. In these activities, various actions were performed to elicit a Subject + Verb + Direct Object construction (e.g.. *La niña lava los platos*). This construction was targeted because it is one of the first types of simple sentence forms used by Spanish-speaking children (González, 1978) (see Table 3–13). All singular person inflection was used in the verb phrase. Singular forms were again chosen, as these are acquired earlier than plural forms (see Tables 3–13 and 3–15). Thus, the clinician, I.B., and another "person" performed a variety of tasks. The third person referent was either a doll or another person. Following the developmental sequence presented in Table 3–13, verb tenses used included present indicative (e.g., *Yo lavo los platos*/I wash the dishes) and simple preterit (e.g., *Yo lavé los platos*/I washed the dishes).

The use of possessive constructions was addressed by contrasting utterances with the use of a possessive pronoun with those with a possessive adjective (*mi casa—la casa mía*). This procedure permitted highlighting word order differences in noun phrase elaboration for *mi* and *mía*. The clinician provided a set of sentences for modeling and the child repeated them, for example, *Es mi casa* and *Es la casa mía*. Games were incorporated where a third person participated; thus first, second, and third person singular forms were targeted (i.e., *mi/mía(o); tu/tuya(o); su/suya(o)*). In addition, items belonging to the clinician and to the child were incorporated into the various activities. The tasks designed for expressive language were very successful. Although intervention focused mainly on articulation, within 9 months, I.B. demonstrated excellent use of possessive forms and simple sentence structures for word order and person verb inflection.

I.B. communicates primarily using complete sentences with frequent use of coordinated sentences with *y* (and). Although he used complete sentences, certain morphosyntactic errors were noted. Of special significance were the consistent omission of the prepositions and the clitic pronouns. This, in addition to his difficulties with embedding, made it difficult to follow his conversations and narrations.

At present, language therapy for I.B. entails teaching him the use of clitic pronouns and prepositions. The developmental data available for both aspects aided in establishing order of presentation for intervention. The use of clitic pronouns has focused on their use as direct objects (e.g., *Yo te peino*/I comb you). Initially, first and second person clitic pronouns were targeted, as these are acquired earlier than third person forms (see Table 3–15). As specific order of acquisition of reflexive and nonreflexive use of clitics has not been established, these were used in both reflexive and nonreflexive constructions (e.g., *Yo me peino*/I comb myself; *Yo te peino*/I comb you). Third person direct objects were targeted following consistent use of first and second person forms. Structured play activities, where the child and clinician are engaged performing various actions to each other and themselves, were incorporated in the therapy. Through these activities, the deictic use of first and second person forms was presented to I.B.

Prepositions are also taught in a contrastive manner. Pairs of prepositions are taught together. Following the developmental hierarchy presented in Table 3–13, the prepositions *en* (in) and *a* (to) were chosen as the initial contrasting pair. In these activities, various dolls visit different sites (e.g., home, school, supermarket). The clinician presents the doll going towards ("to") a location and that doll, after arriving, "in" the setting. The clinician provides both verbal models and the child is asked to imitate. These activities have proven effective. I.B. is beginning to use both prepositions and clitic pronouns in spontaneous speech in other clinical activities. Other prepositions to be targeted include *con, para,* and *de* (see Table 3–13). Future goals will address the development of embedding and coordination.

⌐

CONCLUSION

The purpose of this chapter was to present clinicians with basic information pertaining to morphology and syntax in Spanish-speaking children. Salient features of Spanish grammar were discussed and developmental data on Spanish were summarized. Morphology is an important aspect of Spanish and must be part of the assessment of Spanish-speaking children. It is through inflection that meaning is frequently conveyed in Spanish. Developmental data demonstrate that

Spanish-speaking children evidence the use of inflectional morphology for verbs, pronouns and nouns at a very early age and that many forms are well established by 4 years of age. Syntactic development also indicates that Spanish children demonstrate correct use of simple sentence structures and question transformations by 3 years of age. In addition, embedding and subordination is apparent during the period of 3 to 4 years of age.

Two case studies describing how specific morphosyntactic structures were chosen for intervention and the procedures used for facilitating the children's acquisition of them were presented. A developmental hierarchy inferred from the data available for Spanish-speaking children was used for this procedure.

Clinicians working with Spanish-speaking children need to assess morphosyntactic skills. As part of this assessment, they need to consider issues pertaining to dialectal differences and English contact when evaluating and remediating language form in Spanish-speaking children. Information concerning Spanish language input and community use of the language should be obtained, and diagnostic and intervention decisions should conform to community norms. Furthermore, clinicians must have an understanding of Spanish morphosyntactic structure and development. Without this knowledge base, it would be difficult to analyze children's use of morphosyntactic structures and to develop intervention strategies to facilitate learning. Consultation of texts and readings on Spanish linguistics, as well as studies on morphosyntactic development in both typical and atypical Spanish-speaking children, are recommended to clinicians to help their decision-making process with language-impaired Spanish-speaking children.

⊔

REFERENCES

Anderson, R. T. (1987). *Personal pronoun development in two- and three-year-old monolingual Spanish-speaking children*. Unpublished doctoral dissertation, Northwestern University, Evanston, IL.

Bowerman, M. (1985). What shapes children's grammar? In D. Slobin (Ed.), *The cross-linguistic study of language. Volume 2. Theoretical issues* (pp. 1257–1319). Hillsdale, NJ: Lawrence Erlbaum.

Brown, R. (1973). *A first language: The early stages*. Boston, MA: Harvard University Press.

Connell, P. J. (1986). Teaching subjecthood to language-disordered children. *Journal of Speech and Hearing Research, 29*, 481–492.

Connell, P. J., & Stone, C. A. (1992). Morpheme learning of children with specific language impairment under controlled instructional conditions. *Journal of Speech and Hearing Research, 35*, 844–852.

Cziko, G. A. (1989). A review of the state-process and punctual-nonpunctual distinctions in children's acquisition of verbs. *First Language, 9*, 1–31.

García, E. (1975). *The role of theory in linguistic analysis: The Spanish pronoun system*. New York: North Holland.

Gili Gaya, S. (1943). *Curso superior de sintaxis española* (Advanced course on Spanish syntax). Mexico City: Ediciones Minerva.

Gleitman, L. (1990). The structural sources of verb meaning. *Language Acquisition, 1*, 3–55.

González, G. (1978). *The acquisition of Spanish grammar by native Spanish-speaking children*. Rosslyn, VA: National Clearinghouse for Bilingual Education.

González, G. (1983). Expressing time through verb tenses and temporal expression in Spanish: Age 2.0–4.6. *NABE Journal, 7*, 69–82.

Hochberg, J. G. (1986). Functional compensation for /s/ deletion in Puerto Rican Spanish. *Language, 62*, 609–621.

Hodson, B. W. (1986). *The Assessment of Phonological Processes—Spanish*. San Diego, CA: Los Amigos.

Hyams, N. (1986, October). *Core and peripheral grammar and the acquisition of inflection*. Paper presented at the 11th. Annual Boston University Conference on Child Language, Boston, MA.

Hyams, N. (1992). Morphosyntactic development in Italian and its relevance to parameter-setting models: Comments on the paper by Pizzuto and Caselli. *Journal of Child Language, 19*, 695–710.

Kernan, K. T. & Blount, B. G. (1986). The acquisition of Spanish grammar by Mexican children. *Anthropological Linguistics, 8*, 1–14.

Kvaal, J. T., Shipstead-Cox, N., Nevitt, S. C., Hodson, B. W., & Launer, P. B. (1988). The acquisition of 10 Spanish morphemes by Spanish-speaking children. *Language, Speech, and Hearing Services in Schools, 19*, 384–394.

Langacker, R. (1970). Review of Spanish case and function by Mark Godin. *Language, 46*, 167–185.

Leonard, L. B., Sabaddini, L., & Leonard, J. S. (1987). Specific language impairment in children: A cross-linguistic study. *Brain and Language, 32*, 233–252.

Leonard, L. B., Sabaddini, L., Volterra, V., & Leonard, J. S. (1988). Some influences on the grammar of English- and Italian-speaking children with specific language impairment. *Applied Psycholinguistics, 9*, 39–57.

Linares-Orama, N., & Sanders, L. J. (1977). Evaluation of syntax in three-year-old Spanish speaking Puerto Rican children. *Journal of Speech and Hearing Research, 20*, 350–357.

López-Ornat, S. (1988). On data sources on the acquisition of Spanish as a first language. *Journal of Child Language, 15*, 679–686.

Lund, N. J., & Duchan, J. F. (1993). *Assessing children's language in naturalistic contexts.* Englewood Cliffs, NJ: Prentice-Hall.

Máez, L. F. (1983). The acquisition of noun and verb morphology in 18–24 month old Spanish speaking children. *NABE Journal, 7*, 53–68.

Merino, B. J. (1992). Acquisition of syntactic and phonological features in Spanish. In H. W. Langdon & L. L. Cheng (Eds.), *Hispanic children and adults with communication disorders* (pp. 57–98). Gaithersburg, MD: Aspen.

Morales, A. (1986a). *Funciones básicas y formas verbales en la adquisición del lenguaje* (Basic functions and verb forms in language acquisition) . Unpublished manuscript, University of Puerto Rico, Río Piedras.

Morales, A. (1986b). *Manifestaciones del pasado en niños puertorriqueños de 2-6 años* (Past tense use in 2-to-6-year-old Puerto Rican children). Unpublished manuscript, University of Puerto Rico, Río Piedras.

Otero, C. (1973). Agrammaticality in performance. *Linguistic Inquiry, 4*, 551–562.

Paul, R., & Alforde, S. (1993). Grammatical morpheme acquisition in 4-year-olds with normal, impaired, and slow late-developing language. *Journal of Speech and Hearing Research, 36*, 1271–1275.

Pérez-Pereira, M. (1989). The acquisition of morphemes: Some evidence from Spanish. *Journal of Psycholinguistic Research, 18*, 289–311.

Peronard, M. (1985). Spanish prepositions introducing adverbial constructions. *Journal of Child Language, 12*, 95–108.

Pizzuto, A., & Caselli, M. C. (1992). The acquisition of Italian morphology: Implications for models of language development. *Journal of Child Language, 19*, 491–558.

Romero, M. (1985). *Verb acquisition in Spanish as a native language in Puerto Rico.* Unpublished doctoral dissertation, New York University, New York.

Sera, M. D. (1992). To be or not to be: Use and acquisition of the Spanish copulas. *Journal of Memory and Language, 31*, 408–427.

Schnitzer, M. L. (1993). Steady as a rock: Does the steady state represent cognitive fossilization? *Journal of Psycholinguistic Research, 22*, 1–20.

Schroten, J. (1972). *Concerning the deep structures of Spanish reflexive sentences .* The Hague: Mouton.

Schum, G., Conde, A., & Díaz, C. (1992). Pautas de adquisición y uso del pronombre personal en la lengua española: Un estudio longitudinal (Acquisition and use of personal pronouns in Spanish: A longitudinal study). *Estudios de Psicología, 48*, 67–86.

Silva-Corvalán, C. (1986). Bilingualism and language change: The extension of estar in Los Angeles Spanish. *Language, 62* , 587–608.

Slobin, D. I. (1985). Crosslinguistic evidence for the language-making capacity. In D. I. Slobin (Ed.), *The crosslinguistic study of language. Volume 2: Theoretical issues* (pp. 1157–1256). Hillsdale, NJ: Lawrence Erlbaum.

Solé, Y., & Solé, C. (1977). *Modern Spanish syntax: A study in contrast.* Lexington, MA: Heath.

Terrell, T. (1978). Sobre la aspiración y elisión de /s/ implosiva y final en el español de Puerto Rico (Aspiration and elision of postvocalic /s/ in Puerto Rican Spanish). *Nueva Revista de Filología Hispánica, 27,* 24–33.

Werner, E. O., & Kresheck, J. D. (1989). *Spanish Structured Photographic Expressive Language Test—Preschool.* Sandwich, IL: Janelle Publications.

APPENDIX 3A

VERB CONJUGATION FOR E- AND I- STEMS

TABLE 3A–1
Verb e- stem simple conjugation (*comer*/to eat).

Tense	Singular			Plural		
	1st	2nd	3rd	1st	2nd	3rd
Present indicative	como	comes	come	comemos	comen	comen
Imperfect indicative	comía	comías	comía	comíamos	comían	comían
Preterit	comí	comiste	comió	comimos	comieron	comieron
Future	comeré	comerás	comerá	comeremos	comerán	comerán
Conditional	comería	comerías	comería	comeríamos	comerían	comerían
Present subjunctive	coma	comas	coma	comamos	coman	coman
Imperfect subjunctive	comiera/ comiese	comieras/ comieses	comiera/ comiese	comiéramos/ comiésemos	comieran/ comiesen	comieran/ comiesen

TABLE 3A–2
Verb stem i- conjugation of simple tenses (*subir*/to climb).

Tense	Singular			Plural		
	1st	2nd	3rd	1st	2nd	3rd
Present indicative	subo	subes	sube	subimos	suben	suben
Imperfect indicative	subía	subías	subía	subíamos	subían	subían
Preterit	subí	subiste	subió	subimos	subieron	subieron
Future	subiré	subirás	subirá	subiremos	subirán	subirán
Conditional	subiría	subirías	subiría	subiríamos	subirían	subirían
Present subjunctive	suba	subas	suba	subamos	suban	suban
Imperfect subjunctive	subiera/ subiese	subieras/ subieses	subiera/ subieses	subiéramos/ subiésemos	subieran/ subiesen	subieran/ subiesen

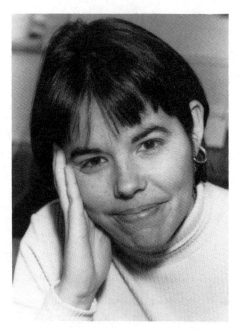

RAQUEL ANDERSON, PH.D.

Dr. Anderson is an Assistant Professor in the Department of Speech and Hearing Sciences at Indiana University, Bloomington. She received her bachelor's degree in 1980 from Oberlin College, her master's degree in 1982 from the University of Puerto Rico-Medical Sciences Campus, and her doctorate in 1987 from Northwestern University. Her primary interest is in typical and atypical language development in Spanish-speaking and bilingual children, with special focus on grammatical acquisition. Her previous positions and employment include speech-language pathologist for Head Start, Archdiocese of San Juan, Puerto Rico; bilingual consultant for the Board of Education, City of New York; Assistant Professor at the University of Puerto Rico-Medical Sciences Campus; and Co-director of the Bilingual Program in Speech-Language Pathology at Texas Christian University-Fort Worth.

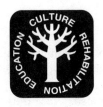

CHAPTER 4

"EARLY INTERVENTION? QUÉ QUIERE DECIR ÉSO?"/... WHAT DOES THAT MEAN?

ROSEMARY QUINN, Ph.D., CCC-SLP

This chapter deals with early intervention (which inherently focuses on the very young child with disabilities and the family) and the issues of culturally based values and beliefs that this focus engenders. Cultural differences become particularly salient as early interventionists respond to the family focus of recent legislation (Public Law 99-457). Values about child rearing and parental roles are two areas where parents and professionals have been shown to differ (Winton & Turnbull, 1981), and where disagreements often are due to differences in life experiences between professionals and the parents with whom they work.

Let us begin by noting that traditional cultural/ethnic minorities (i.e., African Americans, Hispanic Americans, Asian Americans, and Native Americans) are and will continue to be proportionally *over-rep-*

resented in statistics which place their infants at higher risk for disabilities or developmental delay (National Center for Clinical Infant Programs, 1986; U.S. Bureau of the Census, 1988; U.S. Department of Health and Human Services, 1985). Hispanics (the second largest minority in the United States) currently constitute the majority in many communities throughout the United States (most notably, California, Texas, Florida, New Mexico, New York, and New Jersey).

In contrast, individuals from cultural/ethnic minorities are grossly *under-represented* in all early intervention professions, including speech-language pathology. According to the American Speech-Language-Hearing Association (ASHA), self-identified minorities represent approximately 4% of the membership (ASHA, 1987), and less than 1% of the membership self-identify as fluent speakers of a language other than English (ASHA, 1991). Thus, most speech-language pathologists engaged in early intervention are likely to encounter culturally based values and beliefs which differ from their own.

Finally, the assumptions and practices of the majority of early interventionists are derived from a knowledge base that is narrowly focused and provides them with little practical guidance in dealing with such cross-cultural encounters. As a result, large numbers of (minority/Hispanic) infants with disabilities and their families are underserved or inappropriately served by dedicated, highly motivated professionals who are not prepared for the task. This challenge is of critical concern to our profession, and clearly warrants discussion and practical solutions.

This chapter briefly reviews the traditional knowledge base on early language socialization practices and presents related literature and research for Hispanics. Next, ways that the cross-cultural literature and literature on best practices may be used to generate culturally sensitive early interventions are discussed. This is augmented by a case study of early intervention involving a low-income Puerto Rican family from the Northeastern United States.

⅂⅂

TOWARD A BROADER KNOWLEDGE BASE

A careful review of the early socialization literature highlights the fact that most studies involve small numbers of Anglo American mothers and infants. On this basis, researchers have identified communication and language variables in maternal input which provide language learning experiences for normal learners (Beckwith, Cohen, Kopp, Parmalee, & Marcy, 1976; Bradley & Caldwell, 1976; Broen, 1972; Cross, 1977; Moerk, 1985; Phillips, 1972; Snow, 1977; Tiegerman & Siperstein, 1984). These often-cited variables include: complexity of maternal input relative to the learner's level of comprehension; semantic relatedness of maternal utterances (maternal input is generally child-centered and based in the here and now); redundancy of maternal messages (mothers explain, clarify, or comment on the child's experiences); consistent responses or behaviors from the adult; and reciprocity, meaning that adults interact with infants and young children as if they were independent communicators. In terms of intervention, Cross (1984) concluded from a survey of research in both normal and impaired language development that interventionists should use procedures that will: (a) enhance the semantic contingency of parents' language; (b) reduce parents' directiveness; (c) increase their fluency, intelligibility, and tendency to ask questions; and (d) generally encourage the parents of children with language impairment to talk with them more frequently.

The interactions observed in these studies and the conclusions drawn from them are based on cultural values and beliefs shared by the (Anglo American) subjects and researchers. Consequently, the sociocultural nature of the specific behaviors and principles they represent have not been made explicit. That is, this pattern of interaction socializes children to be members of white, middle class America. In all cultural/linguistic groups, infants learn a set of social and cultural values from their interactions with competent group members through which cultural awareness and cultural membership are constructed. Language is the principle means through which this socialization process is accomplished. Thus, socialization encodes those cultural values and beliefs which influence who talks to an infant, how, and why, as well as what adults teach and infants learn.

The cross-cultural literature demonstrates that these "familiar" language input variables do not constitute universals across cultural/linguistic groups. Although it is beyond the scope of this chapter to review the extensive cross-cultural literature on infant socialization practices, examples that relate to Hispanics are included. (Readers are advised to consult the many widely available sources: Lynch and Hanson, 1992; Nugent, Lester, and Brazelton, 1989; Rogoff, 1990; Schieffelin and Ochs, 1986; van Kleeck, 1994; Whiting and Edwards, 1988.) As a whole, this literature highlights that young children, universally, are spoken to and learn to listen and talk to others according to the particular values and beliefs of their language community.

CULTURAL VALUES AND EARLY LANGUAGE SOCIALIZATION AMONG HISPANICS

Discussions of this nature can be both informative and somewhat dangerous. Assumptions about the behavior of any group or individual based on a cultural label (i.e., "Hispanic") may result in potentially harmful generalizations or stereotypes. The Hispanic population in the United States is characterized by its diversity. Hispanics come from more than 22 countries worldwide, each with a unique sociopolitical history and relationship to the United States.

In a sense, we can discuss cultural values and beliefs as the mean for a particular group, with considerable dispersion around that mean represented by the various life circumstances of the individuals who constitute the group. For example, in general, Hispanic cultural norms and values have been characterized (relative to the mainstream U.S. culture) as more family or group oriented, more accepting and tolerant of children's behavior (with wider latitude in the definitions of "childhood" and its various stages), and more fatalistic or deterministic in terms of causality or future orientation (Vincent, Salisbury, Strain, McCormick, & Tessier, 1990; Zuniga, 1992). These values and beliefs may translate into behaviors such as valuing early gratification, close physical contact, and adherence to the child's rather than the adult's needs. Cooperativeness rather than competitiveness is a goal of child socialization, and families typically place more emphasis on harmony within the family and the larger society than on independence or individual accomplishments (de Valdez & Gallegos, 1982).

It is important to remember that the above describes a group mean and that there is, inherently, dispersion around a mean. Cultural identification cannot be viewed as the sole determinant of one's actions. Many other factors (socioeconomic status, length of residence in the U.S. or in a particular region, availability of family and other support systems, etc.) mitigate the role that culture may play in influencing behavior. Further, individuals vary in the degree to which they identify with a particular cultural group. For example, as a group Mexican Americans are comprised of businessmen, ranchers, university faculty, farmworkers, administrators, clergy, and so on. It would be difficult to describe an exact set of characteristics or practices to encompass this diversity, although certain cultural themes or a unifying strand might be more or less evident among individual members.

There is a paucity of published research on the early language socialization practices of Hispanics. Often-cited sources include Field and Widmayer (1981) (play interactions of Cuban, Puerto Rican, and South American mothers and 3- to 4-month-old infants, residing in Miami); Coles (1977) ("Chicano" children); Heath (1986) (children of recent immigrant Mexican parents); Briggs (1984) (children of Mexican American fieldworkers in New Mexico); and Harkness (1971) (rural Guatemalan mothers and young children). Together, these studies draw a composite of culturally based practices, such as referring to infants/young children as *inocentes* (innocents), who have little volitional control over their own behavior. Thus, adults show great tolerance for and patience with infant misbehavior (Briggs, 1984). Another study reported evidence for "hidden agendas" in parental styles of play with infants, that is, Cuban mothers (who talked the most, using polysyllabic words and long utterances) said parents had a duty "to educate" children, while Puerto Rican and South American mothers engaged in more social,interactive games where mutual enjoyment was the stated goal (Field & Widmayer, 1981). Adults do not ask young children factual questions, and do not encourage them to rehearse information, voice their preferences, or make choices (Heath, 1986). On the other hand, there is more frequent use (relative to the Anglo population) of eye contact, proximity, gestures, and other nonverbal signals to communicate (Coles, 1977; Kayser, 1990).

Recent research adds details to this composite. Results from a study of videotaped play interactions of 12-month-old Puerto Rican infants and mothers (Quinn, 1992) included identification of an interactive profile for this group: mother's frequently focused their infant's attention, demonstrated how to use toys/objects, directed the infants' play, and encouraged them to take their turns in interactions. Mothers and infants tended not to comment on objects or actions (label), and there were low frequencies of use of the maternal categories, request clarification, elicit, or imitate. Deictic terms (it, this, here) were used with relatively high frequency by most of the mothers, reflecting a tendency not to use specific nouns and verbs for visible or ongoing objects and actions. This profile closely resembles the teaching strategies of "Chicano" mothers described by Laosa (1983). These mothers tended to use modeling, visual cue, directive, and negative physical control in interactions with their 5-year-old children. With increasing maternal education level, Chicano mothers' teaching strategies shifted toward praise and inquiry, similar to the study's non-Hispanic mothers.

The following study demonstrates how parental teaching strategies are reflected in early language development. Mata-Pistokache and Quinn (1994) analyzed the receptive and expressive (Spanish/English) language skills of 72, 22-month-old Mexican American children from Southwest Texas, based on parent report, observations of parent-child play, and administration of the *Sequenced Inventory of Communication Development* (SICD) (Hedrick, Prather, & Tobin, 1990). The highest number of single words used by these children fit the category, "family members' names" (i.e., *wela/wita*/oma/grandma, *mama, bebé, chachita* (sister), Sara, Joshie, etc.). This was followed by the categories animal names, household objects, verbs, foods, and social words (thank you). Two-word utterances most frequently coded the semantic relationship, Attentional + X (or X + Attentional) (i.e., *Mira Mami*/Look Mommy, *Este mira*/This look), followed, more predictably, by the semantic relationships Agent + Action and Agent + Object. The cross-cultural language socialization literature demonstrates that children do not, universally, learn the same language skills in the same context or in the same developmental sequence, reflecting differing parenting styles and expectations.

The majority of these children did not complete two receptive items at age level on the SICD: (1) understanding of words ("What kinds of words does [child's name] understand?", by parent report) because the *specific* categories expected (acquaintances' names, household tools, pronouns, names of buildings) differed from those reported/observed; and (2) points to body parts (*specifically*, ears, eyes, hair, mouth, nose). These children tended to identify the body parts: hair, *boca*/mouth, hand, *panza*/belly, and *pata*/foot. Expressively, at age level, the children did not imitate motor acts (put blocks in a box, or stack blocks) or imitate nonspeech sounds (tongue click, cough, car motor) on command, likely reflecting a general unfamiliarity with the unique demands of the testing situation and/or this type of play with an adult, and did not "respond 'hi' when someone else said 'hi' to him/her" (an item testing verbal responsiveness), based on parent report and observation. Interestingly, some parents said they did not know if the child would respond because they never said "hi" to him or her. Nevertheless, most of these toddlers were seen as verbally responsive by their parents and the examiners. They simply expressed this responsiveness through different behaviors. This information is summarized in Table 4–1.

A study by Gutierrez-Clellen and Iglesias (1987) further illustrates how parental expectations affect children's communication. They

TABLE 4–1

Mexican American infants' responses to selected items from the *Sequenced Inventory of Communication Development.*

Item	Expected Response	Subjects' Responses (N = 72)
Receptive Scale		
Understanding words	Acquaintances' names, household tools, pronouns, names of buildings	Other categories reported/observed
Body parts	Ears, eyes, hair, mouth, nose	*boca*/mouth, hand, *panza*/belly, *pata*/foot
Expressive Scale		
Imitate motor acts and nonspeech sounds on command	Put blocks in box, stack blocks; tongue click, cough, car motor noise	Did not imitate; unfamiliar with unique test demands and/or this type of play
Verbal responsiveness	Responds "hi" when someone says "hi"	Did not; many parents did not say "hi" to child

described Puerto Rican mothers' input to (kindergarten and first grade) children as using commands, nonspecific labels for presumably shared referents (i.e., *eso*/that, *este*/this) and object functions. These children tend to use functional descriptions (*para comer*/to eat) as a means of labeling in interactions with their mothers. This also reportedly was prevalent in the responses of a group of Puerto Rican Head Start children on the *Expressive One-Word Picture Vocabulary Test*, which is intended to elicit one-word labels (Peña, Quinn, & Iglesias, 1992).

Again, these studies describe general trends. For example, individual mother-infant dyads (Quinn, 1992) varied in the degree to which they matched the interactive profile identified for the group. One mother, who also had two school-aged children and had worked for Head Start as a "family liaison," used significantly fewer Attentionals, and more Elicits, Labels, and Imitations. Her baby, in turn, used the most single words and was beginning to use jargon speech communicatively. One monolingual Spanish-speaking mother, who left Puerto Rico 3 days prior to participating in the study, was less directive than some mothers who spoke only English, and had been born on the mainland. Variation must be expected and considered, along with central tendencies (or group means), if we intend our understandings to be accurate reflections of the families we serve.

A CULTURALLY INCLUSIVE KNOWLEDGE BASE

Ochs and Schieffelin (1984) suggest that there may be at least two cultural patterns of speech among young children and their caregivers. Among groups that adapt situations to children (as in middle-income, Anglo families), caregivers simplify their talk, negotiate meaning with young children, cooperate with them in making meaning, and respond to their verbal and nonverbal initiations. Among groups that adapt children to the normal situations of the society, caregivers model unsimplified utterances for children to repeat to a third party, direct them to notice others, and build interaction around circumstances to which the caregivers want the children to respond.

Predictably, although this contrast is useful for drawing attention to differing strategies of interaction with children, it, too, does not apply to all cultures or groups. Watson-Gegeo and Gegeo (1986) report that Kwara'ae (Solomon Islands) caregivers speak with children in both of the ways that Ochs and Schieffelin describe. Although the goal of Kwara'ae caregivers is to adapt children to the situation, they argue that it is most effective to start where the baby is functioning. Similarly, differences in parental interaction strategies would be expected among Hispanic families as result of acculturation, socioeconomic status, and other factors previously discussed.

Finally, and most importantly, cross-cultural studies suggest that there are many paths or socialization practices which lead to the universal goal of adult language competence. Different communication skills are considered more or less important, different teaching approaches are valued, and different people and situations are available for their teaching. In a complex, stratified society such as ours, various environments ("barrios," "colonias," "projects") are shaped by and coexist within the framework of larger societal institutions. Child socialization practices encode beliefs and values derived from adaptations to a specific environment, as that environment is perceived by a family. The point, here, is that socialization practices make sense within (or "fit") their contexts. This is best illustrated by the exasperated comment of an inner city African American mother during a meeting with (white, middle income) interventionists to discuss their perception that the way she disciplined and talked to her toddler was too harsh and punitive: "What could you possibly know about what *my* child needs to survive in *our* world?" At the same time, we must be mindful of the critical importance of individualizing each family system in intervention and discussing the extent to which cultural labels and themes are relevant to a particular family.

⊔

FROM KNOWLEDGE TO PRACTICE

This section explores how early intervention practices may be adapted to represent and serve Hispanic families with young children in a culturally sensitive way. These adaptations are discussed in terms of the early intervention program philosophy, service delivery issues, and intervention goals.

PROGRAM PHILOSOPHY

Culturally sensitive intervention begins with an examination of one's own values and the choices they generate. For example, individuals may differ in their views of medicine and health/illness, the meaning and cause of disability, views of change and intervention, or the way family is defined and family decisions are made (Hanson, Lynch, & Wayman, 1990; Harry, 1992). We have seen that families may differ in their beliefs about the ways that caretakers and other adults should interact with infants and young children. Wayman, Lynch, and Hanson (1990) provide a set of guidelines (intended to help interventionists learn about families with cultural backgrounds that differ from their own) which might be used by an early interventionist to examine his or her own values and beliefs. The guidelines include questions in the areas of family structure and child-rearing practices, family perceptions and attitudes, and family language and interaction style.

Suggested questions in the area of family structure and child rearing include: Who is the primary caregiver, and who else participates in caregiving? What is the amount of care given by the mother versus others? What are the mealtime rules? Is there an established bedtime? What are the parameters of acceptable child behavior? In terms of family perceptions, questions include: Are there cultural or religious factors that could shape family perceptions? To what/where/whom does the family assign responsibility for (their child's) disability? Who is the primary medical provider and source of medical information— family members, elders, friends, folk healers, family doctor, medical specialist? From whom does the family seek help, and which family member interacts with outside systems? In the area of interaction styles, the following are some questions for consideration: Does the family tend to interact in a direct/indirect style, quiet/loud manner? Do family members share their feelings when discussing emotional issues? Does the family value a lengthy social time at each home visit (unrelated to the program goals)?

Bernheimer, Gallimore, and Weisner (1990) propose that ecological/cultural or ecocultural theory may help interventionists understand differences in how families think, feel, and react to the same or similar events. This theory explicitly includes the family-constructed meaning of circumstances as "refracted through the lens of family goals and values" (p. 221). Thus, knowledge of family beliefs and values may enhance our understanding of the family's interpretation of and response to a child's disability, professional recommendations, and intervention goals. Similarly, Benson and Turnbull (1986) recommend a philosophy of individualization with regard to families. This means that services are individualized according to the specific needs of the family, as a system with its own structure, cultural style, and ideological style (beliefs, values, and coping behaviors). Winton (1990) proposed adoption of a model which promotes "normalization" of intervention goals and explains individual differences among families in terms of their perceptually based adaptation to stressful events. The challenge is to determine ways to provide support to a family within their definition of normal, based on what they want now for their family and child. A similar strategy, reframing, involves understanding how a family defines events related to their child. For example, understanding that a family has reframed the survival of their very premature infant with disabilities as a gift from God, which they need time to appreciate, will help interventionists think about the perceived "denial" as a normal response and a family strength which, in time, will reinforce intervention goals to address the infant's motor and cognitive disabilities.

SERVICE DELIVERY

Providing services to culturally diverse families, first, requires programs to develop and offer an array of service delivery options (home-based, center-based, hospital-based, and combinations) individually tailored to match family needs and styles. Second, families should be encouraged to participate in intervention at whatever level they choose. Simeonsson and Bailey (1990) describe a six-level hierarchy or continuum of family involvement in early intervention, which reflects qualitative differences in the focus and degree of involvement of the family and interventionists (from Level 0, elective, in which the family rejects available services or elects not to be involved, through Level III, involvement focusing on information and skills needs, to Level VI, psychological involvement, in which family members seek psychological change at the family or personal level). The actual level of family and interventionist involvement will reflect characteristics of both the family and the early intervention program. Factors likely to influence the family's level of involvement include their needs, values, and lifestyle, *and* the nature and comprehensiveness of services and the degree of investment of the interventionists. From this perspective, the program must incorporate a broad-based service delivery model that utilizes all community resources and identifies the specific intervention program as one such resource.

Each of the models mentioned shares a common emphasis in conceptualizing early intervention services in frameworks that are comprehensive in scope and foster the role of family perceptions in the intervention process. This emphasis is critical for culturally/linguistically diverse families that tend to be more isolated from society's medical and helping institutions.

Based on a survey of 536 white, Hispanic, and American Indian parents involved in early intervention, Sontag and Schacht (1994) report several differences among these groups which have implications for service delivery. Hispanic and American Indian parents reported more difficulty in obtaining information about their child's problem or what could be done for their child, were less involved in the coordinating role than were white parents, were less involved with other parents who have children with disabilities, and reported an even higher need to know how to get services, suggesting that they are not sufficiently linked to service agencies. The survey results suggest that these Hispanic and American Indian families differ from families who readily identify with dominant health, education, and social systems and require uniquely tailored strategies to include them more fully in the decision-making process of early intervention.

INTERVENTION GOALS

Families are more likely to be invested in intervention goals congruent with high-priority family goals, and they are more likely to be able to implement professional recommendations that fit with their values and beliefs (Berheimer et al., 1990). Specifically, an intervention goal such as, "Ana will use simple language to talk to Moises throughout daily activities about what he sees and is doing," is not likely to be a priority for a mother who believes that her job is to keep Moises clean, well-fed, and safe and that babies learn by observing what others do (thus, it becomes redundant to talk about what is present and observable). Conversely, a goal that is based on observations of Hispanic mother-infant play, and encourages a Hispanic mother to say "Mira!" each time she lifts her baby into the air and wait for eye contact before lowering him to her lap, is more likely to be implemented. Techniques which programs might use to insure they are sensitive to individual families' goals include gathering ethnographic information to describe the group with which the family identifies, understanding the degree of transcultural identification, and selecting goals that are congruent with family and cultural values (Hanson et al., 1990).

Modifications to traditional early intervention practices have proved successful in providing services to inner-city Puerto Rican families (Bruder, Anderson, Schutz, & Caldera, 1991), including addressing a significant number of family needs, and an increased awareness of culturally based values related to family relationships, child-rearing practices, support networks, and societal responsibilities. At the beginning of the program, goals were primarily in the family support category, followed by information goals and child intervention goals. However, as these families' support and information needs were met, more attention could be focused on child intervention needs. Thus, the importance of prioritizing family and child needs from the family's perspective must be emphasized.

Table 4-2 provides a summary of the issues and adaptations discussed in this section. Next, a case study demonstrates how these

TABLE 4–2
Culturally sensitive adaptations to early intervention practices.

Program Philosophy	
Examine values	Views of health/illness, meaning and cause of disability, change and intervention, the way family is defined/decisions are made, how adults interact with young children, etc.
Ecocultural theory	Family-constructed meaning of events, refracted through the lense of family goals and values
Individualization	Services are individualized for the family as a system
Normalization	Provide support to a family within their definition of normality/ perceptually based adaptation to stressful events
Service Delivery	
Develop array of options	Individually tailored to match family needs and styles
Families participate at level they deem appropriate	Level 0 (rejects services) through Level III (information and skill needs) through Level VI (psychological involvement); comprehensive = utilize all community-based resources
Intervention Goals	
Congruent with high-priority family goals	Professional recommendations fit family values and beliefs; ethnographic information to describe group with which family identifies; understand degree of transcultural identification; prioritize needs

Sources: Benson & Turnbull (1986); Bernheimer, Gallimore, & Weisner (1990); Hanson, Lynch, & Wayman (1990); Simmeonsson & Bailey (1990); Wayman, Lynch, & Hanson (1990); Winton (1990).

issues and adaptations are applied to intervention practices. The case study describes an intervention plan for a low-income, Puerto Rican mother and her son who reside in an inner-city neighborhood in the Northeastern United States.

ᗡ

CASE STUDY

CESAR

Cesar, age 2;10, was referred for an evaluation by a desperate phone call in Spanish from his young mother, Betsy. Betsy said Cesar's behavior was a big problem, and she couldn't take anymore. The evaluation team found Betsy and Cesar living in a two-story building on a narrow street of attached row houses. The sidewalks were littered with trash, broken glass, and crack vials. The house consisted of a living room, dining room, and kitchen downstairs, and two rooms and a bathroom upstairs. In the living room were two folding chairs, an upholstered chair, and a television. In the dining room were a car tire, a rusty tricycle, a laundry basket, and piles of clothes. The kitchen had basic appliances and a folding card table. Despite the intense summer heat, the windows were all closed. The only air came from the screen door. Betsy said she kept the windows closed because she was afraid of the neighbors, and because Cesar had nearly fallen from an open window upstairs.

Betsy said she and Cesar rarely went outside. She described her (mostly African American) neighbors as "bad people," who yelled and cursed at each other night and day. She said she had come from Puerto Rico with Cesar's father when she was pregnant. The father had since left, and she had no contact with him. She was ashamed to let her mother know that Cesar's father was gone and had not spoken to her in months. She said she spoke and understood English, but preferred Spanish over "such an ugly language."

Betsy's main concern about Cesar was that he was too active, never listened/obeyed her (i.e., did not "respect" her), and embarrassed her with his behavior. While the team was present, Cesar repeatedly tried to drag the tricycle outside, while Betsy shouted, pulled him back inside, and slapped his legs. There, apparently, was nothing else for him to play with or do. Betsy said he liked to run up and down the stairs and to hit the walls or floor with a stick (as though he were hammering). The speech-language pathologist noticed that Cesar used only a few single words, and generally did not pay much attention to spoken language. He had frequent ear infections. Betsy said she wasn't concerned about his talking. She always knew what Cesar wanted.

Cesar was found to be eligible for early intervention services. The team's immediate concern was Betsy's fear and isolation from support systems and the effect it was having on her relationship with Cesar. Betsy was put in contact with a community-based Hispanic social service agency. There, she enrolled in a graduate equivalency degree (GED) program and, eventually, English as a second language classes and began to form relationships with other young women her age. The agency provided child care during classes, so Cesar spent the time in supervised play with other children. She also was able to borrow toys from a toy lending library for Cesar. The agency caseworker accompanied Betsy to the children's hospital where Cesar was treated for his ear infections. Through an agency contact, the landlord was convinced to put safety bars on the upstairs windows in compliance with state law.

In time, Betsy began to see that Cesar's problem behavior was largely related to normal, age-appropriate needs for play and activity. She reported that his behavior improved. He began attending Head Start, where a speech and language evaluation revealed a highly communicative little boy, with a moderate delay in expressive language secondary to the history of ear infections.

DISCUSSION

Clearly, Betsy's problems were largely due to poverty. There were apparent cultural themes that the team recognized and acknowledged in designing an intervention: concerns about Cesar's disobedience and lack of respect (*respeto*); his behavior embarrassed her because he appeared *mal educado* (literally "badly educated," but meaning badly raised/brought up); different (later) expectations for Cesar's language development than team members; and rejection of English in order to preserve an endangered cultural identity. The team took care not to evaluate Betsy's seeming lack of concern for Cesar's language development, but saw it within its cultural and environmental contexts (with more pressing issues in the forefront). A holistic, family systems approach emphasized drawing on existing resources, with a primary goal of establishing natural support systems. Betsy's concerns were viewed as expressions of basic human needs for safety, harmony, and social contact, which colored her behavior and her perceptions of Cesar's behavior. The outcome would have been considerably different if these had been compromised by an initial focus on Cesar's language development (in direct conflict with Betsy's perceptions of the problem). Thus, a successful intervention required the team to use culturally sensitive and current best practices in a unique, individualized way.

ᄂᆞ

SUMMARY

Early intervention focuses on the young child with disabilities and the family during a period when values about child-rearing and parental roles are particularly salient. This chapter discussed the critical shortage of minority professionals and demographic trends which indicate that most speech-language pathologists engaged in early intervention are likely to encounter culturally based values and beliefs that differ from their own. We reviewed the familiar or traditional literature on early language socialization practices and compared this to literature and research for Hispanics to expand the knowledge base from which early intervention assumptions and practices evolve. Culturally sensitive adaptations to traditional early intervention practices were presented in the areas of program philosophy, service delivery, and intervention goals to suggest how intervention plans may be individualized in recognition of each family's unique cultural and environmental contexts. Finally, a case study was used to demonstrate application of a broader knowledge base and culturally sensitive practices to an early intervention plan for a low-income, Puerto Rican family.

Essentially, this chapter has been about change. There is a saying, "No pain, no gain," meaning that change is achieved only through considerable effort. For some early interventionists, this is an unappealing dilemma. Others approach the change process with caution or resignation, and some are drawn to the process with a vision of the potential it holds. Regardless of personal preferences, early interventionists today feel strong pressures for change. We have seen how the telephone calls from mothers like Betsy compel us to ensure that change is guided by their realities, perceptions, and rights. My experience and that of my early intervention colleagues has been that the gains, in terms of services delivered, meaningful relationships with families, and personal and professional growth, far outweigh "the pain" associated with the changes discussed and recommended here.

⌐

REFERENCES

American Speech-Language-Hearing Association. (1987). *Multicultural professional education in communication disorders: Curriculum approaches.* Rockville, MD: Author.

American Speech-Language-Hearing Association. (1991). *1991 Omnibus survey results.* Rockville, MD: Author.

Beckwith, L., Cohen, S., Kopp, C., Parmalee, A., & Marcy, T. (1976). Caregiver-infant interactions and early cognitive development in preterm infants. *Child Development, 47,* 579–587.

Benson, H. A., & Turnbull, A. P. (1986). Approaching families from an individualized perspective. In R. H. Horner, L. H. Meyers, & H. D. B. Fredericks (Eds.), *Education of learners with handicaps: Exemplary service strategies* (pp. 127–157). Baltimore, MD: Paul H. Brookes.

Bernheimer, L. P., Gallimore, R., & Weisner, T. S. (1990). Ecocultural theory as a context for the individual family service plan. *Journal of Early Intervention, 14*(3), 219–233.

Bradley, R., & Caldwell, B. (1976). The relation of infants' HOME environments to mental test performance at 54 months: A follow-up study. *Child Development, 47,* 1172–1174.

Briggs, C. L. (1984). Learning how to talk: Native metacommunicative competence and the incompetence of fieldworkers, *Language in Society, 13,* 1–28.

Broen, P. A. (1972, December). The verbal environment of the language-learning child. *American Speech and Hearing Association* (Monograph No. 17).

Bruder, M. J., Anderson, R., Schutz, G., & Caldera, M. (1991). Niños especiales program: A culturally sensitive early intervention model. *Journal of Early Intervention, 15*(3), 268–277.

Cross, T. (1977). Mothers' speech adjustments: The contributions of selected listener variables. In C. E. Snow & C. A. Ferguson (Eds.), *Talking to children* (pp. 128–170). Cambridge, MA: Cambridge University Press.

Cross, T. G. (1984). Habilitating the language-impaired child: Ideas from studies of parent-child interaction. *Topics in Language Disorders, 4*(4), 1–14.

Coles, R. (1977). Growing up Chicano. In R. Coles (Ed.), *Eskimos, Chicanos, Indians* (pp. 112–180). Boston, MA: Little, Brown.

de Valdez, T. A., & Gallegos, J. (1982). The Chicano family in social work. In G. W. Green (Ed.), *Cultural awareness in the human services* (pp. 184–208). Englewood Cliffs, NJ: Prentice-Hall.

Field, T. M., & Widmayer, S. M. (1981). Mother-infant interactions among lower SES Black, Cuban, Puerto Rican, and South American immigrants. In T. M. Field, A. M. Sostek, P. Vietze, & P. H. Leiderman (Eds.), *Culture and early interactions* (pp. 209–242). Norwood, NJ: Lawrence Erlbaum.

Gutierrez-Clellen, V. F., & Iglesias, A. (1987, November). *Expressive vocabulary of kindergarten and first-grade Hispanic students.* Paper presented at the American Speech-Language-Hearing Association national convention, New Orleans, LA.

Hanson, M. J., Lynch, E. W., & Wayman, K. I. (1990). Honoring the cultural diversity of families when gathering data. *Topics in Early Childhood Education, 10*(1), 112–131.

Harkness, S. (1971). Cultural variations in mothers' language. *Word, 27,* 495–498.

Harry, B. (1992). *Culturally diverse families and the special education system.* New York: Teachers College Press.

Heath, S. B. (1986). Sociocultural contexts of language development. In *Beyond language: Social and cultural factors in schooling language minority children* (pp. 143–186). Los Angeles: Evaluation, Dissemination and Assessment Center, California State University.

Hedrick, D. L., Prather, E. M., & Tobin, A. R. (1990). *Sequenced Inventory of Communication Development.* Seattle, WA: University of Washington Press.

Kayser, H. (1990). Social communicative behaviors of language-disordered Mexican-American students. *Child Language Teaching and Therapy, 6,* 255–269.

Laosa, L. M. (1983). School, occupation, culture, and family. The impact of parental schooling on the parent-child relationship. In I. E. Sigel & L. M. Laosa (Eds.), *Changing families* (pp. 79–135). New York: Plenum.

Lynch, E. W., & Hanson, M. J. (Eds.). (1992). *Developing cross-cultural competence: A guide for working with young children and their families.* Baltimore, MD: Paul H. Brookes.

Mata-Pistokache, T., & Quinn, R. (1994, April). *A culturally-sensitive perspective for assessing high-risk Mexican-American babies.* Paper presented at the Texas Speech-Language-Hearing Association state convention, Fort Worth, TX

Moerk, E. L. (1984). *The mother of Eve as a first language teacher.* Norwood, NJ: Ablex.

National Center for Clinical Infant Programs. (1986). *The numbers: Infants can't wait.* Washington, DC: Authors.

Nugent, J. K., Lester, B. M., & Brazelton, T. B. (1989). *The cultural context of infancy.* Norwood, NJ: Ablex.

Ochs, E., & Schieffelin, B. (1984). Language acquisition: Three developmental stories. In R. Schweder & R. A. LeVine (Eds.), *Culture theory* (pp. 276–320). New York: Cambridge University Press.

Peña, E., Quinn, R., & Iglesias, A. (1992). The application of dynamic methods to language assessment: A nonbiased procedure. *Journal of Special Education, 26*(3), 269–280.

Phillips, J. (1972). Syntax and vocabulary in mothers' speech to young children: Age and sex comparisons. *Child Development, 44,* 182–185.

Quinn, R. (1992). *Mother-infant interactions among Puerto Rican dyads.* Unpublished doctoral dissertation, Temple University, Philadelphia, PA.

Rogoff, B. (1990). *Apprenticeship in thinking. Cognitive development in social context.* New York: Oxford University Press.

Schieffelin, B. B., & Ochs, E. (Eds.). (1986). *Language socialization across cultures. Part I.* New York: Cambridge University Press.

Simeonsson, R. J. & Bailey, D. B. (1990). Family dimensions in early intervention. In S. J. Meisels, & J. P. Shonkoff (Eds.), *Handbook of early childhood intervention* (pp. 428–444). New York: Cambridge University Press.

Snow, C. E. (1977). Mothers' speech research: From input to interaction. In C. E. Snow & C. A. Ferguson (Eds.), *Talking to children* (pp. 31–49). Cambridge, MA: Cambridge University Press.

Sontag, J. C., & Schacht, R. (1994). An ethnic comparison of parent participation and information needs in early intervention. *Exceptional Children, 60*(5), 422–433.

Tiegerman, E., & Siperstein, M. (1984). Individual patterns of interaction in the mother-child dyad: Implications for parent interventions. *Topics in Language Disorders, 4*(4), 50–61.

U.S. Bureau of the Census, Ethnic and Hispanic Branch. (1988). *Current population reports: Population characteristics.* (Series P-20, No. 431). Washington, DC: Government Printing Office.

U.S. Department of Health and Human Services. (1985). *Report of the Secretary's Task Force on Black and Minority Health, Volume 1: Executive Summary* (Publ. No. 491-313/ 44706). Washington, DC: Author.

van Kleeck, A. (1994). Potential cultural bias in training parents as conversational partners with their children who have delays in language development. *American Journal of Speech-Language Pathology, 3*(1), 67–78.

Vincent, L. J., Salisbury, C. L., Strain, P., McCormick, C., & Tessier, A. (1990). A behavioral-ecological approach to early intervention: Focus on cultural diversity. In S. J. Meisels & J. P. Shonkoff (Eds.), *Handbook of early childhood intervention* (pp. 173–195). New York: Cambridge University Press.

Watson-Gegeo, K., & Gegeo, D. (1986). Calling-out and repeating routines in Kwara'ae children's language socialization. In B. B. Schieffelin & E. Ochs (Eds.). *Language socialization across cultures. Part I* (pp. 17–50). New York: Cambridge University Press.

Wayman, K. I., Lynch, E. W., & Hanson, M. J. (1990). Home-based early childhood services: Cultural sensitivity in a family systems approach. *Topics in Early Childhood Special Education, 10*(4), 56–75.

Whiting, B. B., & Edwards, C. P. (Eds.). (1988). *Children of different worlds: The formation of social behavior.* Cambridge, MA: Harvard University Press.

Winton, P. J., & Turnbull, A. P. (1981). Parent involvement as viewed by parents of preschool handicapped children. *Topics in Early Childhood Special Education, 1,* 11–19.

Winton, P. J. (1990). Promoting a normalizing approach to families: Integrating theory with practice. *Topics in Early Childhood Special Education, 10*(2), 90–103.

Zuniga, M. E. (1992). Families with Latino roots. In E. W. Lynch, & M. J. Hanson (Eds.), *Developing cross-cultural competence* (pp. 151–180). Baltimore, MD: Paul H. Brookes.

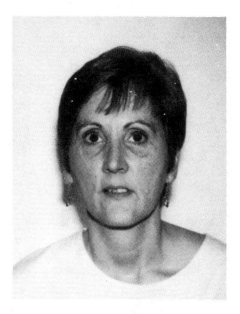

ROSEMARY QUINN, PH.D.

Dr. Quinn is an Assistant Professor in the Communication Disorders Program at the University of Texas-Pan American (Edinburg, Texas). She received her master's degree in 1987 and her doctorate in 1992 from Temple University. Her areas of interest include cross-cultural language socialization practices, the acquisition of preliteracy skills by bilingual children, and early Spanish language development. Her prior experiences include project director for a multi-disciplinary evaluation project serving the birth to three population, co-director of a home-based early intervention project, and adjunct faculty member in the Department of Speech-Language-Hearing at Temple University.

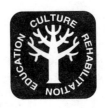

CHAPTER 5

NARRATIVE DEVELOPMENT AND DISORDERS IN SPANISH-SPEAKING CHILDREN: IMPLICATIONS FOR THE BILINGUAL INTERVENTIONIST

VERA F. GUTIERREZ-CLELLEN, PH.D., CCC-SLP

All cultures use narratives to represent and recreate past experience. The study of children's narratives can shed light on the ways culture-specific social knowledge develops, the cognitive frames or schemata children use to make sense of narrative events at a given point in development, and the structure of learning situations that maximize children's narrative development. For example, research

97

with English-speaking children has shown that if we ask a child, "What happens when you go to a birthday party?" the child will produce an account (i.e., a script) organized with a culturally shared, and therefore predictable, temporal, spatial, and causal structure (Slackman, Hudson, & Fivush, 1986). The birthday party script would typically include acts such as going to party or bringing a present, playing games, having birthday cake (singing "Happy Birthday," blowing out candles), opening presents, and going home in temporal and causal sequence. From a very early age, children are also able to respond to the question, "What happened when you went to the party?" by providing a personal narrative. Labov and Waletzky (1967) proposed a model for describing personal narratives that has been applied extensively in research and clinical practice on children's narratives (Peterson & McCabe, 1983). According to their taxonomy, a fully developed narrative is organized around a high point or *evaluation* that indicates the "why" a story is told (e.g., I was scared) and contains an *abstract* or summary of the story (e.g., I had an accident), *orientation* or background information about time, place, and so on (e.g., I was in the car), *complicating action*(s) (e.g., A bus crossed the street and my dad crashed into it), *resolution* or outcome of the complicating actions (e.g., I couldn't go to the party), and *coda* or ending (e.g., and that was all).

Script learning, however, is directly related to the child's experience with world events, and therefore the characteristics of scripts may vary across speech communities. For example, *la piñata* might be included as a component of a birthday party script by members of certain Hispanic groups and other acts may not be used by children whose experiences are determined by the characteristics of refugee or migrant camps. Children apply their culturally based knowledge of scripts to the understanding of novel events and to guide the organization of their narratives. For example, a child may be able to anticipate the acts that take place in a friend's birthday party based on his or her previous exposure to a sibling's birthday party. Later, the child's report may focus on novel events experienced at the birthday party and omit information that can be inferred from culturally shared knowledge of birthday-party scripts. Alternatively, children who are unfamiliar with a given script may not be able to fully comprehend or report certain narrative events.

Research with English-speaking children has indicated that the verbal rehearsal of scripts is an important factor that influences learning. Children's script learning is enhanced under the guidance of an adult who provides and prompts verbal descriptions of events before they occur or during the reenactment of events (Lucariello, Kyratzis, & Engel, 1986). A broad understanding of how scripts are learned in the context of adult-child interactions from Spanish-speaking backgrounds is needed to provide a basis for planning culturally and linguistically sensitive interventions. Similarly, the study of personal narratives may be useful in determining children's ability to develop a central theme in their stories, as well as the types of topics or content that will maximize the display of children's narrative skills.

Narrative development is not complete by the time children enter school. Researchers and educators have underscored the significance of narrative development for learning literacy by examining children's fictional stories. Using a story grammar approach, the structure of a fully developed single story episode typically includes a *setting* (e.g., There was a boy named John); an *initiating event* (e.g., One day he found a kitten in the street); a *motivating state* or internal response (e.g., He felt sad because the kitten was lost); an *attempt* (e.g., So he picked it up); a *consequence* (e.g., A big cat came running and meowing); and a *reaction* (e.g., John was happy because the kitten had a mother) (Stein & Glenn, 1982). Children's ability to produce "well-formed" stories is directly related to their experience with literature stories and traditional stories such as fairy tales and fables. For example, in a study with bilingual fourth graders, Jax (1988) found that children's ability to construct a story in English according to the structure of story grammars was significantly correlated with their English reading comprehension scores. Although there was variation in the types of components high and low readers included in their stories (i.e., setting, internal responses, or reactions), the low reading groups were less likely to include initiating events, attempts, or consequences. Thus, analysis of the narratives of school-age children may provide information about their facility with literacy activities, and narrative intervention activities may be significant for the development of children's literacy skills.

There also is evidence that training narrative skills in the native language may have positive effects for the development of narratives in the second language. Carlisle (1986) found that the written narratives and descriptions of children learning English as a second language in a bilingual setting were higher in productivity and syntactic complexity than those of children submersed in a classroom environment where the second language was the only language of instruction. Yet, very few studies have focused on the development of narratives in Spanish-speaking children and, specifically, on how available information can be applied clinically to meet the needs of children with limited English proficiency and language disorders. The following sections attempt to address this issue by describing the development of children's Spanish narratives across various contexts for narrative production from the construction of interactive protonarratives with a parent, to the production of scripts, personal stories, and story retellings in teacher/clinician-child interactions. For each type of narrative context, available developmental research will be used to identify children's narrative skills and to guide the course of intervention for children who experience narrative delays.

ꓶ

THE EARLY STAGES OF NARRATIVE DEVELOPMENT

Clinically, the analysis of young children's language use in their daily routines and interactions with others may provide an index of narrative development during the early stages. The repetitive nature of these interactions allows children to learn that certain events occur in predictable temporal sequences and that events may precede or follow events in a cause-effect relationship. For example, researchers interested in learning how English-speaking children develop scriptal knowledge in the early stages of narrative development (or protonarratives) have examined adult-child use of narrative language across such routines as bathing-time, lunch-time, and play contexts (Nelson, 1986). Children's symbolic play, in particular, may reveal useful information about the development of event representations that later may be utilized in children's narrativization of experience (Seidman, Nelson, & Gruendel, 1986). Their ability to engage and share a situation such as making a telephone call, cooking, or feeding a baby doll may indicate how they organize or sequence events, how they maintain a thematic focus (or topic), their knowledge of social roles, and the types of world experience they apply to their re-enactments. These early event representations or protonarratives are initially guided by a more experienced partner or adult. Thus, parent-child play interactions may be used to maximize children's narrative performance during these early stages.

EARLY NARRATIVES IN CHILDREN LEARNING SPANISH AS A FIRST LANGUAGE

Narrative research with young Spanish-speaking children is scarce. The following observations are based on research conducted as part of a series of studies with children learning Spanish as a first language (Jackson-Maldonado, Thal, Marchman, Bates, & Gutierrez-Clellen, 1993). In the first investigation, reported below, Spanish language samples of 28 children from 11 to 28 months of age were gathered in a play situation between parent and child using sets of predetermined toys (e.g., kitchen pots, pans, dishes, animals, dolls). Parents were asked to play and talk with their children as they would at home to stimulate the child to communicate. All language samples were videotaped, transcribed, and coded according to the following types of narrative interactions:

Symbolic play: Parent and child demonstrate and practice the function or use of everyday objects and actions using toys.

Example:

Mom: Vamos a comer [Let's eat] (showing a spoon or feeding the child or doll)

Child: (grabs the spoon and puts it in her mouth)

Mom: Llama a papi [Call daddy] (giving a toy phone to child)

Child: (grabs phone) ¡Hola! [Hello!]

Mom: Peina a la muñeca [Comb the doll]

Child: (combs the doll)

Event re-enactments: The parent and the child use objects to re-enact and talk about events. Parents demonstrate cause-effect sequences and may talk about future or anticipated events.

Example:

Mom: El nene tiene hambre, dále de comer. [The boy is hungry, give him food]

Child: (feeds the baby)

Mom: Pam Pam le voy a pegar porque se portó mal. [/Pam pam/ I'm going to spank him because he misbehaved]

Child: (spanks teddy bear)

Script: Talk about what usually happens in an event or general event knowledge:

Example:

Mom: ¿Qué haces cuando te levantas de la cama? [What do you do when you get up?]

Child: Me levanto, me lavo los dientes .... [I get up, I brush my teeth]

Mom: ¿Qué pasa cuando vamos a McDonald's? [What happens when we go to McDonald's?]

Child: Me compro una hamburguesa y juego con la arena ... [I buy a hamburger and play with the sand ...]

Story: Talk about a past event (i.e. "there and then" rather than "here and now") Objects are used to support the narration of events displaced in time and space:

Example:

Mom: ¿Te acuerdas qué hizo papi el otro día? [Do you remember what daddy did the other day?]

Child: Me llevó al parque .... [He took me to the park]

Table 5–1 illustrates the average frequency of these types of narrative interactions in normally developing children at the prelinguistic, one-word, and multiword stages of language development. From the prelinguistic to the multiword stages, children demonstrated significantly an increased number of verbal initiations of symbolic play and responses to parent-initiated event re-enactments in their narrative interactions with their mothers (Kruskal-Wallis $H = 6.62$, $p < 05$ and $H = 6.44$, $p < .05$, respectively). Prelinguistic children participated in symbolic play by responding primarily with nonverbal actions. In contrast, the children who used multiword utterances were also capable of initiating verbalizations during symbolic play. It is interesting to note that, across all narrative interactions, there were no instances of script or story, and event re-enactments appeared to be just emerg-

TABLE 5–1
Average number of symbolic play events, event re-enactments, scripts, and stories by children at prelinguistic, one-word, and multiword stages learning Spanish as a first language.

| | Language Development | | |
| | Prelinguistic | One-word | Multiword |
Narrative	(*N* = 8)	(*N* = 11)	(*N* = 9)
Symbolic play			
Child-initiated*	.12	.55	1.89
Parent-initiated	2.25	3.82	4.67
Event re-enactment			
Child-initiated	0	0	.11
Parent-initiated*	0	.36	.56
Script	0	0	0
Story	0	0	0

*Significant at *p* < .05

ing in the interactions of the more advanced children. Similar observations have also been made for English-speaking children (Miller & Sperry, 1988).

IMPLICATIONS FOR ASSESSMENT

It is possible that the play contexts used to sample narrative language did not promote richer parent-child narrative interactions. For example, children may not refer to events or objects not present in the immediate context in play contexts. In contrast, daily routines such as feeding or bathing a baby doll may generate talk about the "there and then" because the predictable structure of these scripts supports the use of more advanced language (Day, French, & Hall, 1985). A longitudinal study with two Mexican-American girls learning Spanish as a first language, from 21 to 32 months and 24 to 38 months, respectively, indicated that parents frequently, elicit conversations about past events at home using the expression *"díle"* (Tell him/her), telling the child what to say to a third participant in the conversation (Eisenberg, 1985). In these home interactions, conversations about past events were also cued by the use of pictures and photographs. Thus, narrative interactions in assessment may need to be elicited using a variety of prompts, activities, and additional participants. The clinician may also ask parents to use specific questions such as "What happen when...?" which may generate more instances of scripts or "What happened when [this] happened?" which may generate more storytelling (Hudson & Nelson, 1984). There is some evidence that by 25 months children may provide general scripts and that in many instances their descriptions of a particular past event (e.g., What happened at Mary's birthday party?) may contain general information common to similar events rather than event-specific information (Eisenberg, 1985). Given that the play interactions in this study did not include specific prompts for eliciting children's narratives, it would be interesting to know whether a more structured play interaction would elicit more and/or different narrative interactions.

In a second investigation, the narrative interactions of six Spanish-speaking children whose vocabulary scores placed them at or below the 10th percentile on the *Fundación MacArthur: Inventario del Desarrollo de las Habilidades Comunicativas* (IDHC) (Jackson-Maldonado, Thal, & Bates, 1992) were compared to the narrative interactions of six children whose vocabulary scores fell between the 25th and 75th percentile. The two groups were matched by age, ranging from 18 to 29 months. As with the first investigation, language samples were gathered in a play situation between parent and child using sets of predetermined toys. The analysis indicated that, although both groups of children were capable of initiating and responding to parent-initiated symbolic play, the language delayed children were less likely to respond to parent-initiated event re-enactments (Mann-Whitney $U = -1.91$, $p < .05$) (see Table 5–2). Differences in children's performance in narrative interactions may suggest a need for increased focus on providing the child with narrative learning experiences. Research with English-speaking children has demonstrated that children who exhibit late language development may be at risk for future language delays (Paul & Smith, 1993).

THE FAMILY AS MEDIATOR OF NARRATIVE LEARNING

One question that may be raised from these observations is the role of the parent as a mediator of language learning and the extent to which their interactional strategies can be applied to clinical interventions. A number of studies with English-speaking children have examined

TABLE 5–2
Average frequency of symbolic play events, event re-enactments, scripts, and stories by language delayed and normally developing children learning Spanish as a first language.

Narrative	Language Development	
	Normal ($N = 6$)	Delayed ($N = 6$)
Symbolic play		
Child-initiated	2.0	1.16
Parent-initiated	4.5	3.16
Event re-enactment		
Child-initiated	0	0
Parent-initiated*	.5	0
Script	0	0
Story	0	0

*Significant at $p < .05$

parental styles in parent-child narrative interactions in an attempt to determine whether there are parental narrative uses more conducive to narrative development. For example, Fivush and Fromhoff (1988) found that a maternal style which they called "elaborative" may facilitate children's descriptions of past events. In this study mothers were told to elicit their children's past events as naturally as possible so that children's personal narratives could be investigated. Two types of maternal style, an "elaborative" and a "repetitive" style, were distinguished. If the child appeared to be motivated to continue a conversation about a past event, the elaborative mothers continued asking more questions than the repetitive mothers. They also provided more information (e.g., using attributes such as "a big fat old pig") to stimulate children's recall. Thus, the elaborative mothers appeared to mediate children's narratives by giving memory cues that included why those events were important to remember (Fivush & Fromhoff, 1988). In contrast, the repetitive mothers appeared to be looking for "the right answer" to their questions, repeating their questions until the child provided a specific aspect of the past event and dismissing "incorrect" responses. The results indicated that children of the elaborative mothers recalled more than children of the repetitive mothers.

Thus, although these parental narrative styles may have an effect on the amount of children's talk, they do not appear to influence the quality of their early narratives.

Parental mediation strategies directed to focus the child on the causes or motives of events may also facilitate the child's later use of this information in their narratives. A longitudinal study of a mother-child narrative interaction from 29 months to 40 months using a storybook showed that information about events, motives, and causes introduced primarily by the mother at the onset were gradually incorporated in the child's descriptions by the end of the study (Snow & Goldfield, 1981). Young children also appear to provide more narrative information to questions directed to elicit specific information about a past event than to general questions directed to elicit a narrative (e.g., Tell me a story). Using the retelling of a fictional narrative, Pratt, Kerig, Cowan, and Cowan (1988) found that 3-year-olds were more likely to generate narrative information when parents used question cues such as "What was X doing?" or "Did X happen?" than when more general questions, such as "Tell me your story," were used. However, parents should be cautioned not to ask too many questions or questions unrelated to the child's own version of a past event. Such questioning may disrupt children's attempts at producing a coherent narrative.

It also has been suggested that the use of requests for clarification or informative expansions (i.e., repetitions of child's incomplete statements with changes) may be more facilitative of children's narrative production than overt corrections because children are given more opportunities for self-correction (McCabe & Peterson, 1991). From 27 to 42 months, parental clarifying questions were found to correlate with an increase in children's immediate use of evaluation and future use of evaluation, orientation, and complicating action statements in their narratives, a few months later (McCabe & Peterson, 1991). This research has also indicated that topic switching may not be a useful strategy to mediate children's narrative learning. McCabe and Peterson (1991) found that the father of a child who had limited language development tended to shift topics in an effort to elicit the child's narratives. Yet, the tactic was not useful because in the initial stages of development a young child may not know how to extend a conversation about the past.

Family mediators may stimulate children's narratives by prompting novel past events. Although talk about shared past events or recounts has been assumed to facilitate the development of decontextualized language (i.e., use of explicit language to represent meanings that can be inferred from context), prompting for unshared experiences (or accounts) has been found to be more helpful to a child's future narrative ability (at least during the early years) than prompts for shared experiences (McCabe & Peterson, 1991). These observations are particularly relevant for planning interventions with children learning Spanish as a first language. Recounts of shared information may not occur in the narrative interactions of some Spanish-speaking groups. A study with Hispanic families in California found a tendency for parents to prompt their children primarily about unshared rather than shared past experiences (Heath, 1986). Thus, there appear to be individual as well as cultural differences in the types of topics (shared, unshared) used in narrative interactions.

Because most research in this area has focused on Anglo families, it is not known whether the mediation strategies just described for adult-child narrative interactions are applicable to Hispanic parent-child narrative interactions. There is evidence that the processes of language socialization vary according to the social status of children in the family and community. Apparent cross-cultural similarities in the narrative contexts available for children's narrative development may be obscured by differences in the rules for participation in those narrative contexts. For example, in a cross-cultural study comparing the narrative interactions of American (working class and middle class) and Israeli families at the dinner table, families in all three groups jointly collaborated in the construction of personal stories. Yet, the American middle class children were less likely than the other groups to participate in the personal stories initiated by other adult speakers (Blum-Kulka & Snow, 1992).

Analysis of narrative interactions in family gatherings indicates that participant structure also may vary according to the types of narratives being told. An ethnographic study of the evening narrative conversations of four Mexican-American families found a wide variety of narratives from traditional folklore *cuentos* (stories), to family *cuentos*, and stories of personal past experience (Vasquez, 1989). For the narration of traditional stories, children were expected to be active listeners. Consequently, they asked for information and commented on the events being told. In contrast, family stories, which revolved around childhood events or family events in Mexico, were typically constructed in collaboration with the audience who shared background information and added elements to the story. Children participated by adding information of their own involvement. Adults tended to challenge the content of their stories through humor (teasing) to engage the child in the creation of conversational stories (Vasquez, 1989). Stories of personal experience were also jointly constructed with the audience asking questions for information to fill in details. Thus, children learned how to produce narratives by being exposed to various types of family conversational narratives. In these interactions, parents appeared to focus on maintaining conversation rather than on "teaching" or correcting children's attempts at describing a past event. These observations are consistent with Eisenberg's (1985) longitudinal research with two Mexican-American families. Parents were found to elicit and respond to children's descriptions of past events ignoring children's inaccuracies. They did not correct the child in instances when the child mentioned elements common to similar events but not present in the specific past event (i.e., when they applied scriptal knowledge to make up their own version of a past event). Furthermore, parents involved their children in conversations about past events, but they did not introduce narrative information about motives and causes in the manner described for Anglo interactions (Snow & Goldfield, 1981). Rather than introducing information about motives and causes in narrative interactions with their children, they asked about motives and causes for the child's own behavior in other conversational contexts (Eisenberg, 1985).

In summary, the literature appears to indicate a number of ways normally developing children learn narratives across families and cultural groups that may guide intervention. Children may have preferred narrative learning styles as well as special needs. For young children with slow language development, narrative skills can be stimulated by applying strategies described in studies with Spanish-speaking families. Parents and other mediators may be asked to promote rich narrative interactions in the home setting by having the child participate and practice descriptions of daily routines and events while focusing on unusual occurrences (e.g., While preparing a meal, talk about something that broke in the kitchen and what would be done next). Participation in triadic interactions with an older sibling or relative using *dile* (Tell her/him) may also be used to generate more narrative interactions . During play the child may be taught how to combine events temporally or causally by instructing the mediator to provide temporal cues (e.g., *¿Ya está?* / All done?, *¿Y después qué hacemos?* / And then what do we do?) and cause-effect cues (e.g., *La nena llora* / *le duele* / The girl cries/It hurts). These early narrative interactions may facilitate the production of narratives during the preschool years. The next section describes the characteristics of preschool narratives, how to assess them using various contexts for elicitation, and how to expand children's narrative repertoire and contextual knowledge.

🗗

PRESCHOOL NARRATIVES

STORIES OF PERSONAL EXPERIENCE

Research with English-speaking children indicates that, during the preschool years, children's narratives develop from a focus on jointly constructed conversational narratives under the guidance of an adult to the production of independent narrations of personal experience (for a review, see Hudson & Shapiro, 1991). However, the narrativization of experience is never context-independent. Children's narratives reflect the child's knowledge of the function of narratives in social contexts and the rules for participation in those contexts. Narrative interactions gathered as part of a large cross-sectional study with preschool and school-age Puerto Rican children demonstrated that the examiner may need to use various question cues to obtain an extended narrative, in particular when using elicited rather than child-initiated topics (Iglesias & Gutierrez-Clellen, 1986). For some groups, narratives about past experience may be constructed in conversation and negotiated in collaboration with an active audience (Gutierrez-Clellen & Quinn, 1993). The following excerpt (translated from Spanish) from a 7-year-old Puerto Rican child illustrates the type of scaffolding needed in the elicitation of a narrative using accidents and visits to the hospital as story prompts:

Examiner:	What happened to your brother? Why did he have to go to the hospital?
Child:	Because he cut his leg.
Examiner:	Oh! Tell me what happened.
Child:	In the park (silence)
Examiner:	What happened?
Child:	When he was running there he fell.

Examiner:	How?
Child:	When he was running.
Examiner:	And?
Child:	And he opened the door and fell.
Examiner:	And then?
Child:	(silence)
Examiner:	And then what happened?
Child:	He cut his leg.
Examiner:	But how?
Child:	(silence)
Examiner:	And then what happened?
Child:	My mom came . . . there and she went away running. (silence)
Examiner:	Running?
Child:	(silence)
Examiner:	She went running? (long silence)
Child:	Back to the hospital.
Examiner:	Oh! She took him to the hospital? And what happened?
Child:	(silence)
Examiner:	What happened there?
Child:	(long pause) They cut his leg.
Examiner:	They cut his leg? What happened?
Child:	They cut his feet.
Examiner:	And?
Child:	(silence)
Examiner:	And then?
Child:	He was taken to the hospital. (silence)

Examiner:	And? And what happened? What happened then when they went to the hospital?
Child:	They operated him.
Examiner:	What did they do to him?
Child:	Mm they saw this.
Examiner:	And?
Child:	And....they something like this on top.
Examiner:	And?
Child:	And they took him home.

In this example the child provides narrative information only when questioned by the examiner. Without the use of question cues, this child's narrative performance might have been limited to one or two narrative statements (i.e., In the park/When he was running there he fell) and judged as immature or below age expectations. Yet, with the use of question cues, the child indicated the basic components of a narrative (i.e., some information about orientation, complicating action, and consequences). Thus, the clinician may need to consider the use of question cues when eliciting children's stories. In a related study using a "Tell me about a scary movie" prompt with 13 Puerto Rican first graders, 5 children were able to tell their stories without assistance while the remaining children required between one to four question cues to complete their stories (Gutierrez-Clellen, 1990). Furthermore, the use of story prompts such as "What happened when you went to the hospital" may generate script information (i.e., what usually happens when you go to a hospital) rather than a true narration of a past event, probably because these are not culturally relevant topics in family narrative interactions. In contrast, even young children may respond to a "Tell me about a scary movie" prompt because the nature of the task (i.e., to narrate unshared or "original" information) may be more conducive to producing a spontaneous narrative. The following excerpt (translated from Spanish) from a 4- year 11 month-old illustrates the child's ability to retell a movie without assistance:

Examiner:	What happened in that movie?
Child:	That what happened is that King Kong climbed a building and and...many helicopters came and

> they shot him . . . He died . . . and and then after
> King Kong fell dead, dead, dead, dead, dead . . .
> Very dead and he had a lot of blood, a lot of blood
> over here . . . A lot and until he died very dead . . .
> And that was what happened and that's all noth-
> ing more.

These observations underscore the need to compare narrative performance across different elicitation contexts (e.g., self-generated vs.
elicited with prompts; spontaneous vs. recalled) and topics before
judgments about children's narrative competence are made. In addition, they suggest that narratives may vary significantly according to
the methods used to assess them.

SCRIPTS AND FILM STORIES

Children's scripts also become increasingly complex with age and
experience. Young children comprehend the possible or optional elements that may be included in script descriptions but they may omit
them in their production of scripts (Gruendel, 1980). For example,
when children are asked "What happens when you go to McDonald's," they may talk about events that usually happen, not events
that may happen. Studies have also suggested that preschool children
are influenced by their knowledge of general event representations or
scripts. Thus, when asked about a unique, specific past event (e.g.,
What happened when you went to McDonald's yesterday?), the
child's recount may contain elements not present in the original past
experience (Hudson & Nelson, 1986) and the narrative may resemble
a script (i.e., a description of what usually happens rather than what
happened). As described earlier, this strategy may be the child's
response to the prompts adults use to elicit narratives.

There are also changes in the structure of preschool children's
narratives. A 3-year-old may narrate a past event by producing a single act (e.g., I ate a cake), a list of acts (e.g., I ate cake, I saw Cathy, I
played), or a sequence of acts (I ate cake, then we opened presents,
and I went home and went to bed) (Applebee, 1978; Hudson & Nelson, 1984). By age 5, the child begins to indicate causal relations by
using such devices as "so" and "because" (e.g., I saw a child was
breaking one of the presents, so I told Cathy's mom, and so she took it
and fixed it) (Hudson & Nelson, 1984). Research has found that
preschool children may include introducers and abstracts in conversa-

tional narratives but not in experimenter-elicited narrative contexts (Hudson & Shapiro, 1991). During the preschool years, children's narratives may consist of complicating actions in additive structure (i.e., a collection of a protagonist's actions or a collection of characters performing the same action), temporal sequence (i.e., actions and events are temporally related), or causal sequence (i.e., actions and events may be connected in cause-effect relationship). There is evidence that from ages 4 to 5 children also increase their use of resolutions (Peterson & McCabe, 1983) and use a wider range of techniques to indicate the point of their stories (Umiker-Sebeok, 1979). The child above introduced the movie story ("What happened is") and provided narrative statements that were connected temporally (i.e., King Kong climbs a building, helicopters come, they shoot him) and causally (King Kong dies). The point of the story was marked by the use of repetitions such as in "King Kong fell dead dead dead dead dead very dead" and in "and he had a lot of blood, a lot of blood over here . . . a lot and until he died very dead" before the story was ended ("And that was what happened and that's all nothing more").

FICTIONAL STORIES

During the preschool years, children also learn to narrate fictional stories using the components specified by story grammars. When asked to tell a make-believe story, preschool children may include setting information but they may omit reference to the internal goals, motivations, or reactions of characters until well into the school years (Stein & Glenn, 1982). Yet, young children may be capable of including information about goals and resolutions when more naturalistic tasks using question cues are used (Peterson & McCabe, 1983). In the Puerto Rican studies described above, young children were able to produce a fictional story when prompted to talk about subjects such as "something really scary." Their stories were about monsters, vampires, or "men that do bad things to children." Thus, narrative performance appears to reflect both contextual knowledge and knowledge of story structure.

In narrating a fictional story, children apply their knowledge of actions and states that may occasion reactions in social interactions and consequences (i.e., what constitutes a problem and how it may be resolved). They may use the recall of a personal past experience or another fictional story in their make-believe narratives. Thus, children's ability to tell a fictional story may depend on their exposure to literature books and traditional story retellings in family interactions. The following example from a 5-year-old Puerto Rican girl illustrates how the child learned about a fictional story. Both Spanish and English versions are included to better capture the prompts used to elicit the narrative:

	Spanish	*English*
Examiner:	¿Mamá te cuenta cuentos a tí?	Does mom tell you stories?
Child:	Sí	Yes
Examiner:	¿Me cuentas tú un cuento a mí?	Would you tell me a story?
Child:	Es de Pinocho pero siempre se me olvida	It's about Pinocchio but I always forget
Examiner:	Bueno, no importa, ¿qué es lo que te acuerdas a ver?	O.K. it doesn't matter. What do you remember? Let's see
Child:	Que un papá quería hacer un hijo/ y hizo un hijo conmadera que se llama Pinocho/ y hay un muñequito que es un sapo	A father wanted to make a son/ and made a son of wood called Pinocchio/ and there was a little doll that is a frog
	que camina camina y todo todo verde/ y era así de chiquito/	that walks walks and all all green/ and it was like this small/
	y después con Pinocho dijo muchas mentiras/ y la nariz se le puso bien grande/ se puso/ y cuando el papá le vio	and then with Pinocchio told many lies/ and the nose got very big/ got/ and when the dad

la nariz/ le contó todo lo que le pasó/	saw his nose/ [he] told [him] every thing that
y el muñeco chiquito el sapo le puso la nariz chiquita/	happened [to him]/and the little doll the frog made his nose small/

This child was able to retell a story from a book (Pinocchio) previously rehearsed with her mother. Yet, for children with limited experience with book-stories, prompts may be initially directed to elicit traditional stories (e.g., stories from their country of origin) told by the family at home. The story of this preschooler included a sequence of temporally and causally related events, a problem, and a resolution. As with English-speaking children, there is still no indication of motives or goals at this young age.

DISTINGUISHING NARRATIVE DIFFERENCES FROM DISORDERS

The findings of these studies suggest that many of the "problematic" narratives children produce during this period may be related to differences in contextual knowledge, rather than ability. Thus, narrative learning may be promoted by teaching the child the function of narratives in a given context and the rules that govern narrative behavior in a given interaction. For example, the child may be given opportunities to make sense of a past event and narrate it in sharing time activities in preschool. Yet, teachers frequently assume children come to these interactions with knowledge of school narratives and deviations from the "norm" may be treated as deviancies. As a result, teachers may not make narrative expectations explicit nor mediate children's narratives during group activities (Michaels, 1991). To address children's diverse narrative experiences, it is imperative that teachers use classroom interactions to provide the scaffolding necessary to support the production of narratives (not to disrupt them) and then encourage the child to independently retell past events (Gutierrez-Clellen & Quinn, 1993). Through these mediated narrative interactions the child will be able to learn that in some contexts they are expected to produce a monologic rather than a conversational narrative. Adult question cues may be directed to generate actions and events in temporal and causal relationship while providing intentionality to the narrative learning activity. The mediator will make the child aware that the purpose of the retelling is to learn and practice different ways of narrativization rather than to penalize the child's narrative style.

For children whose narrative skills are exhibited in only certain contexts, teachers may mediate and stimulate narrations in other types of interactions (e.g., group retellings,teacher-student, peer-assisted) and with various media (e.g., books, pictures, films). Film and TV stories appear to engage the most reluctant storytellers, perhaps because they are action-oriented, and common across homes and income levels. Although book activities may not be very frequent at home, they also provide needed contextual support to stimulate narrative development, in particular for children with limited narrative skills. Children can talk about pictures without relying so much on memory and reducing language processing demands.

DEVELOPING AGE-APPROPRIATE INTERVENTIONS

For children with limited narrative skills, intervention should focus on producing extended and content-oriented (i.e., what, where, when, why) narrative interactions from culturally familiar to more "foreign" contexts and tasks. Although preschool Spanish-speaking children are capable of using complex syntax in conversational samples, there is evidence that young Puerto Rican as well as Mexican-American children prefer simple syntactic structures and use short statements in their story retellings, perhaps as a means to facilitate processing and integration of narrative information (Gutierrez-Clellen & Hofstetter, 1994).

Similarly, during the preschool years, children begin to learn how to introduce and reintroduce characters, objects, and places using appropriate referential devices. New referents are to be introduced using nominal phrases (e.g., There was *a little boy*). Later in the text those referents may be re-introduced by pronouns (e.g., *He* had a frog), phrases containing definite articles (e.g., *The boy* had a frog), demonstratives (e.g., *This boy* had a frog), or ellipsis (e.g., The boy opened the door/ [*he*] grabbed the frog). A study using the retelling of a film with normally developing Puerto Rican children demonstrated that preschoolers may use pronouns and ellipsis for referents introduced for the first time (Gutierrez-Clellen & Heinrichs-Ramos, 1993). This may occur because children assume shared knowledge with their listeners, and they may have difficulty keeping track of newly introduced referents while telling a story. As a result, characters, objects, or places presented in their narratives may be difficult to identify or interpret unless the audience shares background information. The following narrative from a 4-year 6-month old girl illustrates the use of demonstratives *el de esto* (the this) to introduce the story's principal character (the frog) and the use of pronouns *él* (he) to introduce the human protagonist (the boy) for the first time:

Spanish	*English*
Este **el de esto** se fue para morir la rana/	This **the this** went to die the frog/
y se metió en un plato/	and it got on a plate/
y después **él** dijo se acabó la película/	and then **he** said the movie finished/
después se murió/	then [he] died/
se murió con la comida/	died with the food/
y (?) se fue/	and [?] went/
y **el nene** lo cogió/	and **the boy** grabbed him/
y se fue para arriba con la rana al cuarto de **él**/	and went upstairs with the frog to **his** room/
y se fue más para abajo/	and [he] went more downstairs/
y la mamá vino/	and the mother came/
y se rió/	and laughed/
y después la mamá dijo que **lo** bote en la basura/	and then the mother said to throw it to the trash/
y después **él** se fue/...	and then **he** went/...

This typical young child also uses elliptical reference to treat a new referent as given: *[?] y se fue/* (and [?] went/) and definite articles for the introductions of a new referent: *el nene* (the boy). Although young children are capable of providing temporal and causal information in their narratives, their referential cohesion skills appear to develop later during the school years (Gutierrez-Clellen & Heinrichs-Ramos, 1993). Thus, the clinician may focus on the development of referential cohesion once children demonstrate the ability to establish temporal and causal relations in their stories.

ᒪ

THE SCHOOL YEARS

With age, children's script descriptions and narratives become increasingly complex. By 6 and 8 years old, children may indicate preconditions for certain acts (e.g., *If my parents stay at the party we go home late*) and optional acts (e.g., *Sometimes we play with the presents or we have games*) in their script reports (Gruendel, 1980). Children also include more information about events that precede or follow actions in their story episodes, making their narratives more causally cohesive (Gutierrez-Clellen & Iglesias, 1992). Whereas preschool children may connect only one action with a change of state in causal sequence (e.g., He got a present/ He was happy), by age 8 children increasingly intersect statements that explain the character's actions or changes of state interconnecting up to six clauses in causal sequence. These changes in the achievement of causal coherence do not necessarily imply that their narratives will be longer. With age, children adopt individual narrative styles for representing past experiences, and they may use syntactic subordination to condense narrative information (Gutierrez-Clellen & Hoffstetter, 1994). A study with Puerto Rican and Mexican-American children showed that 8-year-olds were capable of using subordination to develop a central theme. For example, they used adverbial clauses to mark when events took place in a movie (e.g., "And *when the man was going to kill the frog* the child came in/ and screamed") and to mark their relationship to the overall plot (i.e., The story was about a pet frog *that escaped from a child's pocket in a restaurant*).

During the early school years, progressions are also apparent in children's referential accuracy. By age 8, children's narratives contain significantly fewer inappropriate references (i.e., introductions of a new referent as given) and ambiguities (i.e., referents that may have more than one antecedent). In addition, children begin to use syntactic devices to disambiguate referents as in "The man *that was carrying the cake* fell down" when competing referents are available in the text (i.e., other men characters were introduced in the story) (Gutierrez-Clellen & Heinrichs-Ramos, 1993). Thus, clinicians may apply these measures to identify children's strengths and weaknesses and to stimulate narrative development in educational and clinical settings. The following case studies will be used to illustrate the narrative skills of two children with language disorders and the intervention strategies that may facilitate their narrative learning.

CASE 1: PEDRO

Pedro is a 6;10 Spanish-speaking child with mild speech and moderate-to-severe language disorders secondary to traumatic head injury at 3 years of age. Spanish is the language spoken at home. A speech and language assessment conducted in Spanish indicated ability to use complete sentences but difficulty producing connected discourse in conversation. In addition, he rarely initiated topics and tended to use gestures or single word utterances in his responses to questions. After 2 months of intervention to increase verbal communication in structured play activities, the child was able to produce the following narrative while turning the pages of a book:

	Spanish	*English*
Child:	[?]Está tomando bibi/	[?] is having the bottle/
Child:	[?]Está peinando/	[?] is combing/
Examiner:	¿El perrito o el osito?	The little dog or the little bear?
Child:	El osito está peinando/	The little bear is combing/
	El bus el bus a la escuela/	The bus the bus to school/
Examiner:	Ajá el autobus se va a la escuela/	Uhu the bus goes to school/
Child:	payaso/	clown/
	galleta/	cookie/
	Santa Claus/	Santa Claus
Examiner:	Santa Claus se mete por la chimenea/	Santa Claus goes into the chimney/
Child:	[?]está llorando/	[?] is crying/

Examiner:	¿está llorando?	is crying?/
Child:	[?]está llorando/	[?] is crying/
Examiner:	El perro, la señora, o el niño, ¿quién está llorando?	The dog, the lady, or the boy who is crying?
Child:	el niño está llorando/ (pause) Colorín colorado este cuento se ha acabado/	the boy is crying/ (pause) And they lived happily ever after/

In this narrative the child exhibits difficulty with establishing temporal or causal relationships interconnecting narrative statements. Structurally, the narrative resembles a collection of unrelated actions in additive relationship as typically found in the narratives of young preschool children. No temporal or cause-effect relationships can be inferred from the narrative actions. The child's use of simple syntax in the narrative may be evidence of difficulty processing and summarizing complex information. There are also problems with the use of appropriate nominal phrases in the introduction of referents ([?] is having the bottle/). In spite of clinician's question cues to elicit explicit referents (as in "the little dog or the little bear? ", the child appeared to have difficulty transferring use of appropriate nominal phrases to the spontaneous introduction of referents six utterances later ("[?] is crying"). The child has learned how to end imaginary stories (i.e., using "and they lived happily ever after"), yet there is a need for further development of narrative structure and narrative coherence relations (i.e., temporal, causal, referential, spatial).

For this child, narrative intervention should focus on stimulating script knowledge and verbalization. Clinic, school, and home activities and routines such as participating in the preparation of meals, crafts, cleaning, shopping, and planning and describing field trips may be used to train sequencing and verbalization of events (i.e., what comes first, second, etc). The contextual support provided by event re-enactments (using dolls or puppets), sequence cards, and picture books may help facilitate learning and production of causes/consequences of actions and events (i.e., discussions about attributes and feelings that may occasion actions and reactions). Initially, the child may be asked to answer questions about well-rehearsed scripts and events, later to verbally reproduce them given a model (or prompts such as pictures), and finally to spontaneously retell a past event with no assistance.

CASE 2: CARLOS

Carlos is an 8;3 bilingual child with mild speech and moderate language disorders secondary to a moderate-to-severe bilateral sensorineural hearing loss. Speech and language deficits are exhibited in both Spanish and English. A speech and language assessment conducted in Spanish indicated ability to use complex syntax to initiate and maintain topics in conversation, yet limited narrative development. The following narrative elicited using a set of five pictures illustrates this child's narrative skills:

Spanish	*English*
Un niño y luego se cayó de la bicicleta/	A boy and then he fell off the bike/
y luego se puso a llorar/	and then [he]started to cry/
y luego el niño corrió a su mamá/	and then the boy ran to his mother/
y luego su mamá le puso bandaid	and then his mother put a bandaid on
donde el niño tiene herido/	where the boy was hurt /

The child's narrative describes a series of actions in temporal sequence explicitly marked by temporal connectives (i.e., and then). However, the narrative does not directly indicate how these actions are causally interrelated. For example, in the action sequence "he fell/ he cried" there is no indication of feeling hurt or scared to explain the character's reaction. The child's narrative performance may be related to a difficulty narrating a story visually shared with the listener using decontextualized language (i.e., as if information were unknown to the audience). Thus, intervention should focus on changing the way the child thinks about the narrative situation. The clinician or teacher can mediate the child's narrative learning by teaching the child to respond to different narrative contexts/rules while validating the child's cultural experience in the joint selection of narrative topics, tasks, and rules for listener participation. In mediated learning, the teacher makes explicit the contextualization processes governing a given narrative situation by (a) modeling narrative content and (b) thinking aloud the purpose of the narration and the strategies for storytelling in the targeted context. (See Feuerstein, Jensen, Hoffman, and Rand, 1985, for a detailed description of the characteristics of mediated learning.) Initially, the child will imitate the teacher's self-talk in directing the production of a narrative (e.g., I need to look at all the pictures and see what's happening; then for each picture I need to give information about who, where, and when things happen even though everybody can see it; then I need to say what happened and why; and finally I need to give an end or resolution to the story). There is evidence that instruction in the structural components of stories increases children's awareness and subsequent use of these elements (Gordon & Braun, 1985). Therefore, the child may be also asked to generate questions about the pictures to help monitor the inclusion of story elements such as setting, initiating event, internal response, attempt, consequence, and reaction or resolution in narratives. Mediation activities may be structured initially with naive peer listeners and later with unfamiliar adults such as a different teacher or aide.

Carlos's narrative performance after a brief mediation session demonstrates the potential outcomes of intervention:

Spanish	*English*
Un día un niño se chocó con un palo/	One day a boy hit a pole/
y luego se cayó de la bicicleta/	and then he fell off the bike/
y luego se asustó mucho/	and then he was very scared/
y luego **un niño** se está sangrando/	and then **a boy** is bleeding/
y luego u**n niño** se puso a llorar/	and then **a boy** started to cry/
y luego **un niño** corría para su casa/	and then **a boy** ran to his house/
luego **un niño** fue con su mamá/	then **a boy** went with his mom/
luego su mamá le dijo: "está bien mi hijo"	then his mom said: "It's okay my son"/
y luego dijo que te haces bien mejor/	and then she said [hope] you get better/
y yo no sé más nada/	and I don't know any more/
y luego says: "con cuidado okey, porque	**and his mother says: "Be careful**

hay muchos palos allí en la calle" okey.	because there are many poles out there in the street" okay/

With the clinician's mediation, Carlos was able to provide more information in his story and include information that was not modeled by the clinician (i.e., that the mother warned the child to be careful because of the many sticks that were out there in the street). This observation indicates he learned to expand the story displayed in the pictures by providing inferences on his own. Second, his narrative shows overuse of indefinite reference ("a boy") rather than use of pronouns (he) or definite articles (the boy) which suggests Carlos is now learning to introduce referents without assuming shared information. Finally, he was able to transfer these new skills to English when asked to retell the story in English. This child showed that when given appropriate model and cues he was able to learn new ways of storytelling. Although the effectiveness of mediated narrative learning may need to be evaluated against other methods such as adult-directed activities related to literature appreciation and drama, the use of mediation techniques may provide valuable information about how children respond to training and in the case of children from diverse backgrounds, their true learning potential.

⊔

CONCLUSION

This chapter described the characteristics of children's narratives from the early stages of development to the school years which may be used to guide the development of clinical interventions. As the examples and the case studies illustrate, a broad range of techniques may be used to facilitate narrative development and can be applied to interventions with Hispanic children. Thus far, there is limited research on the efficacy of the various teaching approaches with Hispanic children. Yet, based on the available narrative research with normally developing children and their families, the clinician may be able to design interventions that recognize diversity and individual differences in narrative learning and experience.

ㄥ

REFERENCES

Applebee, A. N. (1978). *The child's concept of a story: Ages two to seventeen*. Chicago: University of Chicago Press.

Blum-Kulka, S., & Snow, C. E. (1992). Developing autonomy for tellers, tales, and telling family narrative events. *Journal of Narrative and Life History, 2*(3), 187–217.

Carlisle, R. S. (1986). *The writing of Anglo and Hispanic fourth and sixth graders in regular, submersion, and bilingual programs*. Unpublished doctoral dissertation, University of Illinois at Urbana, Champaign.

Day, J. D., French, L. A., & Hall, L. K. (1985). Social influences on cognitive development. In D. L. Forrest-Pressley, G. E. Mac Kinnon, & T. G. Waller (Eds.), *Metacognition, cognition, and human performance* (Vol. 1, pp. 33–56). San Diego, CA: Academic Press.

Eisenberg, A. R. (1985). Learning to describe past experiences in conversation. *Discourse Processes, 8*, 177–204.

Feuerstein, R., Jensen, M. R., Hoffman, M. B., & Rand, Y. (1985). Instrumental Enrichment, an intervention program for structural cognitive modifiability: Theory and practice. In J. W. Segal, S. F. Chipman, & R. Glaser (Eds.), *Thinking and learning skills. Vol 1. Relating instruction to research* (pp. 43–82). Hillsdale, NJ: Lawrence Erlbaum.

Fivush, R., & Fromhoff, F. A. (1988). Style and structure in mother-child conversations about the past. *Discourse Processes, 11*, 337–355.

Gordon, C. J., & Braun, C. (1985). Metacognitive processes: Reading and writing narrative discourse. In D. L. Forrest-Pressley, G. E. MacKinnon, & T. G. Waller (Eds.), *Metacognition, cognition, and human performance* (pp. 1–75). San Diego: Academic Press.

Gruendel, J. M. (1980). *Scripts and stories: A study of children's event narratives*. Unpublished doctoral dissertation, Yale University, New Haven, CT.

Gutierrez-Clellen, V. G. (1990). *The acquisition of causal coherence in Spanish narratives*. Unpublished doctoral dissertation, Temple University, Philadelphia, PA.

Gutierrez-Clellen, V. F., & Heinrichs-Ramos, L. (1993). Referential cohesion in the narratives of Spanish-speaking children: A developmental study. *Journal of Speech and Hearing Research, 36*, 559–567.

Gutierrez-Clellen, V. F., & Hofstetter, R. (1994). Syntactic complexity in Spanish narratives: A developmental study. *Journal of Speech and Hearing Research, 37*, 645–654.

Gutierrez-Clellen, V. F., & Iglesias, A. (1992). Causal coherence in the oral narratives of Spanish-speaking children. *Journal of Speech and Hearing Research, 35*, 363–372.

Gutierrez-Clellen, V. F., & Quinn, R. (1993). Assessing narratives of children from diverse cultural/linguistic groups. *Language, Speech, and Hearing Services in Schools, 24*, 2–9.

Heath, S. B. (1986). The book as narrative prop in language acquisition. In B. Schieffelin & P. Gilmore (Eds.), *The acquisition of literacy: Ethnographic perspectives* (pp. 16–34). Norwood, NJ: Ablex.

Hudson, J. A., & Nelson, K. (1984). Differentiation and development in children's event narratives. *Papers and Reports on Child Language Development, 23,* 50–57.

Hudson, J. A., & Nelson, K. (1986). Repeated encounters of a similar kind: Effects of familiarity in children's autobiographic memory, *Cognitive Development, 1,* 232–271.

Hudson, J. A., & Shapiro, L. R. (1991). From knowing to telling: The development of children's scripts, stories, and personal narratives. In A. McCabe & C. Peterson (Eds.), *Developing narrative structure* (pp. 89–136). Hillsdale, NJ: Lawrence Erlbaum.

Iglesias, A., & Gutierrez-Clellen, V. F. (1986, November) *School discourse: Cultural variations.* Short course presented at national convention of the American Speech-Language-Hearing Association, Detroit, MA.

Jackson-Maldonado, D., Thal, D., & Bates, E. (1992). *Fundación MacArthur: Inventario del Desarrollo de las Habilidades Comunicativas* (IDHC). Developmental Psychology Laboratory, San Diego State University and Universidad de Querétaro, Mexico.

Jackson-Maldonado, D., Marchman, V., Thal, D., Bates, E., & Gutierrez-Clellen, V. F. (1993) Early lexical acquisition in Spanish-speaking infants and toddlers. *Journal of Child Language, 20*(3), 523–549.

Jax, V. (1988). *Narrative construction by children learning English as a second language: A precursor to reading comprehension.* Unpublished doctoral dissertation, California State University, Los Angeles.

Labov, W., & Waletzky, J. (1967)). Narrative analysis: Oral versions of personal experiences. In J. Helm (Ed.), *Essays on the verbal and visual arts* (pp. 12–44). Seattle: University of Washington Press.

Lucariello, J., Kyratzis, A., & Engel, S. (1986). Event representations, context, and language. In K. Nelson (Ed.), *Event knowledge: Structure and function in development* (pp. 137–160). Hillsdale, NJ: Lawrence Erlbaum.

McCabe, A., & Peterson, C. (1991). Getting the story: A longitudinal study of parental styles in eliciting narratives and developing narrative skill. In A. McCabe & C. Peterson (Eds.), *Developing narrative structure* (pp. 217–254). Hillsdale, NJ: Lawrence Erlbaum.

Michaels, S. (1991). The dismantling of narrative. In A. McCabe & C. Peterson (Eds.), *Developing narrative structure* (pp. 303–352). Hillsdale, NJ: Lawrence Erlbaum .

Miller, P. J., & Sperry, L. L. (1988). Early talk about the past: The origins of conversational stories of personal experience. *Journal of Child Language, 15,* 293–316.

Nelson, K. (1986). Event knowledge and cognitive development. In K. Nelson (Ed.), *Event knowledge: Structure and function in development* (pp. 1–20). Hillsdale, NJ: Lawrence Erlbaum.

Paul, R., & Smith, R. L. (1993). Narrative skills in 4-year-olds with normal, impaired, and late-developing language. *Journal of Speech and Hearing Research, 36*(3), 592–598.

Peterson, C., & McCabe, A. (1983). *Developmental psycholinguistics: Three ways of looking at a child's narrative.* New York: Plenum.

Pratt, M. W., Kerig, P., Cowan, P. A., & Cowan, C. P. (1988). Mothers and fathers teaching 3-year-olds: Authoritative parenting and adult scaffolding of young children's learning. *Developmental Psychology, 24,* 832–839.

Seidman, S., Nelson, K., & Gruendel, J. (1986). Make believe scripts: The transformation of ERs in fantasy. In K. Nelson (Ed.), *Event knowledge: Structure and function in development* (pp. 161–188). Hillsdale, NJ: Lawrence Erlbaum.

Slackman, E. A., Hudson, J. A., & Fivush, R. (1986). Actions, actors, links, and goals: The structure of children's event representations. In K. Nelson (Ed.), *Event knowledge: Structure and function in development* (pp. 47–70). Hillsdale, NJ: Lawrence Erlbaum.

Snow, C. E., & Goldfield, B.A. (1981) Building stories: The emergence of information structures from conversation. In D. Tannen (Ed.), *Analyzing discourse: Text and talk* (pp. 127–141). Washington DC: Georgetown University Press.

Stein, N. L., & Glenn, C. G. (1982). An analysis of story comprehension in elementary school children. In R. O. Freedle (Ed.), *New directions in discourse processing, Advances in discourse processes* (Vol. 2, pp. 53–120). Norwood, NJ: Ablex.

Umiker-Sebeok, D. J. (1979). Preschool children's intraconversational narratives. *Journal of Child Language, 6,* 91–109.

Vasquez, O. A. (1989). *Connecting oral language strategies to literacy: An ethnographic study among four Mexican immigrant families.* Unpublished doctoral dissertation, Stanford University, Palo Alto, CA.

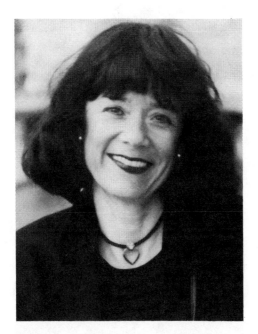

VERA F. GUTIERREZ-CLELLEN, Ph.D.

Dr. Gutierrez-Clellen is an Assistant Professor and Coordinator of the Bilingual Certificate Program in the Department of Communicative Disorders at San Diego State University. Her primary research interest within the area of bilingual speech-language pathology is language development and disorders in Spanish-speaking children and, in particular, the interrelationships between language learning and literacy. This research focused on the precursors of literate language by examining mother-child discourse as well as children's narratives in various Hispanic communities in the United States. Dr. Gutierrez-Clellen has also extensive clinical experience with Spanish-speaking populations in Argentina and Spain.

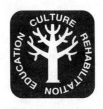

CHAPTER 6

LANGUAGE ASSESSMENT AND INSTRUCTIONAL PROGRAMMING FOR LINGUISTICALLY DIFFERENT LEARNERS: PROACTIVE CLASSROOM PROCESSES

ELIZABETH D. PEÑA, Ph.D.
LUCIANO VALLES, JR., M.S.

For a number of years, educators and researchers have underscored the need for a re-examination of current practices in service delivery to limited English proficient (LEP) and non-English proficient (NEP) Latino-American children. Many programs for LEP and NEP children focus on "basic skills," which prevents them from having opportunities for higher level academic instruction (Reyes, 1992; Reyes

& Laliberty, 1992). This situation is compounded when many LEP children are referred for special education assessment when they do not make adequate academic progress, even though teachers realize that they probably are not impaired (Mehan, Hertweck, & Meihls, 1986; Moecker, 1992), leading to overrepresentation of LEP and NEP children in special education (Figueroa, 1989; Mercer & Rueda, 1991; Ortiz, 1988; Tucker, 1980). Issues that impact service delivery to LEP and NEP Latino American children transcend the single issue of language (L1 vs. L2) use. Children who are language impaired must often first experience failure in learning English before they are referred for special education assessment, leading to underreferral in the early school years (Campbell, Gersten, & Kolar, 1993; Gersten & Woodward, 1994). The following case study illustrates these practices.

⊐

CASE STUDY

Marcos is a 17-year-old Spanish-speaking adolescent in the 11th grade. He has been in a suburban school district since the 8th grade when he immigrated with his family from El Salvador. His educational history indicates that he had a total of 4 years of schooling in El Salvador. He has been receiving resource room support for 2 years. The resource specialist (RSP) states that he has difficulty concentrating and needs extra time to understand assignments. Marcos is failing all subjects. He has had English as a second language (ESL) classes one period a day for 3 years and still does not have enough English to meet the linguistic (reading, writing, and communication) demands of high school. He was referred for special education evaluation because of his school failure and lack of progress in English. At this time psychological and speech-language testing was completed in Spanish by bilingual personnel. Psycho-educational testing indicated that Marcos was having difficulty in the area of language and language learning. IQ testing using the *Weschler Intelligence Scale for Children Revised—Mexican Adaptation* (WISC-RM) indicated normal performance IQ and significantly low verbal IQ. Bilingual language assessment results indicated that Marcos' language development was generally within age range in the social/pragmatic domain. However, he had difficultly with academic language tasks such as single word receptive vocabulary and analogies. These results may, in part, be due to lack of formal educational experiences. Dynamic assessment indicated that Marcos was able to easily learn new tasks with adult intervention. When the IEP team met for program placement, it was stated that no bilingual services were available. Choices for intervention were (1) regular education with ESL; (2) regular education, ESL, speech-language therapy (in English), and continued resource room support; or (3) special day class placement (English only).

Based on Marcos' limited educational experiences, these options may not address his stated needs. The first option, regular education with ESL, does not address his academic needs. The second option, regular education, ESL, and speech-language therapy, has similar limitations. The addition of speech-language therapy in English may help him in his English learning, and because it will be individualized, therapy can focus on some of his academic knowledge. However, resource room support can also address some of the same academic issues. In any case, it is not clear that Marcos is learning or language **impaired**. The final option is also unacceptable, a special day class will not necessarily address Marcos' academic gaps or help him to learn English. In general, the proposed interventions consist of continued decontextualized, discrete skills training, and increased "add on" services or segregated instruction. Although well meaning, none of these interventions is likely to address Marcos' real need: formal educational experiences. These observed trends call for an examination of our pedagogical assumptions in working with LEP and NEP children, the purpose of assessment, and the role and competencies of the speech-language pathologist (SLP). This chapter (1) reviews key issues in working with LEP and NEP special education and regular education "at-risk" children; (2) provides a framework for examining classroom interaction and instruction with LEP and NEP children; and (3) discusses the collaborative role of the SLP in the bilingual classroom.

〓

THE SPECIAL AND REGULAR EDUCATION INTERFACE

Traditionally, education and assessment models have sought to neutralize differences between children and, when they exist, interpret them as deficits (Wolf, Bixby, Glenn, & Gardner, 1991). Assessment typically is used to categorize and to "rule out" impairment (classification), rather than determine the type of intervention the child needs (Lahey, 1990, Leonard, 1991; Lidz, 1991; McCauley & Swisher, 1984; Wang, 1992). The result is referral to a specialist, who has formal training to meet the "different" child's needs (Skrtic, 1991). For non-English-speaking children with impairments, or children with impairments who are in the process of learning English, this process may take more time because more steps are involved. By necessity, LEP and NEP children who are referred for special education must be tested for language proficiency *in addition* to testing for special education classification.

Assessment of children for classification purposes takes place throughout a child's educational program. The nature and timing of assessment influences intervention and programing. For example, surveys are taken to determine the home language of the child, which may lead to a language proficiency testing. Kindergarten readiness tests are given during enrollment or at the beginning of the kindergarten year and may be used to group children within the classroom. On an everyday basis, teachers give criterion-referenced tests to determine progress and assign grades. These more informal measures may lead to classification by "ability" group within classrooms and schools. Children who are not progressing in learning the curriculum are often referred for special testing which may lead to classification into a disability group (e.g., speech-language impaired, learning handicapped, severe impairments of language, communication handicapped, etc.).

Some of the first assessments that bilingual children are exposed to are tests of language proficiency. In individual school districts, the children's language proficiency serves to track them into certain class placements and types of instruction. For example, a child classified as LEP or NEP will likely be placed in English as a second language (ESL) or bilingual education classes. ESL may consist of a number of program options, for example, English vocabulary instruction, exposure to English-speaking peers in nonacademic subjects and activities, formal English instruction consisting of grammar and vocabulary learning, and full immersion with or without formal ESL instruction. Bilingual education may include some to all academic instruction in the primary language with ESL instruction on a pull-out basis, instruction of some subjects in the primary language with others in the second language, or all subjects taught in both languages (see, for example, Cummins, 1984; Hakuta, 1986, 1990; Krashen, 1982; McKay, 1988; Reynolds, 1987 for discussion of bilingual education programs).

Regardless of the program placement, this assessment and placement process is often the first level of classification for ESL students, including language-impaired LEP and NEP children. The assumption that drives this process is that the results of the assessment will ensure proper classification and, therefore, appropriate instruction. Possibly due to lack of trained bilingual special educators coupled with fear of misdiagnosis, LEP and NEP children who have language impairments may not be referred for a speech-language assessment until they experience failure in regular education *as well as* ESL. When children are finally referred, another assessment process is implemented which may result in yet another classification (e.g., speech-language impaired) and intervention (e.g., speech-language therapy). Finally, children who have difficulty learning English but who do not have language impairments may not fit well into either of the two educational categories discussed above. Placement in either regular education (including bilingual education and/or ESL) *or* special education (e.g., speech-language intervention) will occur by default, and individual needs may not be met (Skrtic, 1991). For bilingual children who are language impaired, this linear process often results in a loss of time and an exacerbation of "deficits."

The often used route for special education services for LEP and NEP children—to test for English proficiency, place in ESL if LEP or NEP, and then refer to special education if no progress is observed—has serious implications (Gersten & Woodward, 1994). For children who have a language impairment, waiting for special education services may put them further behind in the regular curriculum. This delay may put them so far behind that they have no hope of catching up with their peers.

LEP and NEP students vary by previous educational experiences (and those of their parents) when they enter the U.S. school system, how quickly they learn interpersonal skills in English, primary and English language and literacy proficiency, prior schooling, and language ability (Cummins, 1989; Faltis, 1993; Ruiz, 1989). In terms of "risk" four major possibilities exist:

1. Formal educational experiences, learns English quickly, has normal language ability. When this student enters the school system he or she may already know some English through community and family support. The student acquires oral English proficiency quickly. The parents have a high degree of formal education and are able to support the child's schooling. Usually within 3 years, the child is transitioned to English-only classes, for which the family is able to provide continued content support. This child is likely not at risk, but may be if oral proficiency is interpreted as academic proficiency and as a result he or she is transferred to English-only classes too soon.

2. Limited formal educational experiences, learns English quickly, has normal language ability. When this student enters the school system he or she may have had limited exposure to English. The student learns oral English quickly. Often within 3 years, the child is transitioned to English-only classes. However, the parents have little formal education and are unable to provide support for school content. Although this child may have normal language ability, she or he may be referred for special education services based on poor academic progress. This student may likely be mislabeled as having a language or learning disability.

3. Range from formal to limited formal educational experiences, easily learns oral English, has a language impairment. When this student enters the school system he or she may or may not have had exposure to English and to formal schooling. Within about 3 years, the child is transitioned to English-only classes based on oral proficiency testing. She or he may be a "borderline" child, but the district policy is to give him or her the "benefit of the doubt." When the child fails in more decontextualized tasks, more support, often through the resource teacher or reading specialist, is provided. It is not until all of these interventions have been attempted that the child is referred for special education services. This procedure may lead to underreferral in the early school years.

4. Range from formal to limited formal educational experiences, has difficulty learning oral English, has a language impairment. When this student enters the school system she or he may or may not have had exposure to English or to formal schooling. If the parents lack formal education, expectations for the child may be low. After approximately 3 years of ESL, and possibly other interventions (e.g., resource room, peer tutoring, parent conferences, after school program), it is noted that little academic progress has been made. This child may be identified and be eligible for special education services, but not until some time has been lost.

Children in risk groups 2, 3, and 4 will need some sort of language intervention at some time. If LEP and NEP students are not provided access to appropriate sociocultural and instructional-communicative opportunities, they may be at risk for academic problems or failure (Gersten & Woodward, 1985; Reyes, 1991; Rosenfield, 1987; Silliman & Wilkinson, 1991; Taylor, 1986; Trueba, 1987; Wallach & Butler, 1994; Willig, 1985). At-risk or potentially at-risk LEP and NEP students may be developing their social language skills appropriately in the first (L1) or second language (L2), but may be failing academically or functioning below grade level.

Many student, home, school, and language variables influence what children know and how they learn (Wallach & Butler, 1994; Wang, Haertel, & Walberg, 1990). A large number of children from low-income and culturally diverse backgrounds may be at risk for academic problems or failure as a function of these factors, some of which include educational inequalities (Freiberg, 1993), mismatches between the socialization practices of the home and the classroom (Heath, 1986; Iglesias, 1985), failure to carefully incorporate the LEP or NEP student's first language as the medium of interactive and meaningful instruction (Cummins, 1986; Fradd & Tikunoff, 1987; Reynolds, 1991), and/or language learning disabilities (Fey, 1986; Nelson, 1993; Wallach & Butler, 1994). If these factors are not addressed appropriately in the classroom, LEP, NEP, and other children at risk will continue to have problems in school. The following case studies provide brief illustrations.

凵

CASE STUDIES

ADRIAN

Adrian, an 8-year-old 1st grader was referred for a speech-language evaluation. The referral indicated needs in the areas of language. His teacher stated that he does well in math and gets extra help in Spanish. Spanish support consists of helping him with math concepts two to three times a week on a pull-out basis. His teacher stated that last year was his first year in school. He was placed in kindergarten where he was not asked to participate in group activities because he did not speak English. He either observed or completed activities on his own during that time. Bilingual speech-language assessment revealed that Adrian has difficulty with sound production and with analogies. All other language areas tested were age-appropriate. Because understanding and using analogies are important academic skills, dynamic assessment procedures were used to teach and then retest in this area. At the end of this session, the retesting indicated normal functioning in this area. This indicated that Adrian had little previous experience with verbal analogies and was able to learn how to solve them with little effort on the part of the examiner. It was recommended that the SLP focus on articulation and monitor classroom language. It was also recommended that the Spanish-speaking volunteer support classroom language concepts in collaboration with the SLP and classroom teacher.

MARISOL

Marisol is a 6-year-old girl in a bilingual K–1 combined class. She was referred by her teacher who stated that she is having academic difficulties, talks very little, and is having difficulty learning. She receives resource help in the classroom twice a week in a small group by a bilingual resource specialist. Speech-language assessment completed in Spanish indicated a significant language impairment. She had difficulty in vocabulary knowledge and learning, verbal reasoning, and planning. Observations in the classroom indicated that she interacted very little with peers and had difficulty transitioning from one activity to another. Therapy will focus on the mentioned areas, in collaboration with the classroom teacher, aid, and RSP.

Adrian's and Marisol's case studies present two approaches for working with at-risk LEP and NEP children. In Adrian's case, he was given little opportunity to learn the class routine and classroom language demands. Spanish support focused on his strength area and was addressed apart from everyday class activities. He needed support in learning classroom language in the classroom. In Marisol's case, support was provided in the classroom context. Although Marisol had significant language and learning difficulties, she was able to function in the classroom with support. These two cases illustrate the diversity of approaches used with LEP and NEP students. Possibly because of assumption that Adrian needed to learn English before including him in group activities, his learning was hindered. A better use of the Spanish support might have been to help Adrian with classroom language concepts in the classroom setting. In Marisol's case, a collaborative approach was used which helped to address her areas of need while participating in classroom activities. Intervention may take many forms and does not necessarily mean special education. However, regular education and special education are often the only two choices. This situation calls for looking beyond special education and bilingual education as mutually exclusive to establishing cooperative, collaborative relationships based on individual children's needs as opposed to classification (Wang, 1992; Wolfram, 1993). In this chapter, we propose that SLPs take a broader approach to working with these risk groups through collaborative relationships with teachers. This implies that SLPs will work within both special education and regular education.

The change-agent role of the SLP in classroom-based models of language intervention requires the SLP to be familiar with certain features of classroom interaction and instruction.

⊔

CLASSROOM INTERACTION AND INSTRUCTION

A broadened role of the SLP is to provide classroom-based language intervention for LEP and NEP children who are at risk for or have a diagnosis of language impairment in a variety possible formats: (1) team teaching in a regular classroom with the classroom teacher and/or other resource specialists (Wang, 1992); (2) providing one-to-one or small group intervention (Nelson; 1989; Wallach & Butler, 1994); (3) providing collaborative consultation with regular or special education teachers and other staff (Despain & Simon, 1987); and (4) providing curriculum or program development (Meyers, Parsons, & Martin, 1979; Nelson, 1989). Within these formats, the SLP assesses and determines whether LEP and NEP students' communicative opportunities are optimal in maximizing students' social and academic language learning potential.

A classroom observation should first examine the classroom method(s) of instruction (Silliman & Wilkinson, 1991). Pedagogy in regular, special, and bilingual education may be classified along two general domains, recitation instruction (passive instruction) and instructional conversation (interactive instruction) (Tharp & Gallimore, 1991). These two approaches may be characterized at opposite ends of a continuum. The type of instructional approach used by an instructor may vary along this continuum and is influenced by the teacher's instructional philosophy. Therefore, teachers' methods may vary along the continuum depending on the task and goal of the interaction, and many teachers may use a mixed approach to teaching. However, for purposes of simplification the two approaches are presented in contrast to each other. In the passive instructional approach, the teacher serves as a transmitter of information and students' conversational participation is inhibited (Goldenberg, 1991). In the instructional conversation (IC) approach, the students' conversational participation is activated and encouraged. IC focuses on group discussion where the teacher and the students transact academic information until the students demonstrate comprehension of the material (Fry, 1992; Tharp & Gallimore, 1991; Vygotsky, 1978).

RECITATION INSTRUCTION

Some researchers have attributed the low academic achievement of some minority language student groups to the predominant use of passive instruction in classrooms characterized by decontextualized, unchallenging, and nonmeaningful teaching (Delgado-Gaitan, 1989; Goldenberg, 1991; Moll & Diaz, 1987). During passive instruction, students are not provided opportunities to become active conversational participants. Children do not participate as conversational creators and negotiators of meaning during classroom lessons (i.e., instruction is teacher-centered and extensive discussion for learning is not encouraged). It is important to recognize that recitation instruction may be needed to explain tasks or concepts or provide instructional directives (e.g., "Open your books to page 63 and look at the second paragraph") as students listen. However, it is also important to recognize that student learning may be stifled if recitation instruction predominates during a major part of classroom lessons (Rogoff, 1990). The following excerpt is an example of recitation instruction in a bilingual Head Start classroom during circle time.

Teacher:	We are going to start with our calendar this morning. OK. I want to hear nice loud voices.
Teacher:	What is this called?
Group:	Calendar
Child 1:	*Calendario*
Teacher:	In English
Child 1:	Calendar
Teacher:	Very good. This is . . .
Group:	The month
Teacher:	Pay attention. And the month is . . .
Group:	October
Teacher:	Very Good. OK. This is a . . . No. This is a . . . What?
Group:	Year
Teacher:	The year, and the year is what, Sean?
Sean:	1991
Teacher:	Very good. Let's do this again. This is called a . . .
Group:	Calendar

In this example it is clear that the children are expected to recite specific information about the calendar. The teacher gives the interaction no context or meaning regarding the purpose or use of a calendar. There is no discussion about calendars and the teacher-student interaction limits the children's linguistic contributions to single word responses. The teacher uses product questions and fill-in-the-blank statements to elicit single word responses from the children. Process questions, which require children to formulate an opinion or interpretation (e.g., Why do we need calendars?), are not used for higher order thinking or to extend their thought processes.

INSTRUCTIONAL CONVERSATION

In contrast, IC involves the teacher's or mediator's subconscious and/or conscious ability to dynamically use a variety of conversational strategies to promote a high level of student conversational participation. The teacher and the students are responsive to the contributions of others in the classroom. This is accomplished during various types of interactions: (1) sequence-initiating actions (e.g., types of questions, informatives, directives, and conversational turn-taking devices) which initiate an instructional interaction; (2) sequence-responding actions by the students, which are in response to the initiating action (e.g., verbal answer, compliance, challenge, disagreement); and (3) sequence-replying actions by the teacher which evaluates the student's response (e.g., positive evaluations such as verbal praise and acknowledgment; negative evaluations such as "no"; partial, full, or extended repetitions; paraphrases; correction; warning; and challenge) (Bloome, 1989; Cazden, 1988; Heap, 1988; Mehan, 1979; Valles, 1994; Wells, 1993). The following excerpt below, from an ethnographic study of a private Christian bilingual kindergarten classroom, demonstrates the teacher's use of an interactive instructional strategy, extending story versions (Valles, 1992). In the (English) excerpt, the teacher is talking about the Passover, in the Old Testament of the Bible. Passover dealt with the shedding of a lamb's blood which represented salvation for the oldest male in each household.

Teacher:	Why did he have to kill this animal?
Miguel:	They have to kill the sheep.
Teacher:	Why did he have to kill the sheep?

Oscar:	Because they have to paint all the doors red.
Teacher:	Why did they put the blood of the sheep on the door?
Luz:	They wanted to.
Teacher:	Who did they want to save? (Several children raise their hands to bid for a response; the teacher calls on Mari to respond).
Mari:	The oldest son.
Teacher:	The oldest son very good. <pause> Remember, God told Pharaoh that the oldest son of every house would die. Remember that the Angel came to every house and said, "the oldest son of every house will die." (pp. 8–9)

The teacher in this interaction provides the children with multiple opportunities to extend their story versions by challenging them to provide more precise/accurate story information. The use of process questions induces the children's conversational participation at the phrase or sentential level of the conversational continuum. If the children's responses are partially correct, the teacher includes part of the children's responses in her subsequent follow-up question to acknowledge the children's conversational participation. This type of interaction continues if the children continue to provide partially correct answers. If this type of interaction continues for several teacher-student conversational turns and the children are not able to provide the correct and complete response, or if a child provides an incorrect response, the teacher uses a single product question with partial answer components. This product question facilitates the child's formulation of a correct and complete response which is partially or fully repeated and verbally praised by the teacher.

The interactive strategy depicted above, extending story versions, is a form of IC. This strategy is used to build on, challenge, and extend students' conversational contributions by using a variety of questions and turn-taking devices that trigger the students' abilities to generate appropriate responses (Cazden, 1988; Lerner, 1993). Turn-taking devices may involve self-selections (students verbalize answers without being called on to respond by the teacher), individual nominations (teacher nominations of students at random which require students to respond to a given question), and teacher selection of bidder (teacher points to or calls out the name of a student who bids to respond). In IC,the teacher's role is to extend the students' thinking related to the academic material, but it is the mutual responsibility of the teacher or mediator and students to co-construct a conversational tapestry whereby meaning is shared. When the students demonstrate difficulty with comprehension of the material, as determined by the teacher, the teacher rewords, simplifies, or clarifies his or her questions or provides instructional directives and informatives to guide the students' comprehension (Rogoff, 1990). Through IC the teacher establishes a common foundation of understanding by incorporating students' prior knowledge channeled through the students' initiations (questions) and responses to the teacher's questions. The teacher or mediator uses IC strategies to extend and challenge students' thinking and learning without threatening or inhibiting students' participation.

LEP, NEP, and English-proficient students from low-income backgrounds who receive interactive opportunities have demonstrated above average academic achievement. Sociocultural instructional contexts such as incorporation of the LEP or NEP student's first language in meaningful, interactive instruction (Cummins, 1986; Fradd & Tikunoff, 1987; Reyes, 1992; Trueba, 1987) and adaptive instructional models that address individual learner differences through active participation with the teacher (Wang, 1992) have been shown to benefit LEP and NEP students. These instructional methods address students' individual learning and cultural differences as well as their social and academic needs in noncategorical (including both impaired and unimpaired students) classrooms (Wang, 1992; Wang, Reynolds, & Walberg, 1990). It is our view that an understanding of classroom interaction and instruction is needed to facilitate the SLP's role as a classroom collaborator and to maximize the language-learning potential of normally developing and language-impaired LEP and NEP students.

⅃

THE CHANGING ROLE OF THE SPEECH-LANGUAGE PATHOLOGIST

Traditionally, the role of the SLP has not involved classroom-based language intervention, but rather the provision of speech-language therapy on a pull-out basis. Based on this approach, children are classified and placed in remediation programs outside of the regular classroom. We advocate a departure from the traditional "classification/placement/pull-out" models which changes the role of the SLP from assessor/remediator (deficient model) to change-agent within the classroom, based on a proactive model of intervention (Fradd & Tikunoff, 1987; Silliman & Wilkinson, 1991; Wallach & Butler, 1994). This change-agent approach to classroom intervention broadens the role of the SLP who serves LEP and NEP children who may be at risk due to their unfamiliarity with classroom culture and genres but who are not language impaired. The application of this model may prevent unnecessary referral of (unimpaired) LEP and NEP students to special education while at the same time meeting their needs and promoting their chances of academic success in the classroom.

Communicative opportunities for LEP and NEP children may be supported, stifled, or denied during individualized, small group or whole class instruction. Thus, language intervention at the classroom level should be proactive in collaboration with the classroom teacher. Problem solving includes the use of ethnographic methods to identify communication demands. Based on the classroom observation, the SLP: (1) examines the targeted child's response to instruction and (2) generates an intervention plan with the teacher based on the child's response to the teacher's instructional methods.

As a participant-observer, the SLP identifies the curriculum-based communicative demands of the classroom and determines the social and academic language needs and learning potential of the LEP and NEP children without undermining cultural and linguistic differences. The children's native language and cultural and individual learning differences are utilized to match and extend their socialization experiences to meet the academic language needs required for academic success.

Additionally, examination of a child's response to instruction may help to determine how much and what type of help the child needs to succeed. A few studies have examined language learning and its ability to predict language impairment in LEP and NEP children. Roseberry and Connel (1991) found that normally developing bilingual children were able to learn and use an invented morpheme, whereas bilingual children with language impairments were unable to do so. Peña, Quinn, and Iglesias (1992) and Peña (1993) found that modifiability measures (examiner effort during mediation, child responsiveness to mediation, and transfer of mediated learning) predicted language ability during a mediated learning experience. The bilingual children developing language normally were able to improve their vocabulary test scores after two 20-minute mediated learning experience sessions; their language-impaired peers had more difficulty. These studies suggest that observation of the learning process may predict language ability. Furthermore, the information yielded during such an observation links directly with intervention.

Determination of a child's response to classroom instruction examines children's ability to learn the task taught by the teacher, given the teacher's input. For example, the SLP may observe the level of questioning that occurs and which types of questions children are able to answer. The SLP may also observe the amount and type of input children receive (language of instruction, modality, instructional method). This observation helps to determine how much of an opportunity the child has had to learn the task. In addition to the classroom observation, the SLP tries alternative methods to teach the child and observes the cognitive/linguistic strategies the child employs to learn the task. Both the teacher and SLP identify emerging skills that may need to be strengthened for the child to experience classroom success. The information from the observation can then be integrated into classroom instruction and individual planning for the targeted child.

For illustration, let us return to the first case presented. Marcos had difficulty with school-based language, even though he seemed to be performing adequately in other language areas, such as interpersonal communication. Based on the classroom demands and Marcos' response to the demands, the teacher, the RSP and SLP together can generate hypotheses about his language learning. According to the ESL teacher, Marcos' verbal skills are very strong, but he lacks reading and writing skills. For example, he has difficulty organizing and sequencing written material. This is not surprising because Marcos has had limited academic experiences. He knows how to read, but does not know the academic expectations of reading tasks. Specifically, Marcos has difficulty remembering what he reads and has difficulty making conclusions. Further probing as to why these are difficult for him should examine the strategies he uses to remember and to infer and the adequacy of these strategies. In addition, the classroom reading content should be examined. Because of Marcos' lack of academic experience, he may have limited exposure to the content used to teach reading. Mediated learning experience (MLE) can be used to teach memory and inferencing strategies to use during reading. Exposure to the content can be ensured through discussion, books on tape, peer tutoring, and class lessons. Finally, a post-MLE observation can be used to judge transfer of targeted skills to the classroom setting.

INTERVENTION

Intervention should be based on the children's response to instruction in the teacher's classroom. Specific targets for intervention might be at the level of the classroom, the child, or both. Focus on the classroom might include introduction of different instructional methods for certain activities to facilitate a specific child's learning. For example, instructional conversation strategies such as use of introductory statements, single questions, extending story versions, cause-effect questions, and inclusion of children's contributions can be introduced. Focus on the child should involve observation of his or her cognitive/linguistic strategies such as planning, attention/discrimination, self-regulation/awareness, transfer, and motivation (discussed further below). Additional support might involve giving the child more time, changing the level of questioning, or providing peer tutoring or other support. Most typically, intervention involves a combination of working with the teacher and environment to facilitate learning for the child and working directly with the child to teach targeted skills.

MLE based on Feuerstein (1979) and Lidz (1991) can be used as an intervention approach with language-impaired children. Research has shown that children with a variety of language abilities and linguistic backgrounds benefit from MLE (Jenson & Feuerstein, 1987; Missiuna & Samuels, 1989; Peña, 1993). MLE is used in the classroom setting to help children become self-regulated and active learners. MLE is characterized by several components which focus on the teacher as mediator including intentionality, mediation of meaning, transcendence, and planning.

Intentionality focuses on the teacher's intent to teach. Specifically, it may include stating the goal so that the children are able to understand and focus their learning toward that goal. The goal focuses on skills or strategies rather than on specific content. For example, during an art activity in which children fill in the colors of the rainbow, the goal is not the rainbow itself. The task is used to introduce the notion of combining primary colors to make secondary colors. In stating the goal the teacher or mediator says, "Today we are going to talk about colors and what happens when certain colors are mixed."

Mediation of meaning helps children to understand why the task is important. Information about the activity and its value is expanded in mediation of meaning. Based on the rainbow example, the meaning of the task can be explained to children as a way to classify colors. The teacher or mediator might state, "If we know which colors to mix, we can make lots of different colors from three basic ones."

Transcendence helps to promote the task or activity to related experiences, moving from the perceptual to the conceptual. These conceptual bridges are used to promote hypothetical, inferential, or cause-effect thinking. For example, the teacher might ask, "Can you think of any other times it's important to pay attention to how colors go together?" "What else do colors tell us?" "They may serve as a warning, or to call attention to something." "What do you think would happen if I mixed all the colors together?"

Finally, **planning** is used to help children learn to generate their own plan to approach a task. This helps children to become active in their learning. The teacher or mediator helps the children to generate their own plans: "What should we do first?" "What do you think would happen if we mixed the paint on the paper instead of the cup?" The teacher, in collaboration with the SLP, can apply MLE to everyday class activities.

Modifiability focuses on child changes. Emerging cognitive/linguistic strategies identified in the assessment phase are strengthened through MLE by the SLP and the teacher. Lidz, (1991) discusses the following cognitive strategies: attention (e.g., ability to initiate and sustain attention to task), discrimination (e.g., selects relevant materials), planning (e.g., identifies problem), self-regulation/awareness (e.g., knows when correct/incorrect), transfer (e.g., uses learned strategy in new task), and motivation (enthusiasm for task). Use of these strategies is stated and expanded during MLE. For example, planning, which includes talking about the goal and talking about the plan, is taught through MLE. The teacher or mediator might ask the child if she or he knows the goal. Similarly, the teacher or mediator might ask the child to talk about the plan to carry out the task. If the child is unable to do so, continued MLE focuses on planning strategies to help the child learn to plan. Focusing on cognitive/linguistic **strategies** represents a shift from content to meta-awareness of the processes needed for a particular task.

For Marcos, intervention should include teaching strategies for learning such as planning, discrimination, and self-regulation. Planning can help him to approach reading in an organized way. For example, if Marcos is assigned to read a short story and then answer some questions about the characters' actions, his plan might be to read the story, focus on the characters, and then answer the questions. Discrimination can be used to help him to know what to focus on in the reading. In this case, it may be the characters' actions versus the character's motivation. Finally, teaching self-regulation will help Marcos to pay attention to when he is off-task or distracted and then to get back to his plan without the teacher asking him to. Teaching these cognitive/linguistic strategies can give Marcos the opportunity to become an active and self-motivated learner.

⊔

CONCLUSION

Many of the issues and examples presented in this chapter are illustrations of problems that confront SLPs working with LEP and NEP children. We have argued that traditional, linear models of assessment, identification, and classification are often inadequate to address the diverse needs of LEP and NEP children. Research suggests that a proactive, dynamic approach can benefit LEP and NEP students in special education *and* regular education. We have proposed a model in which the SLP is an active participant in providing assessment and intervention to Latino children who are at-risk for academic failure and/or may have a language impairment.

Knowledge of instructional methods is critical for assessing children's response to instruction and for providing appropriate, relevant intervention. Although there has been a positive change in terms of inappropriate referral and placement of LEP and NEP children in special education, many students still receive inadequate instruction from classroom teachers (Gersten & Woodward, 1994). It is essential that SLPs become increasingly aware of classroom interaction and instruction to form collaborations with teachers and other personnel who work with at-risk children. There is a need for professionals to close the gap between researcher and practitioner and learn to use ethnographic methodologies to observe classroom interactions (Silliman & Wilkinson, 1991). Based on these observations, MLE has great potential for helping classroom mediators use conversational strategies that promote the social and academic performance of all public school children in multicultural, multilingual, and pluralistic settings.

ᄓ

REFERENCES

Bloome, D. (1989). *Classrooms and literacy*. Norwood, NJ: Ablex.

Campbell, J., Gersten, R., & Kolar, C. (1993). *Quality of instruction provided to language minority students with learning disabilities: Five findings from micro-ethnographies* (Technical Report No. 93-5). Eugene, OR: Eugene Research Institute.

Cazden, C. B. (1988). *Classroom discourse: The language of teaching and learning*. Portsmouth, NH: Heinemann.

Cummins, J. (1984). *Bilingualism and special education*. Clevedon, England: Multilingual Matters.

Cummins, J. (1986). Empowering minority students: A framework for intervention. *Harvard Educaitonal Review, 56*(1), 18–36.

Cummins, J. (1989). A theoretical framework for bilingual special education. *Exceptional Children, 56*(2), 111–119.

Delgado-Gaitan, C. (1989). Classroom literacy activity for Spanish-speaking students. *Linguistics and Education, 1*(3), 285–297.

Despain, A. D., & Simon, C. S. (1987). Alternative to failure: A junior high school language development-based curriculum. *Journal of Childhood Communication Disorders, 11*, 139–179.

Dulay, H., Burt, M., & Krashen, S. (1982). *Language two*. New York: Oxford University Press.

Faltis, C. (1993, December/January). Programmatic and curricular options for secondary schools serving Limited English proficient students. *The High School Journal*, pp. 17–181.

Fey, M. E. (1986). *Language intervention with young children*. Austin, TX: Pro-Ed.

Feuerstein, R. (1979). *The dynamic assessment of retarded performers: The Learning Potential Assessment Device, theory, instruments, and techniques*. Baltimore, MD: University Park Press.

Figueroa, R. (1989). Psychological testing of linguistic-minority students: Knowledge gaps and regulations. *Exceptional Children, 56*, 145–152.

Fradd, S. H., & Tikunoff, W. J. (1987). *Bilingual education and bilingual special education: A guide for administrators*. Boston, MA: College-Hill Press.

Freiberg, H. J. (1993). A school that fosters resilience in inner-city youth. *Journal of Negro Education, 62*(3), 364–376.

Fry, P. S. (1992). *Fostering children's cognitive competence through mediated learning experiences: Frontiers and futures*. Springfield, IL: Charles C Thomas.

Gersten, R., & Woodward, J. (1985). A case for structured immersion. *Educational Leadership, 43*(1), 75–78.

Gersten, R., & Woodward, J. (1994). The language-minority student and special education: Issues, trends, and paradoxes. *Exceptional Children, 60*(4), 310–322.

Goldenberg, C. (1991). *Instructional conversations and their classroom application.* Santa Cruz: National Center for Research on Cultural Diversity and Second Language Learning, University of California.

Hakuta, K. (1986). *Mirror of language: The debate on bilingualism.* New York: Basic Books.

Hakuta, K. (1990). *Bilingualism and bilingual education: A research perspective.* Rosslyn, VA: National Clearning House for Bilingual Education.

Heap, J. L. (1988). On task in classroom discourse. *Linguistics and Education, 1,* 177–198.

Heath, S. B. (1986). Sociocultural contexts of language development. In California State Department of Education (Ed.), *Beyond language: Social and cultural factors in schooling language minority children* (pp. 143–186). Los Angeles: Evaluation, Dissemination and Assessment Center, California State University.

Iglesias, A. (1985). Cultural conflict in the classroom: The communicatively different child. In D. N. Ripich & F. M. Spinelli (Eds.), *School discourse problems* (pp. 279–296). San Diego, CA: College-Hill Press.

Jensen M. R., & Feuerstein, R. (1987). The learning potential assessment device: From philosophy to practice. In C. S. Lidz (Ed., *Dynamic assessment: An interactional approach to evaluating learning potential* (pp. 379–402). New York: Guilford Press.

Krashen, S. (1982). *Principles and practices of second language acquisition.* Oxford: Pergamon Press.

Lahey, M. (1990). Who shall be called language impaired? Some reflections and one perspective. *Journal of Speech and Hearing Disorders, 55,* 621–620.

Leonard, L. (1991). Specific language impairment as a clinical category. *Language, Speech, and Hearing Services in Schools, 22,* 60–64.

Lerner, G. H. (1993). Collectivities in action: Establishing the relevance of conjoined participation in conversation. *Text, 13*(2), 213–245.

Lidz, C. S. (1987). *Dynamic assessment: An interactional approach to evaluating learning potential.* New York: Guilford Press.

Lidz, C. S. (1991). *Practitioner's guide to dynamic assessment.* New York: Guilford Press.

McCauley, R., & Swisher, L. (1984). Use and misuse of norm-referenced test in clinical assessment: A hypothetical case. *Journal of Speech and Hearing Disorders, 49,* 338–348.

McKay, S. (1988). Weighing educational alternates. In S. L. McKay & S. C. Wong (Eds.), *Language diversity: Problem or resource? A social and educational perspective on language minorities in the United States* (pp. 338–366). Boston: Heinle & Heinle.

Mehan, H. (1979). *Learning lessons: Social organization in the classroom.* Cambridge, MA: Harvard University Press.

Mehan, H., Herweck, A., & Meihls, J. L. (1986). *Handicapping the handicapped: Decision making in students' educational careers.* Palo Alto, CA: Stanford University Press.

Mercer, J. R., & Rueda, R. (1991, November). *The impact of changing paradigms of disabilities on assessment for special education.* Paper presented at the The Council for Exceptional Children Topical Conference on At-Risk Children and Youth, New Orleans, LA.

Meyers, J., Parsons, R., & Marti, R. (1979). *Mental health consultation in the schools.* San Francisco, CA: Jossey-Bass.

Missiuna, C., & Samuels, M. (1989). Dynamic assessment of preschool children with special needs: Comparison of mediation and instruction. *Remedial and Special Education, 10*(2), 53–62.

Moll, L. C., & Diaz, S. (1987). Change as the goal of educational research. *Anthropology and Education Quarterly, 18*, 300–311.

Nelson, N. W. (1989). Curriculum-based language assessment and intervention. *Language, Speech, and Hearing Services in Schools, 20*, 170–184.

Nelson, N. W. (1993). *Childhood language disorders in context: Infancy through adolescence.* New York: Macmillan.

Ortiz, A. (1988). *Effective practices in assessment and instruction for language minority students: An intervention model.* Arlington, VA: Innovative Approaches Research Project, Office of Bilingual Education and Minority Languages Affairs, U.S. Department of Education.

Peña, E. (1993). *Dynamic assessment: A non-biased approach for assessing the language of young children.* Unpublished doctoral dissertation, Temple University, Philadelphia, PA.

Peña, E., Quinn, R., & Iglesias, A. (1992). The application of dynamic methods to language assessment: A non-biased procedure. *Journal of Special Education, 26*(3), 269–280.

Reyes, M. de la Luz. (1992). Challenging venerable assumptions: Literacy instruction for linguistically different students. *Harvard Education Review, 62*(4), 42–446.

Reyes, M. de la Luz, & Laliberty, E. (1992). A teacher's "Pied Piper" effect on young authors. *Education and Urban Society, 24*, 263–278.

Reynolds, A. G. (1991). *Bilingualism, multiculturalism, and second language learning.* Hillsdale, NJ: Lawrence Erlbaum.

Rogoff, B. (1990). *Apprenticeship in thinking: Cognitive development in social context.* New York: Oxford University.

Roseberry, C., & Connel, P. J. (1991). The use of an invented language rule in the differentiation of normal and language-impaired Spanish-speaking children. *Journal of Speech and Hearing Research, 34*, 596–603.

Rosenfield, S. (1987). *Instructional consultation.* Hillsdale, NJ: Lawrence Erlbaum.

Ruiz, N. T. (1989). An optimal learning environment for Rosemary. *Exceptional Children, 56*, 130–144.

Silliman, E. R. (1993). *Language and literacy programming across the educational continuum: From inclusive to self-contained settings.* Presentation at the Emerson College Institute in Language Learning Disabilities, Boston, MA.

Silliman, E. R., & Wilkinson, L. C. (1991). *Communicating for learning: Classroom observation and collaboration.* Gaithesburg, MD: Aspen.

Skrtic, T. (1991). The special education paradox: Equity as the way to excellence. *Harvard Educational Review,. 61*(2), 148–194.

Taylor, O. (Ed.). (1986). *Nature of communication disorders in culturally and linguistically diverse populations.* San Diego, CA: College-Hill Press.

Tharp, R. G., & Gallimore, R. (1991). *Rousing minds to life: Teaching, learning, and schooling in social context.* New York: Cambridge University.

Trueba, H. T. (1987). *Success or failure? Learning and the language minority student.* New York: Newbury House.

Tucker, J. A. (1980). Ethnic proportions in classes for the learning impaired: Issues in nonbiased assessment. *The Journal of Special Education, 14*, 93–105.

Valles, L. (1992, November). *Interactive instruction in a kindergarten classroom: An ethnographic study.* Mini-seminar presented at the American Speech-Language-Hearing Association Convention, San Antonio, TX.

Valles, L. (1995). *Teaching as guided participation during small group and whole class reading lessons.* Unpublished doctoral dissertation, Temple University, Philadelphia, PA.

Vygotsky, L. S. (1978). *Mind in society: The development of higher psychological processes.* Cambridge, MA: Harvard University Press.

Wallach, G. P., & Butler, K. G. (Eds.). (1994). *Language learning disabilities in school-age children and adolescents: Some principles and applications.* New York: Merrill.

Wang, M. C. (1987). *The wedding of instruction and assessment in the classroom.* Philadelphia, PA: Temple University Center for Research in Human Development and Education.

Wang, M. C. (1992). *Adaptive education strategies: Building on diversity.* Baltimore, MD: Paul H. Brookes.

Wang, M. C., Haertel, G. D., & Walberg, H. J. (1990). What influences learning? A content analysis of review literature. *Journal of Educational Research, 84*(1), 30–43.

Wang, M. C., Reynolds, M. C., & Walberg, H. J. (1990). *Special education research and practice: Synthesis of findings.* New York: Pergamon Press.

Wells, G. (1993). Reevaluating the IRF sequence: A proposal for the articulation of theories of activity and discourse for the analysis of teaching and learning in the classroom. *Linguistics and Education, 5*, 1–37.

Willig, A. C. (1985). A meta-analysis of selected studies on the effectiveness of bilingual education. *Review of Educational Research, 55*(3), 269–317.

Wolf, D., Bixby, J., Glenn, J., III, & Gardner, H. (1991). To use their minds well: Investigating new forms of student assessment. *Review of Research in Education, 17*, 31–74.

Wolfram, W. (1993). A proactive role for speech-language pathologists in sociolinguistic education. *Language, Speech, and Hearing Services in Schools, 24*, 181–185.

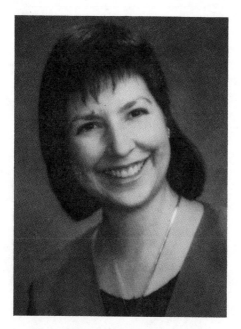

ELIZABETH D. PEÑA, PH.D.

Dr. Peña is an Assistant Professor in the Program of Communication Disorders and Sciences at the University of Texas at Austin. She earned her master's degree in 1984 from San Francisco State University and her doctorate in 1993 from Temple University. Her expertise is in dynamic assessment procedures in speech-language pathology and collaboration in the classroom. She has served as a consultant to several programs offering early intervention and preschool services to multicultural populations. She has made numerous presentations on the topic of assessment.

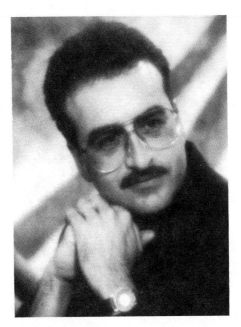

LUCIANO VALLES, JR., M.S.

Luciano Valles, Jr. is an instructor in the Department of Communication Disorders at the University of Massachusetts at Amherst and classroom discourse research assistant at the National Center for Education in the Inner Cities in Philadelphia. Mr. Valles' current interest is in Spanish and English teacher-student discourse with research in conversation analysis and ethnography relative to the role of teaching in promoting inner-city students' academic achievement. His previous positions and employment include assistant professor at Pan American University in Edinburg, Texas and speech-language pathologist at Easter Seals Rehabilitation Center in McAllen, Texas and Mental Health-Mental Retardation Center in Harlingen, Texas. He earned a master's degree in 1984 from Texas Christian University and is currently a doctoral candidate at Temple University.

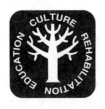

CHAPTER 7

CONSIDERATIONS IN THE ASSESSMENT AND TREATMENT OF NEUROGENIC DISORDERS IN BILINGUAL ADULTS

BELINDA A. REYES, Ph.D., CCC-SLP

Hispanics comprise a significant segment of the population of the United States, numbering approximately 20 million. The major subgroups of the Hispanic population and their proportional representation are: Mexican Americans, 62%; Puerto Ricans, 13%; Central and South Americans, 12%; Cubans, 5%; and other Hispanics, 8% (U.S. Bureau of the Census, 1990). Due primarily to ongoing immigration and high birth rates, Hispanics are projected to surpass the African American population and become the largest minority in the United States within the next decade, numbering more than 30 million (U.S. Bureau of the Census, 1989). In the next two decades, Hispanics are projected to account for one of every three net additions to the U.S. population (U.S. Bureau of the Census, 1990). Thus, it is clear that speech-language pathologists can expect to be faced with increasing numbers of Hispanic individuals requiring services. The purpose of this chapter is to highlight relevant issues for speech-language pathologists interacting with adult bilingual Hispanic individuals. Specifically, demographic information regarding geographic distribution, age, educational level, and income is presented, followed by a discussion of issues regarding health care for the Hispanic population. Subsequently, a discussion of bilingualism and code switching and their implications for assessment and treatment of Hispanic adults is presented. Finally, suggestions for consideration of cultural factors in the management of Hispanic patients with neurogenic communication disorders are discussed.

ᛌᚠ

DEMOGRAPHICS

GEOGRAPHIC DISTRIBUTION

Although Hispanics reside in every state of the union, the largest numbers are located in California (34%), Texas (21%), New York (11%), Florida (8%), and Illinois (4%). A larger proportion of Hispanics than white non-Hispanics live in metropolitan areas and are more likely to concentrate in the inner cities of the largest metropolitan areas (Schick & Schick, 1991). Consequently, speech-language pathologists working in urban settings can expect to see a larger proportion of their caseloads comprised of Hispanic individuals, whereas professionals employed in rural settings may tend to see fewer Hispanic patients.

AGE

As a whole, the Hispanic population in the United States is younger than the non-Hispanic population, with median ages of 25.5 years and

32.5 years, respectively. Although only 7% of Hispanics are over 60 years old, compared to 17% among non-Hispanics, elderly Hispanics are increasing at a faster rate than non-Hispanics (Schick & Schick, 1991). It is projected by the Census Bureau that the rate of growth among older Hispanics will be 4.5 times the rate of growth for the entire aged population to the year 2000. The elderly Hispanic population has been identified as the fastest growing ethnic minority in the United States (ASHA, 1991; Select Committee on Aging, 1989). These data have several implications for speech-language pathologists. First, currently, adult Hispanic patients with neurogenic disorders can, as a group, be expected to be younger than non-Hispanic patients. Clinicians would be wise to take this into consideration in planning and implementing intervention programs for this population. Second, because the elderly Hispanic population is growing at such a rapid rate and is projected to continue to do so, clinicians can expect to see growing numbers of elderly Hispanic patients requiring services in the future.

EDUCATION

Although absolute gains in educational attainment have been demonstrated by the Hispanic population as a whole over the past 20 years, significant challenges continue to exist. Hispanics are much more likely than other groups to leave school in the early grades (i.e., 6th grade or earlier), and the proportion of Hispanic high school dropouts is at least twice that of non-Hispanics, with Mexican Americans having the highest dropout rate and Cuban Americans having the lowest dropout rate (Schick & Schick, 1991). Approximately 10% of Hispanics 25 years and older have completed 4 or more years of college, compared to 21% of non-Hispanics. Elderly Hispanics are among the most educationally disadvantaged groups in our society by whatever barometer one uses. Elderly Hispanics are six to seven times more likely to be functionally illiterate (i.e., have less than 5 years of schooling) than elderly white non-Hispanics. Approximately 73% of elderly Hispanics have an educational attainment of eighth grade or less, compared to 35% of all elderly individuals (Schick & Schick, 1991). While not all Hispanic individuals are educationally disadvantaged, the speech-language pathologist must pay special attention to premorbid educational level in the assessment and treatment of Hispanic patients. Particularly with elderly Hispanic patients, who are more likely to be functionally illiterate or barely literate, clinicians will need to modify assessment procedures accordingly, so as to not penalize patients for skills not present premorbidly.

INCOME

Below average educational achievement for the Hispanic population is reflected in less favorable occupational status and lower income level. The median family income of all Hispanics lags the median for white non-Hispanics by 35%. Among the total population, 56% of all employed persons fall into the two highest categories of the occupational ladder (professional and technical), whereas only 38% of the Hispanic population does so, except for Cubans (57%) whose working members are classified in the top two categories (U.S. Bureau of the Census, 1990). With respect to the elderly population, only one out of every six Hispanics age 65 and older receives retirement income from a pension or annuity, in contrast to one of every three elderly white non-Hispanics, with aged Hispanics having one of the highest poverty rates among older Americans (Select Committee on Aging, 1989). This high poverty rate, particularly among elderly Hispanics, may result in virtually inaccessible health care, including rehabilitation services. For example, in a study conducted by Marin, Marin, Padilla, and de la Rocha (1983) in California, the primary reason for underutilization of health services by Hispanics was found to be "financial difficulties." Thus, income level may be one factor contributing to the underrepresentation of Hispanics in the caseloads of some speech-language pathology departments.

ᛒ

HEALTH CARE

The educational and socioeconomic characteristics of the Hispanic population, coupled with demographic and epidemiologic determinants of need, result in serious health care inadequacies among this population. Hispanics as a whole, and particularly their largest subgroup, Mexican Americans, are at a higher risk of receiving inadequate or no health care than any other population group in the United States (Furino & Guerra, 1992). For example, studies have shown that Hispanics, particularly Mexican Americans, less often receive prenatal care (Marin et al., 1983; Teller, 1988), dental care (Roberts & Lee, 1980), medical checkups (Marin et al., 1983; Roberts & Lee, 1980), immunizations (Sumaya, 1992), and eye examinations (Roberts & Lee, 1980) compared to the white non-Hispanic population. Many Hispanics are poorly positioned to access the current health care system by virtue of below average family income, above average employment in establishments that do not regularly provide private health insurance, and sizeable numbers living in states with low Medicaid enrollments (Ginzberg, 1992). For example, when compared to the entire population of the U.S., Hispanics are more than twice as likely not to be covered by health insurance, and only 21% of the Hispanic elderly have private insurance to supplement Medicare, compared to 69% of the total population (Schick & Schick, 1991). Another reason for the difficulties experienced by Hispanics in obtaining adequate health care is their underrepresentation in the health professions. Hispanic dentists, registered nurses, pharmacists, and therapists only account for approximately 2 to 3% of the totals in these professions. Although the proportion of physicians is somewhat higher (approximately 5%), reflecting the considerable number of physicians being trained abroad and subsequently immigrating to the United States, this percentage still reflects a paucity of Hispanics in this profession (Ginzberg, 1992).

With respect to health status, the literature indicates that certain causes of neurological impairment disproportionately affect minority individuals, including Hispanics (Anderson & Cohen, 1989; Council on Scientific Affairs, 1991; Sotomayor & Randolph, 1988; Wallace, 1993; Yatsu, 1991). These causes and risk factors include cardiovascular disease and stroke, diabetes, trauma, and infectious diseases, and may be associated with communication disorders, thus being of particular interest to speech-language pathologists.

CARDIOVASCULAR DISEASE

Cardiovascular disease is believed to be a leading cause of death among Mexican Americans as it is among the general population. However, a lack of knowledge regarding the impact, nature, and control of cardiovascular disease among Mexican Americans, a key prerequisite to adopting risk-reducing behaviors, has been documented in the literature (Sotomayor & Randolph, 1988). For example, an investigation conducted by the American Heart Association (1984) found that 80% of white non-Hispanics were able to identify at least three behavioral habits or characteristics associated with increased risk of cardiovascular disease, but only 54% of Mexican Americans were able to do so. Similarly, Hazuda and Stern (1985) documented that, regardless of socioeconomic status, Hispanics were less informed than their Anglo counterparts regarding heart attack prevention. Only 30% of Hispanic respondents were able to name one or more warning signs of heart attack, whereas more than 50% of the Anglo respondents were able to do so. A variety of cardiac conditions including atrial fibrillation, atherosclerotic heart disease, rheumatic heart disease, acute myocardial infarction, and bacterial endocarditis have been found to predispose patients to cerebral emboli (Netter, 1992). This in turn puts these patients at a higher risk for neurogenic communication disorders.

DIABETES

Hispanics, particularly Mexican Americans and Puerto Ricans, have a two- to threefold higher incidence and prevalence of type II diabetes (adult onset, noninsulin dependent) than the white non-Hispanic population (Furino & Guerra, 1992), and approximately one-third higher prevalence than African Americans and American Indians (Jacobson, 1994). In addition, it is suspected that millions more Hispanics unknowingly have the disease (Jacobson, 1994). Moreover, Hispanics are at a higher risk of succumbing to traditional diabetic complications, such as severe retinopathy and end-stage renal disease, than their white non-Hispanic counterparts. A combined earlier age of onset and the younger age structure of the Hispanic population results in many individuals being afflicted in the prime of life, and makes diabetes a major pubic health problem among this population (Stern & Haffner, 1992). Because diabetes is associated with an increased risk of stroke, which in turn is a leading cause of aphasia, the preponderance of this disease may ultimately result in significant increases in numbers of Hispanic stroke patients requiring speech-language therapy.

TRAUMA

Trauma, the fourth most costly health hazard in the United States, is believed to disproportionately affect minority Americans. Although very little data exist on the incidence and prevalence of trauma across ethnic boundaries in the U.S., a study conducted by Muñoz, Tortella, Sakmyster, Liveronese, McCormac, Odom, and Torres (1992) at a large urban level 1 trauma center in the Northeast found that African Americans and Hispanics had a disproportional share of admissions relative to the non-Hispanic white population. That is, African Americans and Hispanics comprised the majority of trauma admissions, a proportion much greater than their representation in the general population. In addition, Hispanics were found to have distinct mechanisms of injury compared to both blacks and whites. Specifically, Hispanics were found to have a lower rate of penetrating injury (such as stab or gunshot wounds) than blacks (25% vs. 51%), but a higher rate than whites (13%). Secondly, Hispanics were found to have a higher rate of blunt trauma (i.e., motor vehicle accidents) compared to blacks (75% vs. 49%), but a lower rate than whites (87%). These data suggest that Hispanics may suffer a distinctly different pattern of trauma compared to African Americans and white non-Hispanics.

INFECTIOUS DISEASE

Despite limitations in information, sufficient data are currently available in the medical literature to indicate that Hispanics suffer disproportionately from a number of infectious diseases such as rubella, syphilis, tuberculosis, and acquired immunodeficiency syndrome when compared to the non-Hispanic white population (Novick et al., 1989; Rieder, Cauthen, Kelly, Bloch, & Snider, 1989; Schoenbaum, Hartel, Selwyn, & Klein, 1989; Snider, Salina, & Kelly, 1989; Sumaya, 1992). Due to the growing pervasiveness of AIDS and the resulting myriad of neuropsychological deficits often referred to as AIDS dementia complex, this disease has particular consequences for clinicians. Specifically, dysphagia, motor speech impairment, memory loss, reduced concentration, impaired problem solving, and reduced processing speed are some of the sequelae of AIDS that are of concern to speech-language pathologists (ASHA, 1989; Butlers, 1990; Navia, Jordan, & Price, 1986; Navia & Price, 1987; Price & Brew, 1988; Sliwa & Smith, 1991; Tucker, 1989). The number of minority individuals (particularly African Americans and Hispanics) diagnosed as having AIDS greatly exceeds the expected rate based on overall representation in the population (Centers for Disease Control, 1990). In addition, Hispanics are overrepresented in the proportion of women and children with AIDS (Sumaya, 1992). A demographic finding that has received less attention in the literature is the difference in statistics for AIDS and HIV infections that exists among Hispanics according to geographic location in the country. In general, the rates of AIDS cases for Hispanics in the Northeastern states (particularly New York and New Jersey) are particularly high; the rates among Hispanics in Florida are at intermediate levels; and the rates for Hispanics in the Southwestern states are at expected or at underrepresented numbers given the proportion of this group in the general population (Sumaya, 1992; Sumaya & Porto, 1989).

In summary, it is evident that the Hispanic population is disproportionately affected by certain causes of and risk factors associated with neurological impairment, including cardiovascular disease and stroke, diabetes, trauma, and infectious diseases. These causes of neurological impairment are also associated with communication disorders, and thus have a direct impact on speech-language pathologists. Given the increased risk for neurological impairment among the Hispanic population, speech-language pathologists should be aware of this increased risk and of linguistic and cultural factors to consider in the delivery of services to this population. These issues will in turn be discussed.

⊔

BILINGUALISM

Extensive studies of language use among ethnic groups in the United States indicate that the Spanish language is the most persistent of all foreign languages and has the greatest possibility for continued use (Romo, 1992). According to Schick and Schick (1991), it is estimated that a minimum of 11 million people in the U.S. speak Spanish in the home setting, and of these, one fourth do not speak English well or do not speak it at all. In fact, the United States has been identified as the fifth largest Spanish-speaking nation in the world (Romo, 1991; U.S. Bureau of the Census, 1990). Although not all Hispanics are bilingual, many Hispanics maintain that the Spanish language is inseparable from their cultural identity, and seek to remain bilingual. A discussion of bilingualism and code switching will in turn be presented, followed by specific questions to be asked by the speech-language pathologist and factors to consider in the assessment and treatment of bilingual patients with neurogenic impairments.

BILINGUALISM DESCRIBED

To date, no universally accepted definition of bilingualism exists, although numerous definitions have been proposed by individuals across various disciplines. For example, Bloomfield (1935) suggests that a bilingual must have native-like control of two languages, whereas Haugen (1969) defines a bilingual as one who can produce meaningful sentences in a second language. MacNamara (1967), on the other hand, proposes that the possession of at least one of the language skills (listening, speaking, reading, or writing) in a second language, even to a minimal degree, constitutes bilingualism. It is clear that the term "bilingualism" is interpreted and defined differently by different people. Baetens-Beardsmore (1986) suggests that, rather than attempting to delineate a definition of bilingualism, typologies or descriptive labels be used. The reader is referred to Kayser (Chapter 8) for a discussion of typologies of bilingualism. It is recommended that speech-language pathologists working with bilingual patients with neurogenic communication disorders gather as much information as possible regarding premorbid bilingualism, particularly in reference to these typologies, and use this information in the implementation of assessment and therapeutic procedures. For example, expectations for performance in the second language post- insult would be very different for the premorbid incipient bilingual than they would for the equilingual, one who has equal abilities in both languages. A discussion of patterns of language use in the adult bilingual Hispanic population will in turn be presented.

PATTERNS OF LANGUAGE USE

Numerous investigators have examined patterns of language use among normal adult bilingual speakers. Those studying the bilingual Hispanic population have focused primarily on the Mexican American segment of the Hispanic population. In an investigation conducted by Keefe and Padilla (1987), "language ability" was determined for Mexican American adults living in southern California. These investigators found that, for first generation Mexican American adults, 83% spoke primarily Spanish, 14% were bilingual, and 3% spoke primarily English. Of the second generation individuals, 15% spoke primarily Spanish, 42% were bilingual, and 42% spoke primarily English. Finally, for third generation subjects, 7% spoke primarily Spanish, 30% were bilingual, and 63% were found to speak primarily English. This study indicates a high rate of maintenance of the Spanish language for first generation Mexican Americans, with subsequent generations becoming more bilingual and more proficient in English. A similar finding has been observed by Peñalosa (1980) with Mexican American adults in San Bernardino, California. Peñalosa found that, when speaking to their parents, 68% of Mexican American adults spoke primarily in Spanish, 11% spoke both English and Spanish equally, and 21% spoke primarily in English. Speaking to their spouses, 41% of the subjects spoke primarily in Spanish, 24% used both English and Spanish, and 36% spoke primarily in English. Finally, speaking to their children, 26% of the individuals spoke primarily in Spanish, 20% spoke both English and Spanish equally, and 54% spoke primarily in English. Penalosa (1980) suggests that "the dropoff in the use of Spanish by generation is obvious from these figures" (p. 201).

Perhaps one of the most comprehensive descriptions of patterns of language use among Mexican American adults has been provided by Sanchez (1983). Sanchez suggests that factors such as nativity or place of birth, length of residence in the United States, socioeconomic status, age, residence in urban versus rural areas, residence in integrated versus segregated neighborhoods, and domains of activity all influence the patterns of language use exhibited by individuals. In her investigation, Sanchez delineated four generations of subjects: (1) those born in Mexico (first generation in the United States), (2) those born in the United States, with parents and grandparents born in Mexico (second generation), (3) those born in the United States with one parent born in Mexico and one in the U.S., and the grandparents born in Mexico (mixed parentage: second-third generation), (4) those born in the United Stated with native-born parents and foreign-born grandparents (third generation), and (5) those born in the United States with parents and at least one set of grandparents born in the United States (fourth generation). Sanchez was interested in examining language proficiency and use in relation to generation, language proficiency of parents, area of residence (rural or urban), type of residential area (segregated or integrated), socioeconomic status, and domain of activity. Results of this investigation yielded several interesting findings. First of all, as a whole, although most first generation individuals were more proficient in Spanish, succeeding generations tended to shift to English, with third and fourth generations being either primarily bilingual with greater proficiency in English or English speaking monolinguals. Secondly, Sanchez distinguished between middle and working class individuals. As a whole, middle class Hispanics tended to participate primarily in English in all domains (i.e., home, neighborhood, recreation, work, media, government), although first and second generation speakers retained some use of Spanish in the home. The pattern of language use exhibited by working class subjects was different and was influenced by area of residence (urban versus rural). For working class Mexican Americans living in rural areas, Spanish was maintained to some degree in all domains except for government, which was always in English. For the urban working class individuals, bilingualism was the rule except for third and fourth generation speakers who functioned primarily in English in all domains. Thus, it is evident that various factors influence the pattern of language use among Hispanic adults. The speech-language pathologist will want to take all of these factors into consideration in assessing and implementing intervention programs with bilingual Hispanic patients who present with neurogenic communication disorders.

CODE SWITCHING

Another linguistic variable to consider in the assessment and treatment of bilingual patients with neurogenic disorders is code switching. Valdes-Fallis (1978) defines *code switching* as the alternating use of two languages at the word, phrase, clause, or sentence level, with a clear break between phonemic systems. Code switching is a commonly observed phenomenon in many bilingual communities. It has been investigated and found to be characteristic of communities bilingual in language pairs such as French and English, Swedish and English, German and English, Yiddish and English, Finnish and English, Greek and English, Japanese and English, and Spanish and English (Gardner-Chloros, 1991; Grosjean, 1982; Grosjean & Soares, 1986; Gumperz, 1982; Jacobson, 1990a; Lipski, 1985; Nishimura, 1986; Poplack, Wheeler, & Westwood, 1989; Sanchez, 1983; Valdes-Fallis, 1978, 1981). An unfortunate yet common misconception is to view code switching as an indicator of deficient language skills in the bilingual speaker. In fact, numerous investigations of code switching have demonstrated just the opposite. Code switching has been shown to be a complex, rule-governed phenomenon that requires a high degree of linguistic competence in more than one language (Auer, 1984; Peñalosa, 1981; Poplack, 1982). In a study of English-Spanish code switching among bilingual Puerto Ricans living in New York, Poplack (1982) found that the most complex form of code switching was produced by the most proficient bilingual speakers. That is, only the speakers with the greatest degree of bilingual ability favored the type of code switching requiring the most skill (i.e., intrasentential code switching). In addition, Poplack found virtually no instances of ungrammatical combinations of first (L1) and second (L2) languages in the 1,835 switches examined, providing additional evidence that code switching is not a random phenomenon, but rather is rule-governed and requires a high level of bilingual competence.

CLASSIFICATIONS

Numerous taxonomies have been proposed in the literature delineating various types of code switching and factors or variables associated with code switching. The classification of code switching which has had perhaps the most enduring influence is that of Gumperz (1976, 1982). Gumperz distinguished between "situational" code switching, in which switches are associated with distinct activities or situations, and "conversational" code switching, in which the switches take place within a single conversation without any change of interlocutors, topic, or other major factors in the interaction (Blom & Gumperz, 1972). Other investigators have distinguished between "intersentential" and "intrasentential" code switching (Hidalgo, 1988; Lipski, 1985). Intersentential switching consists of shifting languages at sentence boundaries, whereas intrasentential switching involves shifting languages in the middle of a sentence, often with no interruptions, hesitations, pauses, or "other indications of a major categorical shift" (Lipski, 1985, p. 2). The latter type of code switching is believed by some to be the most complex and require a high degree of linguistic competence in the two languages being spoken (Poplack, 1981, 1982; Poplack, Wheeler, & Westwood, 1989). Yet other investigators have focused on sociolinguistic, grammatical/linguistic, and functional constraints on code switching (Auer, 1984; Clyne, 1992; Grosjean & Soares, 1986; Lipski, 1985; Nishimura, 1986; Poplack, 1982; Poplack, Wheeler, & Westwood, 1989; Schieffelin, 1994).

VARIABLES AFFECTING CODE SWITCHING

Perhaps more relevant for speech-language pathologists are variables that have been found to affect the type and frequency of code switching in normal bilingual adults. Two major categories of such variables will be discussed in turn: situational variables and stylistic variables.

Language selection by normal adult bilinguals has been shown to be partially determined by various situational variables including *participants* in the speech event, *setting*, and *topic*. In order for code switching to occur, all speech participants must be functionally bilingual in the languages being used to an extent that permits comprehension of bilingual utterances as well as monolingual utterances in each language (Lipski, 1985). For example, Valdes-Fallis (1978) notes that very rarely do Mexican American adult bilinguals code switch in conversations with English-speaking monolinguals or in settings in which English monolinguals may momentarily join in the conversation. Other characteristics of participants that have been found to influence the code switching process include degree of intimacy; personal characteristics shared such as socioeconomic status, age, gender, and ethnic identity; and kinship. A second situational variable found to influence code switching is the *setting*, such as home, church, place of employment, school, and public institutions. Finally, *topics* such as those related to family, child care, religion, business, academic subjects, politics, and professional affairs have been found to differentially influence language selection among bilingual adults.

Numerous stylistic factors have also been found to influence the code switching process in normal bilingual speakers (Gumperz, 1982; McClure, 1981; Valdes-Fallis, 1978). Valdes-Fallis (1978) suggests that stylistic switching is dependent on the speaker's personal preference for one language or the other, provided that the situation in question permits either code. Table 7–1 provides examples of frequently occurring stylistic switches and a brief description of each.

DIFFERENTIATING CODE SWITCHING FROM LANGUAGE IMPAIRMENT

It must be noted that not all bilingual speakers are sufficiently proficient in each of their languages to be able to engage in skilled code switching. Some bilingual speakers switch only when speaking their weaker language in order to add information or emphasis in the stronger language. Others use high frequency words interchangeably in either language without regard to their connotative or affective meanings (Valdes-Fallis, 1978). Yet others engage in noun switching in response to lexical unavailability in one language (Lipski, 1985). Poplack (1982) has delineated four characteristics of skilled code switching in normal bilingual adults: (1) smooth transition between L1 and L2 without false starts, hesitations or lengthy pauses; (2) seem-

Table 7–1
Stylistic code switching.

Function	Description
Quotation	Code switch marks a direct quotation
Repetition	Message in one code is repeated in the second code
Addressee specification	Code switch singles out one of several possible interlocutors
Clarification	Code switch functions to resolve ambiguity or clarify a potential or apparent lack of understanding
Emphasis	Message is emphatically underscored in the second code
Elaboration	Code switch adds additional information to original message
Personalization	Code contrast reflects personal opinion versus known fact
Interjection	Code switch serves to mark an interjection or filler
Topic shift	Code contrast used to mark a desired change in topic
Preformulation	Code contrast marks automatic speech and linguistic routines
Paraphrase	Message in one code is paraphrased in the second code

Sources: Grosjean (1982); Jacobson (1990); McClure (1981); Valdes Fallis (1978).

ing "unawareness" of alternation between the languages (i.e., the switch is not accompanied by metalinguistic commentary, does not constitute a repetition of all of the preceding segment, and is not repeated by the following segment); (3) switches composed of segments larger than single nouns inserted into an otherwise L2 sentence; and (4) code switching used for purposes other than conveying untranslatable items. Although research examining code switching in bilingual patients with neurogenic impairments is virtually nonexistent, Albert and Obler (1978) and Hamers and Blanc (1989) indicate that aphasic polyglots rarely produce language mixing qualitively different from the code switching used premorbidly. This author's clinical experience would support this preliminary finding. Thus, on determination of premorbid code switching ability, the speech-language pathologist may refer to the characteristics of skilled code switching in normal adults outlined by Poplack (1982) and use these as general guidelines to assist in differentiating between switches in codes due to situational or stylistic factors from those due to linguistic impairment post-insult. In addition, the clinician should keep in mind that adult bilingual patients are not likely to code switch when engaged in conversations with monolingual speakers, unless of course they are attempting to compensate for a linguistic impairment.

Lipski (1985) discusses the extent to which lexical unavailability may be responsible for noun switching in some normal bilinguals. Some investigators have indicated that noun switching may occur to fill in lexical gaps in a speaker's repertoire, to shift the overall language of discourse into one temporarily or permanently more comfortable for one or more participants, or due to insecurity regarding the correct usage or pronunciation of a word in one language (Aguirre, 1981; Sanchez, 1983). Although certainly not all lexical switches are indicative of lexical unavailability (as when lexical switches are used to emphasize, clarify, or repeat items; or when certain words, even though known in both languages, may be identified preferentially with one of the languages), switches of single words may be a red flag to clinicians that perhaps the patient is experiencing word retrieval difficulties. This may especially be the case if the patient is also able to produce relatively fluent intrasentential switching.

In summary, code switching is a complex phenomenon observed in many bilingual communities. Numerous situational and stylistic variables affect code switching in bilingual speakers. In working with bilingual patients with neurogenic impairments, it is recommended that speech-language pathologists inquire as to the patients' premorbid code switching abilities and patterns, and systematically examine code switching ability post-insult. Differentiation between "normal" code switching post-insult and language impairment or word retrieval difficulty is a challenging yet necessary task.

ADDITIONAL SUGGESTIONS FOR ASSESSMENT AND TREATMENT

In what follows, admittedly highly personal suggestions will be made for management of bilingual Hispanic patients with neurogenic communication disorders. It is not within the scope of this chapter to delineate general assessment and treatment procedures for the adult neurogenic population. Numerous volumes have been dedicated to this end (Brookshire, 1992; Chapey, 1994; Davis, 1993; Dworkin, 1991; Helm-Estabrooks & Albert, 1991; LaPointe, 1990; Rosenbek, LaPointe, & Wertz, 1989; Wallace, in press; Wertz, LaPointe, & Rosenbek, 1991). Overarching assessment and treatment processes and principles remain consistent regardless of the language(s) spoken by the patient. However, these processes and principles must be couched in a culturally appropriate context to meet the needs of each patient. For example, the assessment process for the Hispanic patient may consist of various components including obtaining a case history; identifying the presence, type, and severity of a communicative impairment; determining patient strengths and weaknesses; making a prognostic statement; and formulating recommendations for treatment. However, specific information to be gathered via the case history, determination of strength and weaknesses, and the nature of the recommendations will vary depending on several factors including the cultural background of the patient. Suggestions for gathering background information and determining which language to use in management of the bilingual patient will in turn be presented.

BACKGROUND INFORMATION

As with any patient presenting with a neurogenic impairment, proper management of the Hispanic patient begins with collection of case history information. With the bilingual patient, however, the case history must be expanded to include information regarding each of the patients' languages. Obtaining the following additional information may be useful in managing the bilingual Hispanic patient:

- Language(s) spoken in the home during childhood and premorbidly
- Language(s) spoken in the environment/community during childhood and premorbidly
- Language(s) in which education was received
- Formal instruction in any other language
- Age and mode of acquisition of each language
- Relative degree of proficiency in each language premorbidly
- Frequency and type of code switching premorbidly
- Attitudes of self, spouse, children, parents, siblings, and any significant others toward bilingualism

- Ability to read in each language premorbidly
- Language(s) of most print media premorbidly (e.g., books, magazines, newspapers, etc.)
- Ability to write in each language premorbidly
- Frequency of written communication in each language premorbidly
- Language(s) in which television, movies and radio programs most often received premorbidly
- Proficiency of spouse, children, parents, siblings and any significant others in each language

Obtaining thorough and accurate background information is an essential step in management of the bilingual patient. This information will in turn assist the clinician in making decisions regarding the most appropriate language(s) in which to conduct therapy.

DETERMINING WHICH LANGUAGE(S) TO USE IN THERAPY

General guidelines and factors to consider in selecting the language(s) in which to conduct therapy with bilingual neurogenic patients will be presented. These are "guidelines" or suggestions resulting primarily from this author's clinical experience with bilingual Hispanic patients with aphasia. Clearly, much remains to be investigated regarding this topic. After obtaining thorough case history information, assessment of *both* of the patient's languages should be conducted. If a bilingual patient does indeed present with a neurogenic communication disorder, it will most likely be observed in both of the languages spoken by the patient. In addition, because traditional assessment of bilingual children as well as adults typically occurs in one language or the other, there is no provision for patients who regularly, predictably, and appropriately code switch. Thus, for the bilingual patient who engaged in code switching premorbidly, it is suggested that the clinician provide opportunity for code switching in the assessment process. Information obtained via the assessment process should be used to help guide the decision as to which language to use in intervention.

The ideal scenario in terms of intervention would be for a bilingual bicultural clinician to work with the bilingual Hispanic patient in the patient's stronger language. However, in the less than perfect world in which we live, this is often not possible. That is, the clinician may only speak one of the patient's languages, and this language may not be the one in which the patient was more proficient premorbidly. On an encouraging note, there is some evidence to suggest that therapy conducted in an aphasic patient's second (or third) language may also lead to improvement in the other language(s) over time (Fredman 1975; Penn, 1993). For example, working only in English with a multilingual aphasic patient who spoke 10 different languages in various contexts premorbidly, and whose most proficient language premorbidly was not English, Penn (1993) found that relative to pretherapy performance, improvement in the target areas was noted in all languages. Thus, although not the best scenario, it may be permissible in some cases for a monolingual clinician to conduct therapy in a language other than the patient's stronger language, particularly if the two languages appear to be impaired to a comparable degree postinsult, and the alternative is no therapy whatsoever. However, it must be emphasized that much care must be taken to ensure that disordered language is indeed being treated, and that therapy is not focusing on language skills not present premorbidly. More preferable options for therapy in this case would be to explore the possibility of establishing cooperatives, networks, and contacts with bilingualbicultural clinicians (ASHA, 1985). Yet another option would be to use an interpreter in the intervention process. The reader is referred to Kayser (Chapter 9) for a discussion of the use of supportive personnel and interpreters in management of bilingual individuals.

It is suggested that the clinician consider additional contextual factors in selecting the language to use in therapy with the bilingual patient. The patient's preferences, needs, strengths and weaknesses, and proficiency in each language post-insult are all contextual factors influencing the selection of the language to be used. Factors influencing premorbid patterns of language use such as place of birth, length of residence in the United States, socioeconomic status, age, residence in urban versus rural areas, residence in integrated versus segregated neighborhoods, and domains of activity should also be considered. In addition, factors such as the language(s) spoken by family members and language(s) spoken in the expected environment on discharge will need to be taken into consideration in determining which language(s) to use in the intervention process with the bilingual Hispanic patient.

Finally, it is recommended that the clinician inquire as to the patient's premorbid code switching ability. If code switching characterized the patient's premorbid communication style and the patient is able and willing to code switch post-insult, this aspect of communicative behavior may be incorporated into the therapeutic process.

In summary, bilingualism and code switching have been described. In addition, suggestions for assessment and treatment of bilingual Hispanic patients with neurogenic communication disorders have been presented, with the ultimate goal that the patient become a functional communicator in his environment. The remainder of this chapter will focus on cultural factors to consider in management of bilingual Hispanic patients.

⊔

CULTURAL FACTORS

Although linguistic factors are important in management of bilingual Hispanic patients, cultural factors have greater significance. The professions of speech-language pathology and audiology have become increasingly aware that communicatively impaired individuals from culturally and linguistically diverse populations present with unique clinical needs. The challenge for the clinician is to implement culturally valid management for the individual without imposing Western values and norms on the rehabilitation process. A proper understanding of one's own culture as well as the culture of one's patients is essential in providing appropriate services to communicatively impaired individuals. Unfortunately, assumptions specific to Euro-American culture are frequently made by professionals as they interact with non-mainstream individuals (Pedersen, 1987). These assumptions are usually implicit and taken for granted and, therefore, go unchallenged. One of the consequences of these unexamined assumptions can be cultural bias. It is thus imperative that clinicians make a conscious effort to increase awareness of their assumptions, particularly those reflecting cultural bias. Although each individual must examine his or her own assumptions, three commonly occurring ones will be discussed. Perhaps the most prevalent assumption resulting in culturally biased management of the multicultural patient is that the definition of "normal" behavior is universal. Clinicians often assume that what is normal behavior to them is normal to everyone. That is, we do not ordinarily think of "our" way of behaving as being *one* way of behaving among others, but as *the* way to behave or act. Thus, behavior that does not fit the expected pattern or varies from one's definition of normal must be explained as "disordered." In reality, what is considered to be normal behavior varies according to the cultural background of the individual.

A second assumption that can hinder appropriate management is that clinicians should change the patient to "fit the system." Presuming that one's concept of normal is universal, professionals then assume that they must change the patient's behavior to conform to the mainstream system. Perhaps a more appropriate approach would be to modify the rehabilitation system to best meet the needs of the patient, thus assisting him or her to become an effective communicator in his community.

A third assumption often made by professionals is that they are aware of all their assumptions. It is crucial that clinicians carefully analyze their own behavior and determine which assumptions are motivating that behavior. If clinicians are unable or unwilling to examine their own assumptions, they will be less effective in interacting with persons from other cultures. Thus, continuous awareness and examination of one's assumptions is required for appropriate and effective management of patients from multicultural populations. Although there is much variation among the Hispanic population with respect to cultural beliefs and practices, several of the most prevalent cultural factors influencing management of this population will subsequently be addressed.

LOCUS OF CONTROL

Locus of control is a cultural factor to consider in managing the Hispanic patient, (Chamberlain & Medinos-Landurand, 1991). An external locus of control proposes that events occur independently of one's actions. That is, circumstances are believed to be determined more by external forces (e.g., God, fate, etc.) than by anything the individual can do. On the other hand, an internal locus of control suggests that events are contingent on one's own actions. Thus, people are believed to have control over circumstances and can in turn influence their own destiny. Although many individual differences exist within cultures, in general, Western mainstream culture tends to espouse an internal locus of control, whereas Hispanic cultures—in addition to many other cultures of the world—espouse an external locus of control. This issue is closely related to one's view of illness and concept of medicine. In general, American medicine has been described as aggressive, demanding active treatment, adopting a "can do" approach, and technology oriented (Payer, 1988; Perrone, Stockel, & Krueger, 1989). In addition, Western medicine in many instances assumes that physical illnesses are the sole result of physical causes (e.g., viruses, bacteria, organ malfunctions, genetics, biochemical agents) and that these causes can and should be remediated (Perrone et al., 1989). Medical practice in other cultures, including some Hispanic cultures, tends to be more accepting of illness, focusing on the whole person and emphasizing the role of spiritual and psychological factors in addition to physical ones in the cause of illness (Davitz, Davitz, & Higuchi, 1987; Kraut, 1990; Payer, 1988; Perrone et al., 1989). The issue of locus of control and the concomitant views of illness and medicine may influence whether or not a patient seeks speech-language therapy in the first place. Once in therapy, the issue of locus of control may impact a patient's level of motivation and thus his progress in therapy. In addition, whether a patient adheres to an external or internal locus of control will greatly influence his approach to problem-solving tasks. This should be kept in mind by the clinician particularly when working with the traumatically brain-injured population, and solutions to problems reflecting an external locus of control (although generally not the mainstream view) should be accepted as appropriate.

INTERACTIONS/TIME

Types of interactions and the concept of time are two additional cultural variables to consider in management of Hispanic patients. Hall (1976) has delineated two primary types of interactions exhibited by people across different cultures: monochronic and polychronic. Some cultures (e.g., Western) tend to be primarily monochronic in their interactions. That is, they emphasize schedules, segmentation, and promptness and tend to be linear in nature, focusing on interactions and activities one at a time. Other cultures are primarily polychronic in their interactions, handling several interactions and activities at the same time, going back and forth between tasks with great ease, and stressing involvement of people and completion of transactions rather than adherence to present schedules. The assessment and therapeutic processes may need to be structured differently depending on whether the patient exhibits a propensity for monochronic or polychronic interactions. For example, for patients favoring monochronic interactions, assessment and treatment tasks would ideally be highly structured and compartmentalized with one task being completed in its entirety prior to beginning a new task. For patients favoring poly-chronic interactions, on the other hand, working on several tasks or activities at a time and allowing for participation back and forth between tasks may be more appropriate. In addition to variations in interactions, the clinician should be reminded that the concept of time varies across cultures, and different cultural groups have different rules regarding the use of time. For example, Western mainstream culture tends to place much emphasis and importance on adherence to stringent schedules, whereas in other cultures time is viewed as a relative concept with the quality of interpersonal relationships taking priority over schedules and punctuality. Lingenfelter and Mayers (1986) suggest that Americans and Germans belong to "time-ori-ented" cultures, whereas Hispanic and Yapese cultures are more "event-oriented." People who are time-oriented tend to express great concern about punctuality, the length of time expended, and utiliza-tion of time to its maximum potential. In contrast, people who are event-oriented tend to show concern that an activity be completed regardless of the length of time required and emphasize unscheduled participation, focusing on the event itself. Again, therapy may need to be structured differently for the time-oriented versus the event-ori-ented patient. In the latter case, for example, a patient may become very involved in a therapy task (i.e., event), wanting to spend more time working on a particular deficit area or task than the clinician had originally allotted, thus warranting flexibility on the part of the clini-cian. In addition, for the event-oriented patient, the establishment and maintenance of personal relationships is of great importance. There-fore, it would be wise for the clinician to take time to cultivate a rela-tionship with the Hispanic patient at the risk of sacrificing some efficiency in accomplishment of a particular task. Differences in the concept of time may also present the mainstream clinician with scheduling challenges in interacting with some, although certainly not all, Hispanic patients. Missed outpatient appointments or "late" arrivals may result from differences in the concept of time. Wallace (1993) suggests that creative service delivery options such as home-based treatment may help to address this challenge. In addition, a proper understanding of the patient's perspective may assist the clini-cian in respectfully explaining the importance of "timeliness" as viewed by Western mainstream culture.

RELATIONAL PATTERNS

Clinicians will also want to take relational patterns into consideration in management of Hispanic patients with neurogenic impairments. Cultures vary in their degree of individual versus group orientation. American mainstream culture tends to emphasize individuality, wherein what the individual does and accomplishes is valued, whereas other cultures tend to value interdependence, wherein the good of the group (most often the family) is emphasized. The importance of family is characteristic of many, although certainly not all, Hispanics. In a survey of Mexican American and Anglo adults' family ties, Keefe and Padilla (1987) found that ties with nuclear as well as extended families tended to be much stronger for the Mexican Americans than for the Anglos. As can be seen in Table 7–2, first-, second-, and third-generation Mexican Americans tended to have members of their nuclear and extended families living in the same town much more often than did the Anglo individuals. In addition, a much higher percentage of first-, second-, and even third-generation Mexican Americans had daily or weekly interaction with their nuclear and extended families than did Anglos. Hispanics are often described as

Table 7–2
Family ties.

	Generations			
	First	**Second**	**Third**	**Anglo**
Nuclear Family				
In Town	37%	56%	58%	17%
Interaction				
Daily	19%	19%	23%	7%
Weekly	26%	44%	35%	16%
Extended Family				
In Town	12%	26%	37%	3%
Interaction				
Daily	16%	23%	29%	15%
Weekly	11%	10%	19%	6%

Source: Adapted from *Chicano Ethnicity* by S. E. Keefe, & A. M. Padilla, (1987). Albu-

having a deep consciousness of family, with family members possessing a strong sense of obligation to the family. In addition, *la familia* to the Hispanic generally refers to the extended versus the nuclear family, including the spouse, children, grandparents, aunts, uncles, cousins, in-laws, godparents, and long-time family friends. While the role of the family in the rehabilitation process for patients with neurogenic impairments is always important, it becomes even more so with some Hispanic patients. It is recommended that the clinician encourage and welcome involvement of the patient's family in the rehabilitation process from the beginning, keeping in mind that "family" may very well include members of the patient's extended family. In addition, it may be very appropriate for the patient to have to consult with other family members prior to making important decisions regarding the rehabilitation process.

In summary, consideration of cultural factors is of vital importance in management of the Hispanic patient. Factors such as locus of control, types of interactions, concept of time, and relational patterns must all be examined and considered as the speech-language pathologist interacts with the Hispanic patient.

⌐ᴖ

CONCLUSION

The Hispanic population is a diverse populace consisting of several distinct subgroups. Pertinent information with respect to demographics, including geographic distribution, age, educational level, and income have been provided. In addition, health care among the Hispanic population has been addressed, including a discussion of cardiovascular disease, diabetes, trauma and infectious diseases. Bilingualism and code switching, and their implications for assessment and treatment of Hispanic neurogenic patients, have also been discussed. Finally, cultural factors to consider in the rehabilitation process with Hispanic patients have been highlighted. Clearly, much remains to be learned regarding the most appropriate assessment and therapeutic methodologies to be implemented with this population. It is hoped that this chapter will serve as a point of reference to this end.

⅃ᴛ

REFERENCES

Aguirre, A. (1981). Toward an index of acceptability for code alternation: An experimental analysis. *Aztlan, 11,* 297–322.

Albert, M. L., & Obler, L. K. (1978). *The bilingual brain.* New York: Academic Press.

American Heart Association. (1984). *Heart facts.* Dallas, TX: Author.

American Speech-Language-Hearing Association. (1985). Clinical management of communicatively handicapped minority language populations. *Asha, 27*(6), 29–32.

American Speech-Language-Hearing Association. (1989). AIDS/HIV: Implications for speech-language pathologists and audiologists. *Asha, 31,* 33–37.

American Speech-Language-Hearing Association. (1991). Cultural diversity in the elderly population. *Asha, 33,* 66.

Anderson, N. B., & Cohen, J. J. (1989). Health status of aged minorities: Directions for clinical research. *Journal of Gerontology: Medical Sciences, 44,* M1–2.

Auer, J. C. P. (1984). *Bilingual conversation.* Amsterdam: John Benjamins.

Baetens-Beardsmore, H. (1986). *Bilingualism: Basic principles* (2nd ed.). San Diego, CA: College-Hill Press.

Blom, J. P., & Gumperz, J. J. (1972). Social meaning in linguistic structures: Code-switching in Norway. In J. Gumperz & D. Hymes (Eds.), *Directions in Sociolinguistics.* New York: Holt, Rinehart & Winston.

Bloomfield, L. (1935). *Language.* London: Allen & Unwin.

Brookshire, R. H. (1992). *An introduction to neurogenic communication disorders* (4th ed.). St. Louis, MO: Mosby Year Book.

Butlers, E. A. (1990). Assessment of AIDS-related cognitive changes: Recommendations of the NIMH Workshop on Neuropsychological Assessment Approaches. *Journal of Clinical and Experimental Neuropsychology, 12,* 963–978.

Centers for Disease Control. (1990, May). *HIV/AIDS Surveillance Report.* Atlanta, GA.: Author.

Chamberlain, P., & Medinos-Landurand, P. (1991). Practical considerations for the assessment of LEP students with special needs. In E. V. Hamayan, & J. S. Damico, (Eds.), *Limiting bias in the assessment of bilingual students* (pp. 11–156). Austin, TX: Pro-Ed.

Chapey, R. (1994). *Language intervention strategies in adult aphasia* (3rd ed.). Baltimore: Williams & Wilkins.

Clyne, M. (1992). Linguistic and sociolinguistic aspects of language contact, maintenance and loss: Towards a multifacet theory. In W. Fase, K. Jaspaert & S. Kroon (Eds.), *Maintenance and loss of minority languages* (pp. 17–36). Amsterdam: John Benjamins.

Council on Scientific Affairs, American Medical Association. (1991). Hispanic health in the United States. *Journal of the American Medical Association, 265*(2), 248–252.

Davis, G. A. (1993). *A survey of adult aphasia and related language disorders* (2nd ed.). Englewood Cliffs, NJ: Prentice-Hall.

Davitz, L. L., Davitz, J. R., & Higuchi, Y. (1987, April 14). Cross-cultural inferences of physical pain and psychological distress. *Nursing Times,* 521–558.

Dworkin, J. P. (1991). *Motor speech disorders: A treatment guide.* St. Louis, MO: Mosby Year Book.

Fredman, M. (1975). The effect of therapy given in Hebrew on the home language of the bilingual or polyglot adult aphasic in Israel. *British Journal of Disorders of Communication, 10,* 61–69.

Furino, A., & Guerra, F. A. (1992). The issues: An overview. In A. Furino (Ed.), *Health policy and the Hispanic* (pp. 3–11). Boulder, CO: Westview Press.

Gardner-Chloros, P. (1991). *Language selection and switching in Strasbourg.* Oxford: Clarendon Press.

Ginzberg, E. (1992). Access to health care for Hispanics. In A. Furino (Ed.), *Health policy and the Hispanic* (pp. 22–31). Boulder, CO: Westview Press.

Grosjean, F. (1982). *Life with two language: An introduction to bilingualism.* Cambridge, MA: Harvard University Press.

Grosjean, F., & Soares, C. (1986). Processing mixed language: Some preliminary findings. In J. Vaid (Ed.), *Language processing in bilinguals: psycholinguistic and neuropsychological perspectives* (pp. 145–179). Hillsdale, NJ: Lawrence Erlbaum.

Gumperz, J.J. (1976). *The sociolinguistic significance of conversational code-switching* (Working Paper 46). Berkeley: University of California Language Behavior Research Laboratory.

Gumperz, J.J. (1982). *Discourse strategies.* Cambridge: Cambridge University Press.

Hall, E. T. (1976). *Beyond culture.* Garden City, NY: Anchor Press.

Hamers, J. F., & Blanc, M. H. (1989). *Bilinguality and bilingualism.* Cambridge: Cambridge University Press.

Haugen, E. (1969). *The Norwegian language in America: A study in bilingual behavior* (2nd ed.). Bloomington: Indiana University Press.

Hazuda, H. P., & Stern, M. P (1985). Ethnic differences in health knowledge and behaviors related to the prevention and treatment of coronary heart disease. *American Journal of Epidemiology, 117*(6), 717–728.

Helm-Estabrooks, N., & Albert, M. L. (1991). *Manual of aphasia therapy.* Austin, TX: Pro-Ed.

Hidalgo, M. (1988). *Perceptions of Spanish-English code-switching in Juarez, Mexico* (Research Paper Series No. 20). Albuquerque: University of New Mexico Press.

Jacobson, A. R. (1994). Health: Fighting diabetes. *Hispanic, 7*(2), 58.

Jacobson, R. (1990a). Introduction. In R. Jacobson (Ed.), *Code switching as a worldwide phenomenon* (pp. 1–13). New York: Peter Lang.

Jacobson, R. (1990b). Socioeconomic status as a factor in the selection of encoding strategies in mixed discourse. In R. Jacobson (Ed.), *Codeswitching as a worldwide phenomenon* (pp. 111–139). New York: Peter Lang.

Keefe, S. E., & Padilla, A. M. (1987). *Chicano ethnicity.* Albuquerque: University of New Mexico Press.

Kraut, A. (1990). Healers and strangers: Immigrant attitudes toward the physician in American. *Journal of the American Medical Association, 263*(13), 1807–1811.

LaPointe, L. L. (1990). *Aphasia and related neurogenic language disorders.* New York: Thieme Medical.

Lingenfelter, S. G., & Mayers, M. K. (1986). *Ministering cross-culturally.* Grand Rapids, MI: Baker Book House.

Lipski, J. M. (1985). *Linguistic aspects of Spanish-English language switching.* Tempe, AZ: Center for Latin American Studies.

MacNamara, J. (1967). The bilingual's performance: A psychological overview. *Journal of Social Issues, 23*, 58–77.

Marin, B. V., Marin, G., Padilla, A. M., & de la Rocha, C. (1983). Utilization of traditional and non-traditional sources of health care among Hispanics. *Hispanic Journal of Behavioral Sciences, 5*(1), 65–80.

McClure, E. (1981). Formal and functional aspects of code switched discourse in bilingual children. In R. P. Duran (Ed.), *Latino language and communicative behavior* (pp. 69–94). Norwood, NJ: ABLEX.

Muñoz, E., Tortella, B. J., Sakmyster, M. A., Liveronese, D. S., McCormac, M., Odom, J. W., & Torres, R. (1992). Traumatic injury in Hispanic Americans: A distinct entity. In A. Furino (Ed.), *Health policy and the Hispanic* (pp. 126–131). Boulder, CO: Westview Press.

Navia, B. A., Jordan, B. D., & Price, R. W. (1986). The AIDS dementia complex: Clinical features. *Annals of Neurology, 19*, 517–524.

Navia, B. A., & Price, R. W. (1987). The acquired immunodeficiency syndrome dementia complex as the presenting or sole manifestation of human immunodeficiency infection. *Neurology, 44*, 65–69.

Netter, F. H. (1992). *CIBA collection of medical illustrations. Vol. I, Nervous system Part 2, Neurologic and neuromuscular disorders.* Caldwell, NJ: CIBA

Nishimura, M. (1986). Intrasentential code switching: The case of language assignment. In J. Vaid (Ed.), *Language processing in bilinguals: Psycholinguistic and neuropsychological perspectives* (pp. 123–143). Hillsdale, NJ: Lawrence Erlbaum.

Novick, D. M., Trigg, H. L., Des Jarlais, D. C., Friedman, S. R., Vlahov, D., & Kreek, M. J. (1989). Cocaine injection and ethnicity in parental drug users during the early years of human immunodeficiency virus (HIV) epidemic in New York City. *Journal of Medical Virology, 29*, 181–185.

Payer, L. (1988). *Medicine and culture: Varieties of treatment in the United States, England, West Germany, and France.* New York: Penguin.

Pedersen, P. (1987). Ten frequent assumptions of cultural bias in counseling. *Journal of Multicultural Counseling and Development, 15*, 16–24.

Peñalosa, F. (1980). *Chicano sociolinguistics: A brief introduction.* Rowley, MA: Newbury House.

Peñalosa, F. (1981). *Introduction to the sociology of language.* Rowley, MA: Newbury House.

Penn, C. (1993). Aphasia therapy in South Africa: Some pragmatic and personal perspectives. In A. L. Holland & M. M. Forbes (Eds.), *Aphasia treatment: World perspectives* (pp. 25–53). San Diego, CA: Singular Publishing Group.

Perrone, B., Stockel, H. H., & Krueger, V. (1989). *Medicine women, curanderas, and women doctors.* Norman: University of Oklahoma Press.

Poplack, S. (1981). Syntactic structure and social function of code switching. In R. P. Duran (Ed.), *Latino language and communicative behavior* (pp. 169–184). Norwood, NJ: ABLEX.

Poplack, S. (1982). "Sometimes I'll start a sentence in Spanish y termino en español": Toward a typology of code switching. In J. Amastae & L. Elias-Olivares (Eds.), *Spanish in the United States: Sociolinguistic aspects* (pp. 230–263). Cambridge: Cambridge University Press.

Poplack, S., Wheeler, S., & Westwood, A. (1989). Distinguishing language contact phenomena: Evidence from Finish-English bilingualism. In K. Hyltenstam & L. K. Obler (Eds.), *Bilingualism across the lifespan* (pp. 132–154). Cambridge: Cambridge University Press.

Price, R. W., & Brew, B. J. (1988). The AIDS dementia complex. *Journal of Infectious Disease, 158*(5), 1079.

Rieder, H. L., Cauthen, G. M., Kelly, G. D., Bloch, A. B., & Snider, D. E., Jr. (1989). Tuberculosis in the United States. *Journal of the American Medical Association, 262,* 385–389.

Roberts, R. E., & Lee, E. S. (1980). Medical care by Mexican Americans: Evidence from the human population laboratory studies. *Medical Care, 18,* 266–281.

Romo, O. I. (1991). *Missions in ethnic America.* Atlanta, GA: Home Mission Board of the Southern Baptist Convention.

Romo, O. I. (1992). *America's Hispanics.* Atlanta, GA: Home Mission Board of the Southern Baptist Convention.

Rosenbek, J. C., LaPointe, L. L., & Wertz, R. J. (1989). *Aphasia: A clinical approach.* Boston: College-Hill Press.

Sanchez, R. (1983). *Chicano discourse: Socio-historic perspectives.* Rowley, MA: Newbury House.

Schick, F. L., & Schick, R. (1991). *Statistical handbook on U.S. Hispanics.* Phoenix, AZ: Oryx Press.

Schieffelin, B. B. (1994). Code-switching and language socialization: Some probable relationships. In J. F. Duchan, L. E. Hewitt, & R. M. Sonnenmeier (Eds.), *Pragmatics: From theory of practice* (pp. 20–42). Englewood Cliffs, NJ: Prentice-Hall.

Schoenbaum, E. E., Hartel, D., Selwyn, P. A., & Klein, R. S. (1989). Risk factors for human immunodeficiency virus infection in intravenous drug abusers. *New England Journal of Medicine, 321,* 874–879.

Select Committee on Aging, House of Representatives, 100th Congress. (1989). *Demographic characteristics of the older Hispanic population.* Washington, DC: Government Printing Office.

Sliwa, J. A., & Smith, J. C. (1991). Rehabilitation of neurologic disability related to human immunodeficiency virus. *Archives of Physical Medicine and Rehabilitation, 72,* 759–762.

Snider, D. E., Jr., Salina, L., & Kelly, G. D. (1989). Tuberculosis: An increasing problem among minorities in the United States. *Public Health Reports, 104,* 646–653.

Sotomayor, M., & Randolph, S. (1988). The health status of the Hispanic elderly. In M. Sotomayor & H. Curiel (Eds.), *Hispanic elderly: A cultural signature* (pp. 203–225). Edinburg, TX: Pan American University Press.

Stern, M. P., & Haffner, S. M. (1992). Type II diabetes in Mexican Americans: A public health challenge. In A. Furino (Ed.), *Health policy and the Hispanic* (pp. 57–75). Boulder, CO: Westview Press.

Sumaya, C. V. (1992). Major infectious diseases causing excess morbidity in the Hispanic population. In A. Furino (Ed.), *Health Policy and the Hispanic* (pp. 76–96). Boulder, CO: Westview Press.

Sumaya, C. V., & Porto, M. D. (1989). AIDS in Hispanics. *Southern Medical Journal, 72,* 943–945.

Teller, C. A. (1988). Physical health status and health care utilization in the Texas borderlands. In S. R. Ross (Ed.), *Views across the border.* Albuquerque: University of New Mexico Press.

Tucker, T. (1989). Central nervous system AIDS. *Journal of Neurological Sciences, 89,* 119–133.

U.S. Bureau of the Census. (1989). Projections of the Hispanic population: 1989–2080. *Current Population Reports* (Series P-25, No. 995). Washington, DC: Government Printing Office.

U.S. Bureau of the Census, (1990). The Hispanic population in the United States. *Current Population Reports.* Washington, DC: Government Printing Office.

Valdes-Fallis, G. (1978). *Language in education: Theory and practice: Code switching and the classroom teacher.* Arlington, VA: Arlington Center for Applied Linguistics.

Valdes-Fallis, G. (1981). Code switching as deliberate verbal strategy: A microanalysis of direct and indirect requests among bilingual chicano speakers. In R. P. Duran (Ed.), *Latino language and communicative behavior* (pp. 95–107). Norwood, NJ: ABLEX.

Wallace, G. L. (in press). *Adult aphasia: Clinical management for the practicing clinician.* Reading, MA: Andover Medical.

Wallace, G. L. (1993). Adult neurogenic disorders. In. D. E. Battle (Ed.), *Communication disorders in multicultural populations* (pp. 239–255). Boston: Butterworth-Heinemann.

Wertz, R. T., LaPointe, L. L., & Rosenbek, J. C. (1991). *Apraxia of speech in adults: The disorder and its management.* San Diego, CA: Singular Publishing Group.

Yatsu, F. M. (1991). Strokes in Asians and Pacific-Islanders, Hispanics, and native Americans. *Circulation, 83*(4), 1471–1472.

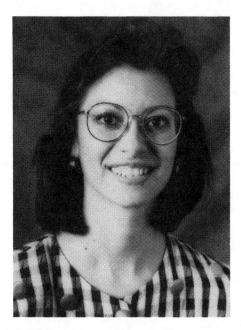

BELINDA A. REYES, Ph.D., CCC-SLP

Dr. Reyes is an Assistant Professor in the Department of Speech-Language Pathology at the University of Texas at El Paso. She received her master's degree in 1984 and her doctorate in 1989, both from The University of Texas at Dallas. Her primary interest in speech pathology is aphasia, with research in adult neurogenic communication disorders among Spanish-speaking and bilingual (Spanish-English) populations. Dr. Reyes' previous employment settings include Texas Christian University, Dallas Rehabilitation Institute, and the Callier Center for Communication Disorders.

PART II

ASSESSMENT ISSUES AND CONSIDERATIONS

Part II addresses issues that affect the assessment of Spanish- and English-speaking children. These issues include the myths that surround bilingualism in children and how they affect the assessment process, the utilization of interpreters during the evaluation, and intelligence testing for Hispanic children. Recommended practices in speech and language assessment as well as language elicitation and the analyses procedures for language samples also are discussed.

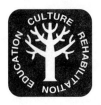

CHAPTER 8

BILINGUALISM, MYTHS, AND LANGUAGE IMPAIRMENTS

HORTENCIA KAYSER, Ph.D.

I think that (bilingualism) has to be a positive for any child. A little first grader can look and have two different perceptions of their world you know, that an adult can't have . . . And these kids just know it naturally. And they can go back and forth. But they make the mistakes of pronouns and the "ings, but the fact is they have that cognitive knowledge that perception that other kids don't have. So it's positive but it turns out unfortunately in the system negative because they don't have all the, you know, the perfect little finishing touches on it. So people look at 'em as that kid's a less of a communicator because instead of looking at their perception (that) the two languages gives them. They look at the fact . . . they make all those errors in syntax. (Kayser, 1985, p. 84)

S peech-language pathologists are becoming increasingly aware that bilingualism among their clients is a phenomenon that affects their clinical practice. Their knowledge about children's acquisition of two languages is central to their effectiveness in assessment and intervention with these children. When clinicians are unfamiliar with the literature on child bilingualism, hypotheses, beliefs, and myths are developed to fill this void. These beliefs may come from discussions with other clinicians, their work experiences, or possibly workshops. As in any community, the belief system or myths may not be completely accurate and may be based on an individual's perceptions concerning another culture and language. If there are misconceptions concerning bilingual behaviors, they will impact the assessment and perceived progress of bilingual children who are identified as language impaired. Thus there may be confusion and difficulty in determining what is a language impairment versus what is a language difference.

The purpose of this chapter is to assist clinicians in understanding some basic concepts about bilingualism and how they may be mistaken for language impairments. This will be accomplished through a discussion of some myths among speech-language pathologists about bilingual children and the literature concerning language impairments in Hispanic children. The third section will be a presentation of a study of three Mexican American students who were identifed as language impaired and how two of these children were mislabeled.

⊔

MYTHS AND BELIEFS

Although we would like to believe that all speech-language pathologists base their understanding concerning second language acquisition on the research literature, clinicians are not exposed to this literature in language development courses. Therefore, myths and a belief system do develop concerning children who learn two languages. Kayser (1985, 1990) identified four beliefs concerning bilingual children that were predominant among 20 speech-language pathologists. The clinicians were interviewed with open-ended questions to initiate in-depth discussion concerning bilingualism and the Hispanic children they served. During these conversations all of the clinicians described four beliefs: (1) bilingualism is equal knowledge of two languages; (2) the optimum time for learning two languages is before the age of three; (3) the preferred method of learning a second language in the home is to have one person speak language A and one person speak language B; and (4) code switching, the alternating use of two languages, is a reflection of inadequate vocabulary in both languages or word finding problems. The objective of this section is to provide a brief discussion concerning what is known about the definition of bilingualism, optimum time for learning two languages, home language environments, and code switching among children.

BELIEF 1: BILINGUALISM IS EQUAL KNOWLEDGE OF TWO LANGUAGES

Baetens-Beardsmore (1986) stated that definitions of bilingualism have continued to be offered without a feeling of some progress or resolution. The term "bilingual" has different meanings to different individuals and has had a varying degree of strictness to the definition. For example, Bloomfield (1935) defined "bilingual" as an individual who has native-like control of two languages and where there is no loss of the native language. A less strict definition is suggested by Halliday, McKintosh, and Streven, (1972) who stated that a bilingual is one who can speak only one language but who can switch register, styles, and functionally differentiated language varieties to coincide with place, topic, and interlocutor. MacNamara's (1967) definition stated that a bilingual individual possesses at least one of the language modalities in the two languages to a minimal degree (i.e., listening, speaking, reading, or writing). Considering the inadequacy of these definitions to encompass all of the ranges possible for bilingual speakers, Baetens-Beardsmore (1986) suggested that definitions are exclusive and do not provide a realistic and accurate statement that describes the degree and variability in the use of two languages by bilingual individuals.

Equal knowledge of two languages is rare (Baetens-Beardsmore, 1986). Very few individuals would meet the strictness of the clinicians' definition of "bilingual." Realistically, bilingual speakers develop language domains of competence in each language. For example, a child who has learned to speak the home language enters the English-speaking classroom with a reference of experiences that may not be similar to children from monolingual English-speaking homes. The natural bilingual, the individual who learns the second language because of circumstances, does not usually have the same lexical development in both languages (Baetens-Beardsmore, 1986). Arnberg (1987) states that the rate of language development of both languages in a bilingual child may not be equal to that seen in a monolingual speaking child. This may be due to a favored language environment which then leads to a slower rate of learning of the second language. The expectation for children to speak Spanish and English with equal ability is unrealistic especially because they are still acquiring communicative competency in both languages.

Just as researchers in child bilingual studies must define for themselves "bilingual," clinicians may also define for themselves what is true bilingualism among the children they serve. We may each personally define "bilingual" differently based on our experiences. Monolingual clinicians who do not speak a second language and some bilingual clinicians may expect proficiency levels for children that are comparable to monolinguals for each language. Native or natural bilinguals may have a different perspective about children's abilities in two languages. Native speakers may recognize that it is not the proficiency level that makes a competent speaker, but rather the ideas communicated that makes a bilingual accepted within his or her community. If we continue to look only at the surface features or proficiency level of children's language, we misidentify children as language impaired. Equal ability in two languages is unrealistic for children.

BELIEF 2: THE OPTIMUM TIME FOR LEARNING TWO LANGUAGES IS BEFORE THE AGE OF THREE

The acknowledged age range in childhood bilingualism research is through preadolescence (Haugen, 1953). Therefore, researchers have studied the linguistic abilities of children at different ages as well as in different language situations. We know that children do learn second languages at different ages. For example, Leopold (1939–1949) studied his daughter's development of English and German until she was 16 years of age and reported that Hildegard did not have complete grammatical control of both languages until she was 5 years of age. Semantic knowledge in the two languages was described as unequal. Hakuta (1974) documented the English language development of a Japanese 5-year-old child who resisted learning English but eventually did begin to use English in the preschool setting. Kessler (1972) studied Italian-English bilingual children ranging in age from 6 to 8 years. Fantini (1985) detailed his son's bilingualism from 18 months to

10 years of age and provided details of his child's development of English and Spanish after age three. The literature has numerous examples of children learning two languages after age three.

The circumstance for many first and second generation Spanish-speaking children is use of Spanish in the home and English for school and community. The family may not use two languages in the home; therefore, learning two languages before the age of three would be virtually impossible for many of these children. Hispanic children from age 3 years to adolescence are brought daily into the mainstream of American education through Head Start programs, the public schools, and secondary institutions such as churches and other organizations. These children bring language experiences and cognitive strategies that help them learn a second language. What is important to remember is that optimum language learning is not limited to below age three (McLaughlin, 1984). Look at the language environments that the child is presently experiencing and build on his or her knowledge.

BELIEF 3: THE PREFERRED METHOD OF LEARNING A SECOND LANGUAGE IN THE HOME IS TO HAVE ONE PERSON SPEAK LANGUAGE A AND ONE PERSON SPEAK LANGUAGE B

The literature in child bilingualism describes researchers' efforts to separate the languages for the child by using the one person/one language system. These authors were linguists who were fortunate to have cooperative spouses to control the early language environment of the children (Grosjean, 1982). But this type of environment is difficult to maintain. Leopold (1939–1949) moved his family to Germany for 6 months when Hildegard began to prefer English. She quickly developed her German abilities, but when the family returned to the United States, Hildegard quickly regained her English proficiency and consequently lost some abilities in German. Saunders (1982) states that attempts to maintain a one person/one language home environment is difficult because of encounters with the children's friends and relatives. Families cannot insist that extended family members, friends, and community members speak a specific language in front of the child.

Harding and Riley (1986) describe five types of bilingual families (see Table 8–1). Each of these families' language use differ on the basis of the language of necessity and the community language. Only two

TABLE 8–1

Types of bilingual familes.

Family Type	Language Spoken			
	Mother	**Father**	**To Child**	**Community**
I	B	A	B	A
II	B	C & A	B & C	A
III	B	B	B	A
IV	B	C	B & C	A
V	A	A & B	A & B	A

Key: A = Dominant Community Language; B = Native language; C = Second Native language.

Source: Adapted from *The Bilingual Family: A Handbook for Parents* by E. Harding and P. Riley, 1986. New York: Cambridge University Press.

of the five types could possibly use the one person/one language strategy. Arnberg (1979) suggests that this is just one method families may use to develop two languages in their children. Schmidt-Mackey (1971) described four strategies: (1) one person/one language; (2) one language and one place; (3) one language and one time, topic, and activity; and (4) a combination of any of the other strategies. All of these methods appear to produce bilingual speakers.

The Spanish and English environments of children are important considerations. But, the bilingual family or the monolingual Spanish-speaking family is only one of many influences on the language development of children. Bilingual speakers also have societal and individual influences that determine how the person will learn the second language and whether either language is maintained or lost (Kayser, 1993). Societal influences include external factors that impinge on the life of the individual (Conklin & Lourie, 1983). These societal influences include distance and frequency of visits to the home country. The closer and more frequent the visits, the more likely that the home language will be maintained. Rural settlement will maintain the language, whereas urban settlement may help the acquisition of English because of increased numbers of majority language speakers. Greater numbers of Spanish speakers in the community will increase the likelihood of Spanish maintenance. Smaller numbers of Spanish speakers in a community may shift the community into complete assimilation and use of only English within one generation.

Depending on the model of the local educational system, Spanish may be lost within the first year of the child's schooling. Different bilingual program models may result in native language maintenance, bilingualism, or monolingualism in the majority language (Hakuta, 1986; MacLaughlin, 1984). Other factors that work toward maintaining the language include ethnic schooling, Spanish church services, radio, television, and newspapers (Conklin & Lourie, 1983). The family's strategy for bilingualism is only one factor that will determine the child's development and proficiency in two languages (Fishman, 1966; Miller, 1984).

Individual influences are internal factors that may be innate or chosen by the bilingual individual and will vary from person to person (Conklin & Lourie, 1983). Each child will bring affective variables such as a unique personality, motivation, attitudes toward the two cultures, and emotional attachment to the home language. Innate factors may include intelligence, language aptitude, and cognitive strategies. The suggestion that the family is the sole basis of success in learning two languages in addition to limiting the learning environment to a one person/one language model is oversimplifying a dynamic and complex process. Families are important models for attitudes and beginning language learning experiences, but children also learn from peers, siblings, teachers, and other community members.

BELIEF 4: CODE SWITCHING, THE ALTERNATING USE OF TWO LANGUAGES, IS A REFLECTION OF INADEQUATE VOCABULARY IN BOTH LANGUAGES OR WORD FINDING PROBLEMS

Valdes-Fallis (1978) defined code switching as the alternating use of two languages at the word, phrase, clause, or sentence level where there is a clear recognition of each language in pronunciation and form. Code switching among many Hispanic bilinguals is a style of communication where the functions and linguistic ability will vary among speakers. It clearly is a reflection of the culture.

Children who code switch are dependent on the community's acceptance and use of this form of communication. If they are exposed to code switching, they learn the rules of use from the community of adults and other children. For example, we know that normally developing bilingual children will not alternate between two languages with persons who speak only one of the languages (Valdes-Fallis,

1978). Genishi (1981) stated that children generally will choose the language that the interlocutor, child, or adult speaks more fluently. Therefore, a child may switch languages when she or he recognizes that the other speaker has linguistic limitations. They perceive the language choice of the situation, topic, and the language preference of the listener.

Many bilingual children carry the stigma of being incompetent users of two languages (DeBois & Valdes, 1980). It can only be assumed that the expectations and belief system of clinicians concerning child bilingualism may affect and negatively impact the diagnosis and intervention of speech and language impairments in this population. Clinical bias in the form of clinician expectations and beliefs before the tests are selected and administered only support the myth that bilingual children are incompetent users of two languages. It is important to recognize and accept that learning two languages may occur at any age and that each individual has varying linguistic abilities that are functional for their bilingual environments. And finally, bilingualism is the functional use of two languages (Baetens-Beardsmore, 1986) and not the equal knowledge of two languages. A definition of bilingualism that is descriptive of how the languages were developed (e.g., academic versus natural) and to what extent (e.g., active versus passive) will assist clinicians in the assessment and intervention processes more than a broad and exclusive definition such as equal knowledge of two languages.

⊔

LANGUAGE IMPAIRMENTS
IN HISPANIC CHILDREN

A *language disorder* is defined as a significant impairment in the use of language, whether in its representational-cognitive function, communicative-relationship function, or both (Hubbell, 1981). Lahey (1988) has described language disorders as any disruption in learning or use of language content, form, or use in the interacton among these components. The child with a disruption in content may have well-developed form and use interaction but a poorly developed content component. The child may be articulate and fluent, but his or her utterances are inappropriate. The child with a disruption in form will have ideas about world knowledge, and abilities to communicate these ideas are more intact than their abilities to use the linguistic system. The child with a disruption in use will talk about ideas that are out of context and either ramble repetitively or tangentially associate ideas without regard to the listener. Lahey (1988) states that these components may be distorted or separated from each other. Thus children's language impairments can be specific or occur in combination with the other components and be mild, moderate, severe, or profound in severity.

In addition to these types of language impairments, there may also be sequencing problems at any or all levels of language, language processing and word retrieval difficulties, auditory agnosia, echolalia, and perseveration. With these varying possibilities, a child will be unique and have child-specific language impairments (Hubbell, 1981).

Taylor (1986) defines a language disorder among culturally and linguistically different populations as communicative behaviors that are deviant from the norms and expectations of the language community of the individual. Among the heterogeneous bilingual population, Linares (1983) broadly states that a language impairment exists when comprehension and/or expression is unlike the language used by peers and interferes with communication. Omark and Watson (1983) suggested that among bilingual children there are significant delays in receptive and expressive language abilities, delayed association and memory, articulation errors, and problems with code switching.

The research on Spanish-English speaking children has not taken into consideration the wide range of possibilities of language impairment. There have been group as well as individual case study descriptions of language impairments. These children have been described as not having the ability to associate sounds with objects or experiences; discriminate tones, phonemes, and morphemes; remember words; and understand who, what, where, and why questions (Ambert, 1986; Langdon, 1983). Ambert (1986) described Spanish-speaking Puerto Rican language impaired children who had difficulty with the phonemes /s/, /l/, /r/, and /rr/. They substituted, omitted, and distorted sounds, reversed the order of sounds in words and shortened the length of words (i.e., coalescence). In syntax, these children omitted articles, pronouns, prepositions, copulas *ser* and *estar*, auxilliary *estar*, reflexive pronoun *se*, plural endings, and conjunctions. There was incorrect word order, substitutions of the schwa for grammatical structures, difficulty with noun-verb and article-noun agreement, and confusion of verb tenses. In the area of semantics, these children had inappropriate labels for objects, actions, and persons. They circumlocuted when they had retrieval difficulties. The Spanish-speaking children did not retell stories or narrate personal experiences. They could neither correct grammatical errors in a sentence presented to them or problem solve situations.

Bilingual clinicians would probably agree that monolingual Spanish-speaking children are readily identified when the impairment affects the linguistic form, content, and/or use. The problem of describing a language impairment in a bilingual child becomes more difficult because of the possibility of a number of factors, such as second language acquisition that might affect the form, content, and use of the second language and possibly language loss that would affect the form, content, and use of the first language.

The child's comprehension of English and Spanish is often used to identify semantic impairments in children. But this may be misleading because bilinguals do not have the same lexical development in both languages, nor do they achieve comprehension levels comparable to monolingual speakers of either language (Beatens-Beardsmore, 1986). Carrow (1955, 1972) studied normal preschool and school-age bilingual children to determine their comprehension of English using language samples and an experimental version of the *Test for Auditory Comprehension of Language* (Carrow, 1973). She determined that bilingual preschoolers had greater frequency of errors than the monolingual group in all areas tested except in the comprehension of verbs, plurality, is/are, and verb tense (Carrow, 1972). Carrow (1955) also reported a study of 55 normal third grade bilingual and monolingual students, who were similar in socioeconomic status and intelligence, in which no differences were found in the oral language functioning of the monolingual and bilingual children as measured by length of clause, number of words used during a time period, index of subordination, and complexity of sentence structure. Carrow's study did find a significant difference between the two groups in hearing and speaking vocabulary and articulation skills.

Miller (1984) noted that bilingual children frequently will know a word for an object in one language, but not in the other. When they do not know a word, he observed that children with normal language development use gestures, substitute a word in the other language, or circumlocute. The child with difficulties often reacted with silence. Kayser (unpublished data) tape recorded eight bilingual Hispanic children, four normal and four language impaired, matched for age and gender, in a first-grade classroom. Table 8–2 summarizes the chil

Table 8–2
Frequency of words and utterances, range of utterances, and mean length of response for 4 normal and 4 language-impaired bilingual children in a 1-hour classroom language sample.

Measure	Normal	Language Impaired
Number of utterances	614	238
Number of different words	2,537	729
Mean number of utterances	153.5	59.5
Range of utterances	123–186	26–126
Mean length of response per child	4.13	3.06

dren's expressive language skills as they interacted freely with their peers in the classroom. The data reflect 1 hour of classroom interactions. The normal bilingual children had more utterances and words but their mean length of response (MLR, see Chapter 12 for definition) was not different from the language-impaired group of children. Further analysis of the language samples indicated that children in the normal group asked more questions of peers (69 versus 31 for the language-impaired group) and used circumlocution (6 times), whereas children in the language-impaired group did not circumlocute during the 1-hour sampling. For these children, circumlocutions were used to clarify and did not indicate a problem with expression.

What is lacking in these few studies is an acknowledgement that individual bilingual children have specific difficulties that cannot be compared with other children. Studying large groups of Spanish-speaking children and clustering the language difficulties does not clearly describe the uniqueness of the impairment that each child may present. No two children will be identical in their bilingual language proficiency, nor will any two children be identical in their language impairment.

⊔

CASE STUDIES

The following case studies are an attempt to describe the communicative abilities of three bilingual children who were identified as language impaired. The purpose of this section is to illustrate the importance of in-depth knowledge about a child's background, community, and language experiences in assessing the status of a child's communicative competency and determining whether a language impairment truly exists.

Ethnography has been recommended as the research methodology of choice for children from culturally and linguistically different backgrounds (Saville-Troike, 1986; Taylor, 1986). This methodology is time-consuming, but the information that is acquired will assist clinicians in differentiating language differences from language impairments. The children studied were observed and tape recorded, and their parents, teachers, and community members were interviewed over a 4-month period.

THE CHILDREN

Lupita (first grade), David (second grade), and Pete (third grade) are bilingual Mexican American children who were labeled as language impaired. They entered school speaking only Spanish but later lost their ability to speak the home language. The children had similar economic and social backgrounds, and were similar in their testing profiles. All had been retained once, and were receiving language intervention.

Each child also tried to follow classroom rules and, therefore, did not talk loudly (Kayser, 1985, 1987, 1990). They understood that loud and too much talking would eventually mean the elimination of their privileges with friends. Lupita and David were very similar in their interactions with school friends. Pete had a different relationship with the children in his classroom. Both Lupita and David had friends who were in low- and high-achieving reading groups. They had peers who initiated talk with them; therefore, they were not always the initiators of conversations with classmates. Both were observed to organize games outdoors and with small groups in the classroom. Both were discreet in their use of their hands or body so not to call attention to themselves when speaking to their friends in the room. Nonverbal communication with friends was frequent and included smiles; frowns; eye movements to direct the listener to an object; person, or activity; and head nodding or shaking.

Pete, on the other hand, did not show these interaction patterns with his peers. All of his friends were low-achieving students. Pete talked to himself and this visibly annoyed the children around him.

Other children did not initiate conversation with him, rather he joined the ongoing conversations of the children and/or just listened. He did attempt to contribute to their conversations, but the intent of his comments was critical and therefore negatively received by the other children. He was not observed to organize play among his friends. Pete used overt behavioral movements for requesting and controlling the behavior of male friends.

Although there were distinct differences in the peer relationships and behaviors in and out of the classroom, academically, Lupita and David were both seen by the teachers as needing language intervention while Pete was viewed to be like any other child in the classroom. Lupita and David were poor readers; Pete was an average student who academically was on grade level. The teachers' perceptions of these children did not appear to be substantiated by the children's communicative behaviors in and out of the classroom.

LUPITA

Lupita did not talk readily to strangers and appeared at first to be in a world of her own. She went through the motions concerning classroom routines, following the teachers' instructions, slightly delayed in reaction time, but she did eventually follow through. She appeared to prefer coloring her papers, rearranging crayons in her crayon box, or sending signals to one of her five girlfriends in the classroom. Their favorite meeting place to exchange a few words was the water fountain near the class restroom door. There the girls could talk before one returned to her seat and the other entered the restroom.

Lupita received language intervention in a group session with two boys from her classroom. Lupita's mother stated that Lupita hated boys. There were primarily male siblings in her home, so she did not enjoy being placed in therapy with more boys. She considered them *mocosos* (snotty) and would not play with them in the neighborhood or playground. Lupita did not receive any special services other than oral language development from an English as a Second Language (ESL) aide. Because the teacher believed that she was getting sufficient language development assistance from the speech-language pathologist, the teacher eventually requested that Lupita exit the ESL aide program. Thus, Lupita received language instruction for 15 minutes per day and had been in therapy for 1 year.

Lupita's teacher was bilingual, but she did not use Spanish for classroom instruction. She considered Lupita's English language skills as "terrible." Lupita was described as low achieving in spelling, writing, and reading. The teacher considered Lupita to be a low level student who had a difficult time with academics.

Lupita and her mother both expressed Lupita's dislike of school. She would get up in the morning upset because she had to get dressed and face the day. The mother reported that at least once a week Lupita would ask for a day off from school, and attendance records confirmed Lupita's high absenteeism. Her mother and grandfather spoke of several instances when Lupita went to the bus stop and hid behind the large tree next to her home. The bus driver could not see Lupita, so the bus passed the house.

Lupita did not appear to like using Spanish. The mother and uncle expressed how Lupita would get upset with her brothers and uncles because they all spoke Spanish to her. She told them that they would never get ahead or learn anything unless they stopped speaking Spanish. The mother was concerned about this attitude because it had affected Lupita's relationship with the rest of the family. Lupita loved her father and would speak to him in Spanish and had conversations with him about his work.

DAVID

David was a gentleman and went out of his way to open doors for the teacher and other students. He followed all of the rules in the classroom and had many friends in the classroom.

The teacher, who was monolingual English-speaking, considered David to be low average. She stated that he was courteous and polite. He tried very had to do his work but still had problems with reading and understanding the assignments. David also was in the special education resource room for 2 hours a day for reading and spelling. His mother and teacher reported that he disliked the resource room because he did not like the work and strict environment. The resource teacher believed that David needed to be in a self-contained special education classroom because he did not do any of the work in her room, and she, therefore, assumed that he could not do the work. The regular classroom teacher did not agree, because he worked well in her classroom. David also received language intervention for conversational language usage for 30 minutes twice a week. He had been in therapy for 2 years.

David did not like speaking Spanish. His mother and sister reported that he would become upset with his mother because she used Spanish in the house and with her friends. When the family visited Mexico, David did not try to communicate with relatives, but relied on his mother to interpret for him. He loved his grandparents who lived in the house next door. They spoke only Spanish and he understood them and enjoyed their company. They did not require him to speak the language.

PETE

Pete enjoyed talking with his friends but frequently was not understood by the other children in his classroom. He talked to himself while he worked, and this annoyed the students who sat around him. He also was a gentleman to the girls in the room. With the boys he knew who had authority and would exercise his power over the boys who did not have peer status in the social hierarchy of the classroom.

Pete had a bubbly personality. Everything that came his way was taken in stride. If his papers were completed incorrectly, he would redo the assignment without an argument or complaint. The teacher described Pete as a hard worker and a strong average student. She did not know why he was receiving language intervention. He did all of his work, he read at grade level, but he did have difficulty with writing. Pete received speech-language intervention for syntax and question development twice a week and had been in therapy for 5 years. He did not receive any other special service.

What was interesting about Pete and his siblings was that they were all receiving speech-language services. They made fun of each other and talked about how they used to say words. They would practice saying new vocabulary and laughed at their own attempts at pronouncing multisyllabic words. Even Pete's 5-year-old sibling, corrected his speech.

The parents stated that they both used Spanish in the home. Pete enjoyed speaking Spanish and would listen to the adults in the neighborhood and attempted to use the language with them. He also enjoyed visiting Mexico and attempted to use his limited Spanish skills with his extended family. His attitude toward Spanish was positive, and he actively initiated interactions with adults who could speak the language.

THE DIAGNOSES

Pete was orginally identified as language-impaired through a kindergarten screening and was considered to be high risk because of a language delay and familial history. The parents had an Rh-negative blood factor that required blood transfusion for the first child but only injections of medication for Pete when he was born. All of Pete's siblings and he himself had a history of high fevers and scarlet fever. His mother described him as being slow in talking, *se tardo mijo* (my son was late).

Lupita and David both had normal births with no problems during their mothers' pregnancies. Both were viewed as normal in physical and language development by their parents. When the parents were informed that their children had a language impairment at the end of the first grade, neither set of parents could understand how their child could have problems with language because they perceived the child as a good communicator.

All three children had average intelligence. Lupita and David had below average skills in academics. The language tests supplied by the speech-language pathologists indicated that David had a large battery of tests with most scores indicating "average skills." *The Test of Language Development* (Newcomer & Hammill, 1988) and the *Test of Early Language Development* (Hresko, Reid, & Hammill, 1981) indicated "within normal range skills," but the other two tests, the *Token Test for Children* (DiSimoni, 1978) and the *Clinical Evaluation of Language Functions* (Semel, Wiig, & Secord, 1989) rated David poorly in receptive language abilities. A language sample was not obtained so David was placed on the basis of receptive or auditory language disabilities. No Spanish tests were administered.

Lupita, on the other hand, had received only one language test. She did not do well on this instrument, and no other tests were administered. Although Lupita was bilingual and her home language was Spanish, she was not tested in Spanish. A language sample was not obtained, but her conversational skills were judged informally and assessed to be inadequate. Her language impairment was determined to be expressive and receptive in nature.

Pete was the only child who was referred in kindergarten for speech difficulties. There were more references in his file to inability to express himself, difficulty with articulation, and problems with moving the oral mechanism, all of which were verified by the parent in the case history. The parents reported that he continued to have difficulty expressing himself.

The test data for each of these children were not systematically or uniformly obtained. The children had taken different batteries of tests, and the results were interpreted by the clinicians' judgment. David and Lupita had no measures of their Spanish comprehension and expressive abilities on file, although Spanish was their home language. Additionally, their parents did not believe anything was wrong with their children's speech and language development. On the other hand, Pete's family recognized that he had speech and language difficulties, and his developmental and medical history supported and confirmed those observations.

LINGUISTIC COMPETENCY

As clinicians we often examine a child's language form to determine whether a language impairment exists. Tests and language samples often serve as measures. Among bilingual children, the focus on form may be problematic because the majority of second language learners may have difficulty with English form, especially with morphology. Therefore, observation may be necessary to ensure that what is measured and how a child communicates with the clinician are not factors of an unknown social interaction (e.g., the testing situation or lack of experience with English) (Kayser, 1989; Taylor, 1986). Second language learners do have a variety of linguistic skills, and how these are viewed by clinicians, teachers, and parents is critical to the accurate identification of a language impairment.

Although all three children described here had some difficulty with syntax and morphology, Pete's use of language form was different. What made Pete's expressive language different? His linguistic form was telegraphic, lacking prosody. He omitted morphological markers, irregular forms of verbs and plurals, conjunctions, prepositions, pronouns, and auxiliary verbs. He appeared to want to say more and often began his utterances with a starter phrase, but his messages were never completed (e.g., "I'm gonna make-ummmm, Who gots the-ummmm"). This lack of fine-tuning in Pete's expressive language could be viewed as part of second language learning, but it was more his difficulty in learning new forms and lack of generalization from his intervention sessions that made his use of form appear impaired.

For example, when Pete asked questions in class and in therapy, his inability to correctly phrase his questions was not typical of a second language learner. Gestures also often accompanied his questions. In a game of 20 questions during one therapy session, Pete did not appropriately use the targeted question form.

Pete: Is it something for you put money in?

Clinician: Let's say it again.

Pete: It is something that money put money in?

Pete: It is something your eat?

Clinician: No.

Pete: Is it something made out a a ice?

Clinician: Made our *of* ice?

Pete: (nods)

Note that Pete had already been in therapy for 5 years, and this procedure had been used for two academic semesters.

Determining whether a language impairment exists in a bilingual child should be confirmed through information obtained from the parents, teachers, and the clinician's testing. Pete's parents and the clinician recognized that a language impairment existed, but the teacher related Pete's language impairment with academic classroom difficulty. The teacher defined language impairment differently from what the clinician was assessing. Pete was an average student, and therefore, the teacher did not believe Pete was language impaired. For Lupita and David, the teachers and clinicians believed they had language impairments, but the parents did not confirm or agree with the diagnoses.

⊔

CONCLUSIONS

As speech-language pathologists, we are ready to assess the speech and language abilities of bilingual children, but often fail to look at the child as a person who has been affected by society and individual choices. The societal influences in the communities of these three children were extremely different and did have an effect on the children's use of English and Spanish. Lupita, who lived in a Spanish-speaking community and home environment, refused to participate in that environment. She used English whenever possible and thereby isolated herself from the family. Her English skills, as described by the teacher and clinician, were poor. The formal and informal evaluations by these professionals may have had an effect on Lupita's own attitude toward her home language. She did not want to participate in speaking Spanish at home and looked for English speakers to improve her English language. David, who was in an English-speaking community and a Spanish-speaking home, also did not attempt to use Spanish. He did not want his mother to use Spanish in their home but was in daily companionship with his Spanish-speaking grandparents. David had support in the use of English from school, neighborhood friends, and merchants. Although he had good English skills, David was assessed and judged on his auditory processing and vocabulary skills. Both of these areas would be greatly affected by his bilingual environment. Pete, on the other hand, lived in a bilingual community and home. His parents had a positive attitude toward both languages, and Pete enjoyed speaking both languages.

All three children had different attitudes and opportunities to use English and Spanish; therefore, their abilities in the two languages were different. They lived in different environments. None of the children began their bilingualism before the age of 3 years and they did not have equal ablities in both languages. None were fortunate to have the one parent/one language environment, and none of the children used code switching.

Pete was the only child who could, with certainty, be labeled as language impaired. His case history, familial background, siblings' difficulties with language, kindergarten referral, and peer interactions all point to a diagnosis of language impairment.

In contrast to Pete, there is uncertainty about whether David and Lupita were indeed language impaired. Both children had questionable and incomplete evaluations, parents who insisted that they had appropriate language skills for their age and community, case histories that were medically uneventful, and referrals that were based on academic performance in an English-only environment when both were primarily Spanish-speaking when they entered school. It is likely that both David and Lupita were victims of language loss, lack of bilingual education, and inappropriate testing procedures.

The purpose of this chapter was to present the complexity of factors that must be considered when determining whether a language impairment exists in children who speak two languages. Testing children with a few tests does not adequately sample the scope and depth of what children learn in their homes and school environments. This chapter reviewed some of the myths clinicians may have concerning bilingualism in children and how these myths may affect the clinicians' approaches to the assessment process and ultimately the differential diagnosis. These were countered with a brief discussion of what is known about bilingualism in children and language impairments in Hispanic children. Finally, three case studies were presented to illustrate the complexity and contribution of the child's language environment to the child's communicative competency, attitude toward language, and academic achievement.

⊔

REFERENCES

Ambert, A. N. (1986). Identifying language disorders in Spanish-speakers. In A. C. Willig & H. F. Greenberg (Eds.), *Bilingualism and learning disabilities* (pp. 15–33). Princeton, NJ: American Library.

Arnberg, L. (1979). Language strategies in mixed nationality families. *Scandinavian Journal of Psychology, 20,* 105–112.

Arnberg, L. (1987). *Raising children bilingually: The pre-school years.* Philadelphia, PA: Multilingual Matters.

Baetens-Beardsmore, H. (1986). *Bilingualism: Basic principles.* London: Treto, Ltd.

Bloomfield, L. (1935). *Language.* London: Allen & Unwin.

Carrow, M. A. (1955). *A comparative study of the linguistic functioning of bilingual Spanish-American children and monolingual Anglo-American children at the third grade level.* Unpublished doctoral dissertaion, Northwestern University, Evanston, IL.

Carrow, E. (1972). Auditory comprehension of English by monolingual and bilingual preschool children. *Journal of Speech and Hearing Research, 55,* 299–306.

Carrow, E. (1973). *Test for Auditory Comprehension of Language.* Allen, TX: DLM Teaching Resources.

Conklin, N. F., & Lourie, M. A. (1983). *Host of tongues: Language commnities in the United States.* New York: The Free Press.

DeSimoni, F. (1978). *The Token Test for Children.* Hingham, MA: Teaching Resources.

Dubois, B. L. & Valdes, G. (1980). Mexican-American child bilingualism: Double deficit? *The Bilingual Review, 7*(1), 1–7.

Fantini, A. E. (1985). *Language acquisition of a bilingual child.* San Diego, CA: College-Hill Press.

Fishman, J. A. (1966). *Language loyalty in the United States.* The Hague, Netherlands: Mouton.

Genishi, C. (1981). Codeswitching in Chicano six-year olds. In R. P. Duran (Ed.), *Latino language and communicative behavior* (pp. 133–152). Norwood, NJ: Ablex.

Grosjean, F. (1982). *Life with two languages: An introduction to bilingualism.* Cambridge: Harvard University Press.

Hakuta, K. (1974). A preliminary report on the development of grammatical morphemes in a Japanese girl learning English as a second language. *Working Papers in Bilingualism, 3,* 18–38.

Hakuta, K. (1986). *Mirror of language: The debate on bilingualism.* New York: Basic Books.

Halliday, M. A. K., McKintosh, A., & Strevens, P. (1972). The users and uses of language. In J. Fishman, (Ed.), *Sociology of language* (pp. 139–169). The Hague, Netherlands: Mouton.

Harding, E., & Riley, P. (1986). *The bilingual family: A handbook for parents.* New York: Cambridge University Press.

Haugen, E. (1953). *The Norwegian language in America* (2 vols.). Philadelphia: University of Pennsylvania Press.

Hresko, W. P., Reid, D. K., & Hammill, D. D. (1981). *Test of Early Language Development.* Austin, TX: Pro-Ed.

Hubbell, R. (1981). *Children's language disorders: An integrated approach.* Englewood Cliffs, NJ: Prentice-Hall.

Kayser, H. (1985). *A study of speech-language pathologists and their Mexican American language disordered caseloads.* Unpublished doctoral dissertation, New Mexico State University, Las Cruces.

Kayser, H. (1987). A study of three Mexican American children labeled language disordered. *The Journal of the National Association for Bilingual Education. 12*(1), 1–22.

Kayser, H. (1989). Speech and language assessment of Spanish-English speaking children. *Language Speech, Hearing Services Schools, 20,* 226–244.

Kayser, H. (1990). Social communicative behaviours of language-disordered Mexican-American students. *Child language Teaching Therapy. 6*(3), 255–269.

Kayser, H. (1993). Hispanic cultures. In D. Battle (Ed.), *Communication disorders in multicultural populations* (pp. 114–157). Boston: Andover Medical Publishers.

Kessler, C. (1972). Syntactic contrasts in child bilingualism. *Language Learning. 22,* 221–223.

Kessler, C. (1984). Language acquisition in bilingual children. In N. Miller (Ed.) *Bilingual and language disability.* San Diego, CA: College-Hill Press.

Lahey, M. (1988). *Language disorders and language development.* New York: Macmillan.

Langdon, H. (1983). Assessment and intervention strategies for the bilingual language disordered student. *Exceptional Children, 50,* 37–56.

Leopold, W. F. (1939, 1947, 1949). *Speech development of a bilingual child: A linguist's record* (Vols. 1–4). Evanston, IL: Northwestern University Press.

Linares, N. (1983). Management of communicatively handicapped Hispanic American children. In D. R. Omark & J.G. Erickson (Eds.), *The bilingual exceptional child* (pp. 145–162). San Diego, CA: College-Hill Press.

MacNamara, J. (1967). The bilingual's linguistic performance: A psychological overview. *Journal of Social Issues, 23*(2), 58–77.

McLaughlin, B. (1984). *Second-language acquisition in childhood: Vol. 1 Preschool children* (2nd ed.). Hillsdale, NJ: Lawrence Erlbaum.

Miller, N. (1984). *Bilingualism and language disability: Assessment and remediation.* San Diego, CA: College-Hill Press.

Newcomer, P. L., & Hammill, D. (1988). *Test of Language Development (Revised) Primary*. Austin, TX: Pro-Ed.

Omark, D. R., & Watson, D. L. (1983). *Assessing bilingual exceptional children: In-service manual*. San Diego, CA: Los Amigos Research Associates.

Saunders, G. (1982). Infant bilingualism: A look at some doubts and objections. *Journal of Multilingual and Multicultural Development, 3*, 277–292.

Saville-Troike, M. (1986). Anthropological considerations in the study of communication. In O. L. Taylor (Ed.), *Nature of communication disorders in culturally and linguistically diverse populations* (pp. 47–72). San Diego, CA: College-Hill Press.

Schmidt-Mackey, I. (1971, November). *Language strategies of the bilingual family*. Paper presented at the Conference on Child Language, Chicago. (Eric Document Reproduction, Service No. ED 060 740)

Semel, E., Wiig, E. H. & Secord, W. (1989). *Clinical Evaluation of Language Fundamentals—Revised*. Austin, TX: The Psychological Corporation.

Taylor, O. L. (Ed.). (1986). *Nature of communication disorders in culturally and linguistically diverse populations*. San Diego, CA: College-Hill Press.

Valdes-Fallis, G. (1978). *Language in education: Theory and practice, code switching and the classroom teacher*. Arlington, VA: Center for Applied Linguistics.

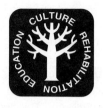

CHAPTER 9

INTERPRETERS

HORTENCIA KAYSER, Ph.D.

Speech-language pathologists have recognized that support personnel are necessary in their profession to meet the growing demands for speech-language and hearing services (ASHA, 1981). Utilization of support personnel with underserved populations, such as American Indians, the economically disadvantaged, remote/rural residents, linguistic minorities, institutionalized, and developing regions, makes it possible for services to be provided where traditional service delivery models have been difficult to implement (ASHA, 1988). As the general population continues to grow with increasing numbers of racially and ethnically different individuals, speech-language pathologists are using support personnel to serve as interpreters and translators in assessment and intervention. The majority of the literature in this emerging service delivery model has focused on the monolingual English-speaking support person working with monolingual clinicians. Little has been mentioned concerning the use of culturally and linguistically different individuals as support personnel with minority language clients. Bilingual support personnel face a different set of issues when they provide support for diagnostic assessments and intervention. Additionally, although bilingual speech-language pathologists normally work alone with bilingual clients, they should also consider using bilingual speech and language assistants to meet the growing demand from Hispanic populations.

This chapter will discuss issues in the selection and training of support personnel, specifically their use as interpreters and translators. A definition of interpreters and translators will be provided and a review of the suggested educational requirements for speech-language assistants, program training models, suggested assistant activities, and best utilization practices will be discussed.

ᛄ

A DEFINITION OF INTERPRETER AND TRANSLATOR

Although, the American Speech-Language-Hearing Association (ASHA) (1981, 1993) has addressed the use of support personnel with English-speaking clients, the roles of interpreter and translator have not yet been defined within the profession. The roles of interpreter and translator must be clearly defined in any work setting because these roles are different and require specialized skills. Langdon (1992a) states that an interpreter conveys information from one language to the other in the oral modality, and the translator uses the written modality. The translator and interpretor each require different abilities in the use of language.

Kayser (1993), Langdon (1992a), and Matsuda and O'Conner (1993) have recommended linguistic and educational qualifications for interpreters or translators. When these individuals have fulfilled the linguistic and educational requirements, their scope of practice may include clinical conferences, assessment, and intervention. Interpreters and translators have a formidable responsibility to convey accurate information from the clinician to the client and, therefore, must have the linguistic, educational, and clinical training that will appropriately meet the needs of culturally and linguistically diverse populations. It cannot be assumed that any individual who speaks two languages has the ability to interpret accurately for families and professionals.

ᄂᄀ

ASHA AND SUPPORT PERSONNEL

The issue surrounding the use of support personnel has been discussed for over 20 years. The American Speech-Language-Hearing
Association first published guidelines for training and supervising
support personnel in the professions in 1981. More recently, guidelines and certification of support personnel have been reviewed by the
membership (ASHA, 1993). Excluded in both of these documents are
the roles of the interpreter and translator.

The primary issues surrounding the use of support personnel as
interpreters and translators must be viewed from the perspective of culturally and linguistically diverse populations with communicative
impairments, the speech-language pathology assistant, and the speech-
language pathologist. There is no question that the clinician's and assistant's knowledge and understanding of their roles will affect the quality
of service provided to clients with speech and language impairments.

Individuals with communicative impairments who come from culturally and linguistically diverse populations must have the highest
quality of service from the best qualified personnel available. Unfortunately, there is a paucity of qualified bilingual speech-language pathologists and audiologists to provide clinical services, although there are
agencies with high numbers of clients from culturally and linguistically
different populations. These agencies must provide services in some
form or the clients will not receive any assessment or intervention programs. In many situations, the individual who is called on to assist the
speech-language pathologist is a secretary, janitor, or a professional in
the agency. When there are bilingual "on call" assistants, the services
that are rendered may be compromised. The client's perceptions of the
professions are based on the interpretation of an untrained volunteer.
The credibility of clinicians does depend on the effectiveness of the
interpreter. Individuals who assist monolingual and bilingual professionals should have training and minimum competencies to more than
minimally serve this growing population (ASHA, 1988).

The assistants who serve as interpreters should have a sense of
reward from their work, but often the individual who assists the clinician may be annoyed, angered, insulted, embarrassed, and possibly a
number of other descriptors. These individuals may not understand the

clinician's professional language and thus become frustrated because of their inability to interpret what is said. If the interpreter does not understand the clinician's explanations to the family, the attempts for clarification may be viewed as the interpreter's difficulties rather than the clinician's abilities to explain matters in a language level suitable for interpretation. Often, interpreters serve in this capacity because they want to serve their own community, therefore, we, as a professionals, have an obligation to train them so that they will be effective assistants. Assistants should have an understanding of the process of interpretation and translation so that they can provide the highest quality of service to multicultural populations, whether in a conference setting, during assessment, or while implementing an intervention program.

In the same regard, speech-language pathologists are asked to implement programs and provide assessments using support personnel, but they may not have received any instruction in the use of assistants. Speech-language pathologists who occasionally or frequently use interpreters have a common concern: the clinician lacks control of the ongoing process and progress of the client because of the language barrier (Roseberry-McKibbin & Eicholtz, 1994). The clinician's inability to understand the client lowers the level of services to clients to the judgment of an assistant. It cannot be assumed that training and utilizing an assistant or interpreter is an easily developed skill for the majority of clinicians. Professionals must be trained to utilize interpreters in the different capacities that are possible when providing clinical services.

The client, the bilingual speech-language assistant, and the speech-language pathologist each has expectations when entering the clinical event (Taylor, 1986). The client expects the best possible service, the assistant expects to provide appropriate services, and the clinician should know what must be accomplished. Ultimately, it is the speech-language pathologist who is responsible for the overall management of the client's progress through the aid of a bilingual speech and language assistant.

⼬

THE WHO, WHAT, AND HOW OF INTERPRETERS AND ASSISTANTS

The focus of discussion for this section will be on the interpreter, because this is the role most often taken by assistants in school systems, clinics, and hospitals. There are three issues or questions that immediately affect the clinician concerning the use of interpreter-assistants: Who may be an interpreter-assistant? What may an interpreter-assistant do? and How may an interpreter-assistant be best utilized? Each of these questions will be discussed briefly.

WHO MAY BE AN INTERPRETER?

There are basic qualifications that ASHA (1981) recommends when hiring support personnel. These include possession of a high school diploma or its equivalent, adequate communication skills, and the ability to relate to the clinical population being served. A draft position statement of the American Speech-Language-Hearing Association (ASHA, 1993) may upgrade these requirements to a minimum of an associate degree or equivalent course work. Practicum experience may be required, and credentialing by ASHA will monitor the assistant's credential renewals, formal examination, and the number of certified clinicians supervising each assistant. Although, these are proposed requirements, a position statement that includes examination and credentialing will benefit clients and clinicians.

In addition to these qualifications recommended by ASHA, Langdon (1988) stated that the interpreter or translator should have a high degree of oral proficiency and literacy in both English and the minority language. They should be able to shift styles depending on the dialect used, be able to memorize and retain chunks of information while interpreting, and have a command of the medical, educational, and speech-language pathology and audiology terminology. Matsuda and O'Conner (1993) recommended that the individual should be able to read passages in English and the second language, translate each passage, and discuss the content of the passage. Additionally, the interpreter should be able to pass an informal cloze test and pass an interview in English. There are language departments in universities that can provide these types of examinations. Some states also offer language proficiency examinations for bilingual educators, and these might be substituted for the recommended tasks.

Finding individuals with the recommended linguistic skills may be problematic, because the majority of bilinguals who were born and educated in the United States are not proficient in reading and writing in Spanish. Native bilinguals may also use a variety of Spanish that is not a standard form of Spanish, yet they are bilingual and actively use the English and Spanish spoken in their communities. The standards for language proficiency may have to be flexible so that interpreter-assistants who are not literate in their home language can still be used for a limited number of activities, defined by the supervising clinician. Recognition of the bilingual assistant's limitations assures the clinician of the appropriateness of the services rendered.

There are professional responsibilities and ethics that need to be developed in addition to having proficiency in two languages. The interpreter must maintain confidentiality, neutrality, accept the clinician's authority, and be able to work with other professional staff. The role and responsibilities of interpreters have to expand to include these areas so that professional standards are maintained in service delivery.

Considering these language and professional competencies, it is recommended that the interpreter not be a client's friend or a family member (ASHA, 1985; Langdon, 1988). Unfortunately, a member of the client's family or a friend is too often asked to interpret. This may lead to a number of problems. Information may be misunderstood, not relayed accurately, or purposely omitted. Reasons for inaccurate interpretation may range from embarrassment concerning the content of the clinician's questions to not understanding the information that is to be interpreted. The next most likely person to be called in to interpret is the bilingual secretary, clerk, or aide. Being bilingual or a native-born speaker of a language does not necessarily qualify an individual to be an interpreter (Baetens-Beardsmore, 1986). Native bilinguals may be able to fluently discuss topics related to home, church, and community, but not have the vocabulary to discuss topics related to medical, educational, and psychological examinations. It cannot be overemphasized that interpreters should be trained and have both linguistic and professional competencies.

If a family member or friend is not appropriate, then who may be an interpreter? If interpreters are used rarely, ASHA (1985) recommends that they may be recruited through professional foreign language schools and universities. Sources for recruiting interpreters also include local churches, educational settings, foreign missions, and cultural centers. Additionally, professional co-workers may be recruited. Paredes-Scribner (1993) suggests that co-workers may be preferable as interpreters when trained support personnel are not available. Individuals within the school, clinic, or hospital already know the policies and programs in the agency. Volunteer interpreters or translators from outside the setting may require training and additional preparation time for a conference or assessment session.

TRAINING

A number of models have been developed for using support personnel but only two models, those proposed by Langdon (1992a) and
Matsuda and O'Connor (1993), train interpreters and translators as
support personnel in speech-language pathology. Both models are
similar in content, except that Langdon proposes that the culture of
the children be part of the training curriculum. Matsuda and O'Connor's program includes instruction in four areas (Table 9–1): (1) basics;
(2) assessment; (3) intervention; and (4) good to know (optional). The
first section introduces the role of the interpreter, functions of the clinician and assistant, protocol, and team dynamics. The assessment
module discusses team assessment, testing procedures, methods, and
principles of assessment, and test administration. The intervention
module has sections concerning team intervention, the learning process, methodology, procedures, and behavior management. The
fourth session is a basic understanding of first- and second-language
acquisition and recognizing different types of communicative disorders. These modules are didactic and presented over the course of an
academic year. Matsuda (personal communication, 1994) stated that
clinical practicum was provided through team assignments with
graduate students in speech-language pathology, thereby providing
both assistants and graduate clinicians specialized team experience in
assessment and intervention.

Langdon (1992a) developed a training manual for interpreters/
translators and special education staff. The manual is a detailed curriculum with a number of activities for training purposes. The manual
has five sections: (1) roles and responsibilities of the interpreter/trans-
lator and professionals; (2) the process of interpreting; (3) training
activities; (4) supplementary information; and (5) sample agendas
(Table 9–2).

Once the speech-language pathologist selects a training program,
the clinician must keep in mind the bilingual assistant's learning and
language differences. Matsuda and O'Connor (1993) gave suggestions
that should increase communication effectiveness during training.
They stated that the clinician should use an elaborated code so that
information is relayed clearly to the interpreter. This may require
explanations of acronyms, professional terms, and figurative uses of
language. Outlines and written information may be helpful to some
interpreter-assistants, thereby giving the trainees a written explanation with the oral presentation. Finally, they suggest that extraneous

TABLE 9–1

Outline of training modules.

Module	Content	Time
I. Basics	Role of interpreter/translator Function of the communication specialist Function of the bilingual paraprofessional Professional protocol Working as a member of a team	3 hrs.
II. Assessment	The bilingual assessment team Testing procedures Methods of assessment Principles of assessment Test administration	3 hrs.
III. Intervention	Intervention team Understanding the learning process Methodology Delivering the lesson Behavior management	3 hrs.
IV. Good to Know	Basic understanding of first and second language acquisition Recognizing different types of communicative disorders	3 hrs.

Source: From "Creating an Effective Partnership: Training Bilingual Communication Aides" by M. Matsuda & L. C. O'Connor, 1993. Paper presented at the California Speech and Hearing Association, Palm Springs, CA.

noises during training do interfere with communication and learning for trainees and should be minimized. The speech-language pathologist should remember that many bilingual individuals need cues and extra assistance in their second language to learn about a new profession. Patience and persistence are critical to the success of their training.

Interpreters and assistants come from different ethnic and racial groups and have differing levels of proficiency in English and Spanish (Matsuda & O'Connor, 1993). They should receive the best possible training to prepare them for the tasks that speech-language pathologists and audiologists may require. Matsuda and O'Connor (1993) noted that these individuals frequently will return to their work settings without extra compensation, receive no recognition for their

TABLE 9–2
Interpreter/translator process in the educational setting.

Section 1. Roles and responsibilities of the assessment team members
Role of the interpreter/translator (I/T)
Qualifications of an I/T
Responsibilities of the special education staff
Responsibilities of the I/T

Section 2. The interpretation process
Dynamics of interpretation
The three basic steps of the interpreting process
How to facilitate the process of interpretation
Advantages/disadvantages of the I/T process and solutions

Section 3. Supplementary training materials
Examples of errors in interpreting
Suggested formats to deliver the content of manual
Study guides
Role play activities

Section 4. Supplementary information
Legal aspects of bilingual and special education
Roles and responsibilities of the special education staff
Cultural notes
Assertiveness training
Translation practice

Source: Adapted from "Interpreter/Translator Process in the Educational Setting" by H. W. Langdon, 1993. Program Curriculum and Training Unit, Special Education Division, California Department of Education. Sacramento, CA.

skills, and yet continue to work in this role to help clients and their families. This pride and need for service to the community should be a major reason for clinicians to always address these persons with respect and gratitude when jobs are well done.

WHAT MAY AN INTERPRETER DO?

The speech-language pathologist or audiologist is the professional responsible for all decisions in assessment, conferences, and intervention (ASHA, 1981, 1988, 1993); therefore, the interpreter's activities should have been reviewed and assigned by the clinician. These activities can be divided into three areas: the assessment, the conference, and the intervention phases.

ASSESSMENT

Omark and Watson (1981) recommend that the interpreter be involved in the total assessment process. The interpreter must have an understanding of the rationale, procedures, and information that is obtained from tests. They should be allowed to review the test questions and examine them for cultural relevancy. Any changes in test stimuli should always be validated through another bilingual from the community. Omark and Watson (1981) also recommend that the interpreter be taught to probe during testing without supplying the client with answers. Interpreters may be trained to administer a variety of tests, obtain questionnaire information, and elicit language samples. In addition, ASHA (1993) suggests that the assistant may be involved in speech-language and hearing screenings, scheduling activities, preparing charts, recording, and displaying test data.

A number of tests are available in Spanish which the interpreter-assistant can be trained to administer (Deal & Rodriguez, 1987). The critical factors are adequate training for the interpreter in the administration of these tests and reliability checks to ensure that the interpreter has the skill necessary to administer and score each test accurately and reliably. An interpreter could first be trained to administer the test instrument in English so that the clinician is assured that the test is administered in a standardized manner. Practice in test administration could be gradual, first scoring a new test with the assistance of videotapes, other personnel, and then with clients. Keep in mind that the trainee's English language proficiency will affect his or her reliability in administering and scoring the tests; therefore, the clinician must use judgment concerning reliability in the minority language. A possible solution to this dilemma is to train two bilingual assistants and have them learn to administer and score instruments using videotapes. They can then score items and discuss acceptable and error responses.

Another possible activity for the interpreter is administering the case history and/or other questionnaires concerning language skills or family background. The experienced assistant also could provide insight into the sensitivity of the questions and assist the clinician in adapting the case history and questionnaires to more reliably obtain family histories.

Language samples may be elicited through, peer- or sibling-child interactions. The interpreter-assistant may then be responsible for transcribing these audio- or videotapes. Analysis and interpretation would be a joint effort. With experience and guidance from the clinician, it is possible for the technician to eventually score tapes independently. This could be accomplished through the use of criterion-referenced lists or categories that are considered to be important for assessment. A reliability check on the accuracy of the transcription and analysis could be performed by another interpreter-assistant until the clinician has confidence in the assistant's work. Interpretation of language samples would always be the responsibility of the speech-language pathologist.

CONFERENCES

The initial conference with the family is critical for understanding the needs of the client. The interpreter serves as the bridge between the agency and the home (Langdon, 1992b). With the interpreter's assistance, rapport may be developed with the family, thereby assisting the clinician in obtaining information concerning the client's communicative competency in the home language. Additionally, information from the family may identify the client's needs in the clinical and educational settings. In this important role, the interpreter must be accurate in relaying questions and responses from the family and the clinician. Unfortunately, there may be miscommunication between the family and the clinician because of interpretation errors.

Langdon (1988) states that there are four common types of changes in information that an interpreter may make during a conference session. The interpreter may omit, add, substitute, or transform the clinician's messages. The omission of information may be at the word, phrase, or sentence levels. The reasons for omitting the utterance may be that the interpreter does not believe a specific word is important to relay, or he or she may not understand the English word, phrase, or sentence. It is also possible that the utterance may not be translatable. More commonly, the interpreter may forget to include the utterance. Additions may be extra words, phrases, or sentences that were not said by the clinician in order to elaborate or to editorialize. Additions also may occur because extra words are needed to explain a concept that is difficult to translate. The interpreter may not remember the specific message, or be confused with words that sound alike; therefore, other words, phrases, or sentences are substituted in place of the clinician's actual message. Transformations are changes in the word order of what was actually said (Langdon, 1988). The clinician must keep in mind that the interpreter-assistant may be concerned with the client's comprehension and therefore may need to elaborate, simplify, and reword.

These possible errors during the conference are avoidable. Langdon (1988) suggests that the professional keep the language simple and short, without professional jargon and extra wording. The professional should watch the interpreter's body language and listen for the use of too many or too few words compared to the clinician's utterances. Langdon also suggests that the interpreter should be free to request that the speaker rephrase unclear messages. Listening carefully, taking notes, consulting a dictionary, and knowing one's own limitations as an interpreter also are important guidelines for the interpreter and the professional.

INTERVENTION

An interpreter may be used for fluency, language, voice, and articulation intervention. The assistant should not write, develop, or modify the client's intervention plan in any way without the recommendation, guidance, and approval of the supervising clinician. In addition ASHA (1981, 1993) suggests that the assistant should not counsel the client or family during these sessions.

There are programmed materials for each of these disorder areas that may be used by the interpreter. These programs can be adapted for cultural relevancy and translated by the interpreter before they are used with the client. As a precaution, all translated materials should be reviewed by another bilingual, preferably a professional, to ensure the accuracy of the translation. The monolingual clinician could first train the interpreter in English and supervise the interpreter until the clinician feels confident that the interpreter can follow the program in English. Review of the intervention materials with the interpreter, discussion of the purpose of the procedures, and demonstration by the clinician should be part of training. Training the assistant may require additional time, effort, and patience from the clinician, because the interpreter may need additional time and practice to accurately administer stimuli, judge the client's response, and make modifications when the procedures are not appropriate. Actual supervision of intervention sessions will depend on the client's type of impairment and severity in addition to the experience and competency level of the interpreter/assistant. This may range from 100% supervision at the initiation of intervention to 10% once the assistant and clinician are comfortable with the caseload and procedures. Supervision may be extended to telephone calls and video- or audiotaped sessions, as well as observations. ASHA (1993) suggests that clinician monitoring contact hours should be recorded.

In addition to direct intervention, the interpreter could also record, chart, and graph the client's performance data. The interpreter could also prepare clinical materials, letters, and information handouts in the minority language. Again, all of these materials should be reviewed by a second bilingual individual. Eventually, the interpreter could be a partner in the clinician's inservice, professional, and research projects.

HOW MAY AN INTERPRETER BE BEST UTILIZED?

Once an interpreter/assistant is trained to assist in assessments and intervention programs, their effectiveness will also depend on how the monolingual clinician utilizes the interpreter's skills. An interpreter who is on call and is used by several clinicians may be providing assessments and possibly intervention plans with the clinicians present at all times. These on-call interpreters/assistants, therefore, may not have regular assignments that would allow them some autonomy. For these assistants, Medina (1982) and Langdon (1988) suggest that clinicians have three parts to each conference, assessment, and intervention session: (1) briefing; (2) interaction; and (3) debriefing. The briefing session is the clinician's opportunity to meet with the interpreter and to review the general purpose of the session, whether it is for an initial conference or testing session. The briefing should include background information about the client to be tested or the family to be interviewed. The clinician should discuss any previous testing or any unsual circumstances that the interpreter should be made aware of concerning the client. This briefing session should allow the interpreter time to review materials and ask questions.

During the interaction with the client or family, the interpreter should be free to ask questions as needed. The professional should take notes on the interaction of the interpreter and client. These notes could include body language, overuse of verbal or nonverbal reinforcements, cueing, and excessive or minimal talking. The debriefing follows the interaction and allows the clinician and interpreter to discuss the client's responses, errors, the interpreter's observations, test scoring, and difficulties during the session. The clinician will receive an interpreters' best efforts with reliable results if these three procedures are routinely practiced.

⌐ᵧ

CONCLUSIONS

There are many activities for a full-time interpreter in a school district, clinic, hospital, or agency. For centers that may have a bilingual speech-language pathologist, several individuals could be easily trained and supervised by both the monolingual and bilingual clinicians.

Interpreters are seen as a necessity for many school districts, agencies, clinics, and hospitals so that they can better serve minority language clients. Until more bilingual clinicians are in the work force, speech-language pathologists should be ready to provide the necessary training and supervision of interpreters and translators who can communicate with these clients. The expense and commitment of time and energy to develop the linguistic and professional competencies of these bilingual assistants should be priorities for our profession.

⌐ᵧ

REFERENCES

American Speech-Language-Hearing Association (1981). Guidelines for the employment and utilization of supportive personnel. *Asha, 23*(3), 165–169.

American Speech-Language-Hearing Association, Committee on the Status of Racial Minorities. (1985). Clinical management of communicatively handicapped minority language populations. *Asha, 27*(6), 29–32.

American Speech-Language-Hearing Association, Committee on Supportive Personnel. (1988). Utilization and employment of speech-language pathology supportive personnel with underserved populations. *Asha, 30*(11), 55–56.

American Speech-Language-Hearing Association, Task Force on Supportive Personnel. (1993, May). Proposed position statement and guidelines for the education/training, use, and supervision of support personnel in speech, language pathology and audiology. Rockville, MD: ASHA.

Baetens-Beardsmore, H. (1986). *Bilingualism: Basic principles* (2nd ed.). San Diego, CA: College-Hill Press.

Deal, V. R., & Rodriguez, V. L. (1987). *Resource guide to multicultural tests and materials in communicative disorders.* Rockville, MD: American Speech-Language-Hearing Association.

Kayser, H. (1993). Hispanic cultures. In D. Battle (Ed.), *Communication disorders in multicultural populations* (pp. 114–157). Boston, MA: Andover Medical Publishers.

Langdon, H. W. (1988, June). *Working with an interpreter/translator in the school setting.* Presentation at State Conference for School Superintendents. Dimensions of appropriate assessment for minority handicapped students: Recommended practices. University of Arizona, June, Tucson.

Langdon, H. W. (1992a). *Interpreter/translator process in the educational sessing: A resource manual.* Sacramento, CA: Resources in Special Education.

Langdon, H. W. (1992b). Speech and language asssessment of LEP/Bilingual Hispanic students. In H. W. Langdon & L. Cheng (Eds.), *Hispanic children and adults with communication disorders: Assessment and intervention* (pp. 201–271). Gaithersburg, MD: Aspen.

Matsuda, M., & O'Connor, L. C. (1993). *Creating an effective partnership: Training bilingual communication aides.* Presentation at the annual convention of the California Speech, Language and Hearing Association. Palm Springs.

Medina, V. (1982). *Interpretation and translation in bilingual B.A.S.E.* San Diego, CA: Superintendent of Schools, Department of Education, San Diego County.

Omark, D. R., & Watson, D. L. (1981). *Assessing bilingual exceptional children: In-service manual.* San Diego, CA: Los Amigos Research Associates.

Paredes Scribner, A. (1993, Spring/Summer). The use of interpreters in the assessment of language minority students. *The Bilingual Special Education Perspective.* 12(2), 1–6.

Roseberry-McKibbin, C. A,. & Eicholtz, G. E. (1994). Serving children with limited English proficiency in the schools: A national survey. *Language, Speech, and Hearing Services in Schools, 25,* 156–164.

Taylor, O. L. (1986). *Nature of communication disorders in culturally and linguistically diverse populations.* San Diego, CA: College-Hill Press.

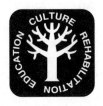

CHAPTER 10

INTELLIGENCE TESTING OF HISPANIC STUDENTS

JOZI DE LEÓN, Ph.D.

Intelligence testing of Hispanic students has greatly impacted on the type of participation and opportunity allowed these students educationally. Intelligence (IQ) test scores have been the "gatekeeper" in allowing minority students into programs for the gifted. IQ scores have also served to label students as deficient and in need of special programs which have often prevented them from maximizing their potential. From an Hispanic viewpoint, examination of historical aspects associated with the development of intelligence tests allows us to put intelligence test scores in their proper perspective. The first intelligence test, the Binet, in 1904 was specifically designed for the purpose of identifying the intellectually deficient student in Paris. In the United States, identification of the "feebleminded" was also of concern. When a test was developed that could identify the mentally deficient segment of the population, it was greeted with great enthusiasm. Issues related to testing culturally diverse populations first became evident around 1910 when tests patterned after the Binet were devised to assess the abilities of large waves of immigrants arriving in the United States (Anastasi, 1982). Because the purpose of testing was to distinguish the "acceptable" from the "unacceptable" immigrant, it was not particularly troublesome to some that certain groups were

223

unilaterally represented as deficient while others were considered normal or even gifted. It was not uncommon to find that individuals from "Western-like" cultures were found to be acceptable on the basis of these tests, whereas individuals from cultures most unlike Western cultures were found repeatedly to function below normal. It is important to note that, had Binet's original intent and cautionary statements been heeded in the adoption of his test and further development of other intelligence tests, some of the problems with their misuse could have been avoided. His statement about the scale makes his thoughts quite clear:

> The scale, properly speaking, does not permit the measure of the intelligence, because intellectual qualities are not superposable, and therefore cannot be measured as linear surfaces are measured. (Binet, as cited in Gould, 1981, p. 151)

Binet established three "cardinal principles" for the use of his scale. These were quickly disregarded by Americans as his tests were imported (Binet, as cited in Gould, 1981). These included:

> (1) The scores are a practical device; they do not buttress any theory of intellect. They do not define anything innate or permanent. We may not designate what they measure as "intelligence" or any other reified entity.

> (2) The scale is a rough, empirical guide for identifying mildly retarded and learning-disabled children who need special help. It is not a device for ranking normal children.

> (3) Whatever the cause of difficulty in children identified for help, emphasis shall be placed upon improvement through special training.
>   Low scores shall not be used to mark children as innately incapable. (p. 155)

In the United States, Binet's intelligence scales found their way into the hands of hereditarians who believed that traits or tendencies were passed on genetically within family lines. If individuals with an inherited low intelligence could be identified, they could then be separated from society where they could do the least damage and no longer propagate. As late as 1969, the hereditarian position was still being argued by individuals like Arthur Jensen and others. Jensen (1969) argued that compensatory education for disadvantaged individuals from different social and racial groups had failed because the low intelligence and achievement scores of these individuals had been attributed to correctable environmental and cultural influences rather than uncorrectable genetically determined mental abilities. His arguments were based on his study of IQ scores of Black and Hispanic individuals and his analysis of the "heritability" factor of IQ scores. With the arguments of individuals like Jensen, the significance of the IQ score was elevated to an unchangeable, indisputable, entity which truly depicted an individual's intellectual capacity. Binet's original intent for the use of his scale had been altered significantly and the era of misuse of intelligence test scores had begun.

In the late 1940s many states passed laws mandating programs for the mentally retarded in the public schools. These programs soon began serving large numbers of low-income, immigrant, and minority children. In my own rural community, there were only two children in the special education program in the early 1960s, a Down syndrome Anglo male and a Mexican American male who was considered normal by the Mexican American community and grew up to be an active member of that community. Although my community was small, and by no means is representative of all communities, it, however, was a microcosm of the general special education picture. The children in special education from the majority culture were moderately to severely disabled, whereas the minority children placed were typically from immigrant, low-income families, and/or from non-English-speaking backgrounds. Males were, and still remain, predominant in special education classes.

As the Civil Rights Movement grew in the 1960s there was great criticism of special education programs which, by that time, had grown in their overrepresentation of minority students, primarily Blacks and Hispanics. Several lawsuits were filed on behalf of Hispanic students to remedy the situation. *Arreola v. Board of Education Unified School District* challenged the placement process. *Covarrubias v. San Diego* also dealt with placement and the consent of parents prior to placement. *Diana v. California State Board of Education* and *Larry P. v. Riles* most directly challenged the misuse of tests in the special education placement process. The use of intelligence testing and poor placement processes were seen as culprits in the misidentification of Hispanic and Black students.

Although more sensitive assessment and placement practices have been implemented, the use of intelligence tests still remains controversial today. School districts have used various means of dealing with the controversy. Some have eliminated the use of intelligence tests with minority students, others have chosen to use nonverbal measures primarily, and the majority have become more careful in the interpretation of intelligence test scores. In all states, however, placement is still driven by test scores. IQ scores still carry a great deal of weight in determining a student's estimated potential and predicted success in school.

⊔

GENERAL FACTORS AFFECTING PERFORMANCE ON INTELLIGENCE TESTS

Five factors that contribute to some of the intelligence test biases for Spanish-speaking students have been identified. They include (a) cultural difference, (b) language difference, (c) norming procedures that do not include representative samples of Hispanic students, (d) the test administration itself, and (e) the interpretation of test scores (Berry & Lopez, 1977; Cummins, 1984; Hamayan & Damico, 1991).

STANFORD-BINET, FOURTH EDITION

The Stanford-Binet (Thorndike, Hagen, & Sattler, 1986) is a derivative of the original Binet scale and a predecessor of many intelligence tests. It is the test against which most of the intelligence tests are validated. It also is one of the most verbally loaded tests of intelligence and, therefore, is probably the least appropriate test for learners of English as a second language. The test developers include a section that addresses the administration of the test with "Limited English Proficient and non-Language Proficient" (not fluent in either their native language or English) students. They state that the test should be administered by a bilingual examiner in the examinee's native language when the examinee does not speak English. They also share some recommendations in the use of translators which restrict the translator to administration of the directions in the item books only and caution against the adding of an instructional component to the directions. Perhaps the most helpful information in the examination of Limited English Proficient students is the specification of which subtests can be administered nonverbally (Bead Memory, Pattern

Analysis, Copying, Memory for Objects, Matrices, and Paper Folding and Cutting). They also suggest modifications for the subtests, Absurdities and Memory for Digits, with Limited English Proficient and non-Language Proficient examinees. In this author's view, despite the modifications, the Memory for Objects, Absurdities, Memory for Digits, and Paper Folding and Cutting require the use of language for full understanding of the task. The scores obtained through the modifications should not be viewed as valid.

WECHSLER INTELLIGENCE SCALE FOR CHILDREN, THIRD EDITION (WISC-III)

The developers of the newly revised third edition of the Wechsler caution examiners against the sole use of test scores derived from the WISC-III (Wechsler, 1991) in the decision-making process. They express the notion that Wechsler's extensive experience in the assessment of children and adults led him to the belief that intelligence is an entity that is greater than what can be measured by cognitive ability tests and that intelligence is a "global capacity" of an individual which is a combined product of genetic makeup and "socio-educational experiences, drive, motivation, and personality predilections" (Wechsler, 1991, p. iii). The test developers state that, although there are many new theories of intelligence, they did not change the basic structure or subtests included in the WISC-III because research has consistently found evidence for a "g factor." The g factor refers to what Spearman referred to as "general intelligence" (Wechsler, 1991, p. 11). Spearman spent the majority of his life examining tests requiring the operation of higher mental process. He found positive intercorrelations among tests requiring such operations, no matter what the task. He hypothesized that all tests that require complex mental processes measure a common factor which he referred to as general intelligence, or simply g (Brody & Brody, 1976).

Examiners of Hispanic children also need to be aware that, although the WISC-R had a Puerto Rican and a Mexican version with norms representing those groups and a Spanish translation with the *Escala Wechsler de Inteligencia para Niños—Revisada* (Wechsler, 1982) which used the WISC-R norm tables, there are presently no Spanish translations or Spanish versions of the WISC-III. Although the translations and Spanish versions have not been perfect in the past, they nonetheless allowed diagnosticians and school psychologists to assess Spanish-dominant children.

The WISC-III is designed to assess the intellectual ability of children aged 6 years to 16 years, 11 months. Like its predecessors, the WISC and WISC-R, it is by far the most frequently used intelligence test for school-age populations. It yields three composite scores, the Verbal, Performance, and Full Scale IQs. Most examiners find them useful because it allows them to gain a sense of a child's cognitive ability through verbal and nonverbal expression. The test developers claim that the WISC-III includes tasks that tap different areas of general intellectual ability such as abstract reasoning, memory, perceptual skills, and other skills valued by "our culture" and relate to skills generally associated with intelligent behavior. In a pluralistic society like the United States it is erroneous to believe that a test that focuses on a singular cultural perspective can adequately assess cognitive ability across all American cultures.

The test includes 12 subtests. Table 10–1 provides a description of what each subtest measures and the subscale it belongs to.

TABLE 10–1
Description of Verbal and Performance subtests of WISC-III.

Verbal

Information—Includes questions which the child is asked orally about events, objects, people, and places.

Similarities—Pairs of words are presented orally for a determination of the similarity between the two words/objects named.

Arithmetic—Arithmetic problems are administered orally and figured out without the use of paper and pencil.

Vocabulary—Words are presented orally and the student defines orally. Responses are scored with two, one, or zero points based on the complexity and completeness of the response.

Comprehension—Questions are presented orally in which the student determines the appropriate response based on knowledge of social rules and concepts. Responses are scored with two, one or zero points based on the completeness of the response.

Digit Span—A sequence of numbers is presented orally and must be repeated by the student. A set of numbers is administered forwards and a set is administered backwards.

TABLE 10-1 *(continued)*

Performance

Picture Completion—Pictures are presented individually to the student in which he or she determines what important part is missing within a 20 second time limit.

Coding—The student prints the corresponding symbol to the shape (Coding A) or number (Coding B) within a 2 minute time limit. Coding A is designed for younger children and Coding B for older children.

Picture Arrangement—Picture cards depicting a story sequence are presented in a certain order and require that the student reorder them in appropriate sequence within a certain time limit.

Block Design—A printed geometric pattern is presented to the student who must then duplicate the design using two-color cubes within a certain time limit.

Object Assembly—A series of puzzles of objects are given to the student to put together within a given time limit.

Symbol Search—A new optional subtest added to the WISC-III. A series of paired groups are presented in which the student determines whether the target group appears in the search group. The student marks a yes or no response for each set and is given a 2 minute time limit for the subtest.

Mazes—The student works his way through an increasingly more difficult set of mazes by marking his way out from beginning to end. Each maze is timed.

Students whose primary language is not English have consistently demonstrated significantly lower verbal subtest scores on intelligence tests compared with performance scales (Altus, 1953; Chandler & Plakos, 1969; Cummins, 1984; Hamayan & Damico, 1991; Munford & Munoz, 1980; Oplesch & Genshaft, 1981). The Hispanic student's lower Verbal IQ will decrease his or her Full Scale IQ which can then be interpreted as an indication of lower cognitive ability. A significant Verbal and Performance IQ discrepancy has also been considered an indication of a language deficit. For students who are bilingual and whose primary language is not English, it is not uncommon to find Verbal IQ scores that are significantly lower than the Performance IQ. Such low scores are generally characteristic of the nature of the test rather than always indicative of a student deficit that merits language intervention or some other form of special placement due to a language-related disability. A lower Verbal IQ does point to the need to build stronger English language skills, but not necessarily to label the child deficient or language impaired.

When the different verbal subtests are examined, one can obtain a sense of the cause of lower Verbal IQ scores among bilingual students whose primary language is not English. The Similarities subtest, for example, requires a high level of understanding of the English language to make the connection between the two terms compared and to be able to verbally articulate the similarities. For the Information subtest, the bilingual student may need to be able to translate the acquisition of certain facts into English if they were learned in a language other than English. In addition, the student needs to understand some advanced vocabulary and be able to use higher level vocabulary in responding. Some of the facts assessed by this subtest may not have been learned by a student who was schooled in another country, for example, "Who was Christopher Columbus?" and "How far is it from London to New York?" The Vocabulary subtest also requires the student to understand higher level vocabulary than he or she might have been exposed to. In responding, the student needs to be able to use more complex language and expanded responses in explaining the meanings in order to obtain maximum points for the response. For example, in defining "mimic" if the student responded with terminology like "imitate," "mock," or "impersonate," he or she would receive 2 points; however, if he or she said "to act like someone" they would be queried and if they did not clarify with a response that indicated that it means to copy or repeat what someone else does, he or she would be given only 1 point for the response. Such linguistic subtleties may be difficult for bilingual students to understand and/or articulate.

The Comprehension subtest requires not only the knowledge of social rules and behavior in mainstream American society, but it also requires students to articulate responses using more complex language. For example, on a question about why the government inspects meat before it is sold, if the student responds that it is "to make sure the meat isn't bad and can be sold to the public" he or she obtains 2 points, but if the response is "meat could be spoiled," it receives only 1 point. In addition, the more the student elaborates on the response the more likely it is that he or she will obtain maximum points per response. On some questions, if two thoughts are expressed concerning the general idea the student receives 2 points, but if only one thought is expressed the student receives only 1 point. Although individually the number of points obtained per question may not make a difference, collectively a series of 1 or 0 responses may greatly influence the Verbal IQ and, ultimately, the Full Scale IQ. Knowledge of vocabulary, the ability to manipulate the English language, and the ability to use English extensively in complex forms are vital in achieving a high score on the verbal subtests of the WISC-III.

The Performance subtests are not as problematic for bilingual and English as a second language learners. In fact, bilingual Hispanic students might have a chance to redeem themselves on the Performance subtests. This does not mean that the Performance subtests do not require caution in interpretation. Despite less reliance on language for the Performance subtests, if a student is limited in his or her English speaking ability, the directions can be above the student's level of understanding. In addition, the time constraints of most of the subtests may penalize students who are not used to functioning within such constraints. It is not uncommon for diagnosticians to rely on the Performance IQ as a better indicator of potential when the Verbal IQ is significantly lower. Such a practice should be used cautiously because the Performance IQ may not merit such confidence.

NORMS

The test developers used the 1988 Census data in the selection of a standardization sample that would reflect the United States population. The representation of the sample closely matches the 1988 Census statistics in socioeconomic status (determined through years of parents' education), racial/ethnic makeup, and region of the United States. Out of a total norming sample of 2200 approximately 11% (242) of the norming sample is Hispanic. One hundred and nineteen are Hispanic males and 123 are Hispanic females. One hundred ninety-four of the Hispanic sample had parents with a high school education or less. Two hundred and four of the Hispanics included came from the Southern or Western regions of the United States and only 37 came from Northeastern or North Central regions.

The norming sample is adequate for most Hispanic groups except those living in the Northeastern or North Central portions of the United States. A very small number of individuals whose parents had a post-secondary education were included. It is not known what percentage of the individuals tested fell at either extreme of the socioeconomic scale. This is a concern for those testing children from low socioeconomic backgrounds. Another aspect to keep in mind is that, because Hispanics are one of the fastest growing minority groups in the country, the 1988 Census as an indication of population profiles will quickly become outdated and so will the norms.

KAUFMAN ASSESSMENT BATTERY FOR CHILDREN (K-ABC)

The K-ABC (Kaufman & Kaufman, 1983) was first published in 1983. It was designed for children ages 2½ to 12½. Kaufman states that intelligence as measured by the K-ABC is "an individual's style of solving problems and processing information" (p. 2). It examines two styles of processing information, sequential and simultaneous. Sequential processing places emphasis on serial or ordering of stimuli when problem solving. The individual has to break stimuli down into subparts in order to problem solve. Simultaneous processing involves the wholistic integration of stimuli. The individual looks at the stimuli as a whole rather than breaking them down into smaller steps or parts. Kaufman's development of the K-ABC borrows from neuropsychology and cognitive psychology. The Kaufmans claim that the subtests have been purposely designed to rely less on language and verbal skills and to include stimuli that are gender fair and less biased for individuals from diverse backgrounds. To the Kaufmans' credit, they have deliberately created an instrument that separates learned skills (vocabulary, certain language skills, academic information, etc.) from skills involving rational and logical thought. Although one still might ask, "whose logical and rational thought?", the fact remains that they have earnestly made an attempt to make their intelligence instrument look less like an achievement test and more like an instrument designed to assess cognitive processing. The Kaufmans state that they had six primary goals in mind when they developed the K-ABC:

1. to measure intelligence from a strong theoretical and research basis
2. to separate acquired factual knowledge from the ability to solve unfamiliar problems
3. to yield scores that translate to educational intervention
4. to include novel tasks
5. to be easy to administer and objective to score
6. to be sensitive to the diverse needs of preschool, minority group, and exceptional children. (p. 5)

The K-ABC includes a Sequential Processing Scale, Simultaneous Processing Scale, and an Achievement Scale. The Sequential and Simultaneous Processing Scales are the only two used to determine the Mental Processing Composite (typically referred to as an IQ score by other tests). In designing the instrument in this manner, the Kaufmans have separated acquisition of learned facts from the determination of cognitive ability. In addition, a Nonverbal Score can be derived which is often useful in the assessment of Spanish-dominant limited English-speaking students. The directions for the subtests included in the derivation of the Nonverbal Score have also been standardized to be administered in Spanish. This is very helpful to practitioners who are interested in obtaining a measure of cognitive ability but do not want to use a nonverbal intelligence test and find the Stanford-Binet or WISC-III too verbally loaded for Spanish-speaking students they are testing. Table 10–2 describes the subtests of the K-ABC.

NORMS

One hundred and fifty-seven Hispanic children between the ages of 2;6 to 12;5 were included in the norming sample. Eighteen of the Hispanic sample came from the Northeast, 8 from the North Central section of the United States, 23 from the South, and 108 from the West. Forty of the Hispanic children included in the norming sample had parents with less than a high school education. The only problem with the norming sample is that a lower percentage with less than a high school education than occurs in the Hispanic population at-large was included while a higher percentage of Hispanics with higher education made up the sample. According to the Kaufman's own definition of socioeconomic status, the Hispanic sample came from a higher socioeconomic level than the United States Hispanic population. This indicates that scores obtained by children from low socioeconomic backgrounds must be interpreted with caution.

NONVERBAL INTELLIGENCE TESTS

There are several nonverbal intelligence tests available which are used with Spanish-speaking students due to their limited demands on English language use. Some practitioners see nonverbal intelligence tests as the answer to some of the problems previously discussed con-

TABLE 10–2
Description of the K-ABC subtests.

Sequential Processing Scale

Hand Movements (ages 2;6 to 12;5)—The examinee repeats a series of hand movements after the examiner has performed them.

Number Recall (ages 2;6 to 12;5)—The examinee orally repeats a series of digits from memory after the examiner presents them.

Word Order (ages 4;0 to 12;5)—The examinee touches a series of silhouettes of common objects in the same order the examiner has named them. At the more difficult level, the examinee is presented a stimulus page with colored dots which they name before recalling the order of the previously named silhouettes.

Simultaneous Processing Scale

Magic Window (ages 2;6 to 4;11)—The examinee identifies a picture as it is rotated for 5 seconds and partially shown through a narrow window.

Face Recognition (ages 2;6 to 4;11)—The examiner exposes a picture of a person(s) briefly and the examinee chooses the correct person from a picture on the next stimulus page in which the person is pictured in a group with other individuals.

Gestalt Closure (ages 2;6 to 12;5)—The examinee names the partially completed inkblot object.

Triangles (ages 4;0 to 12;5)—The examinee assembles colored foam triangles to duplicate a design presented. The task is timed.

Matrix Analogies (ages 5;0 to 12;5)—The examinee selects the appropriate item to complete the visual analogy.

Spatial Memory (ages 5;0 to 12;5)—The examinee recalls the position of a picture on a page after it has been exposed for 5 seconds.

Photo Series (ages 6;0 to 12;5)—The examinee sequences photographs of a common event in the order that it would logically occur.

---

cerning verbally loaded intelligence tests. Unfortunately, we cannot find our panacea in the assessment of cognitive ability using nonverbal instruments. In some cases, nonverbal tests may even present more problems than they solve. Verbal intelligence tests are better predictors of academic achievement. In addition, Oller (1991) cautions that nonverbal tests of intelligence require just as much verbal manipulation as verbal tests. Because language is culturally based, these tests often also present their own measure of cultural bias.

The *Leiter International Performance Scale* (Leiter & Arthur, 1955, 1979) is designed to assess individuals 2 years to adulthood and takes 40 minutes to an hour to administer. The Leiter is often recommended for use with non-English-speaking students because of its limited language use and because it has been considered to be a culture-fair intelligence test. First, the notion that a "culturally fair" test can exist is questionable. Second, examiners often assume that, because the norms were developed using ethnic Hawaiian groups and the test was used in studies of native Africans, it is appropriate for all non-Western cultures. The Leiter has just been renormed, but the renormed version is not yet available. Only time will tell whether it will be an improvement on the earlier version.

The Leiter can be useful in providing supplemental information on cognitive functioning when other measures seem inappropriate; however, it should not be used as the sole measure. The norms are outdated and inappropriate for culturally and linguistically diverse populations.

The *Raven's Progressive Matrices* (Raven, Court, & Raven, 1986) were developed in Great Britain to assess abstract reasoning, concept formation, spatial ability, and classification. It is simple to administer and compared to all the other cognitive ability tests requires the least amount of training. It can be administered individually or to a group; however, it is best to administer this test individually to Hispanic students, especially those with limited school experience. Very little information is included in the manual about the technical aspects of the test. This instrument should be used as a supplemental measure of cognitive ability and should not be the sole measure of cognitive processing.

The *Test of Nonverbal Intelligence* (TONI) (Brown, Sherbenou, & Johnsen, 1982) is one of the most recently developed nonverbal intelligence measures. It is simple to administer, and many examiners like it because they can derive a score of cognitive ability in 15 to 20 minutes. This author suggests caution in interpretation of the score and advises that not too much weight be placed on the score, given the limited abilities assessed by this instrument. The TONI should be used only as a screening instrument and a gross indicator of intellectual functioning.

ᛃ

LANGUAGE PROFICIENCY AND THE MEASUREMENT OF COGNITIVE ABILITY

An examination of the Hispanic student's language proficiency and language profile is often the most critical first step in any evaluation process, but it is especially critical when intellectual ability will be assessed. By examining language proficiency, first and foremost, we can determine: (1) the appropriateness of certain tests for second language learners; (2) whether to use an interpreter or a Spanish translation of a test; and (3) how to interpret the test results (De Leon, 1990). This is important in all areas of assessment, but is perhaps even more important when we examine intelligence. The score that intelligence tests derive still carries a great deal of weight in the psychoeducational evaluation process. With the intelligence test we determine "estimated potential." We derive a score indicating the student's expected level of functioning in all other areas. Decisions about special placement are dependent on the comparisons made between the expected level of functioning and low scores noted on various other tests. If the intelligence test score we obtain is faulty and not valid, then our whole premise about the child's expected level of functioning and the rationale for placement is also faulty.

Table 10–3 addresses the different questions that an examiner needs to address in order to perform appropriate evaluations of bilingual Hispanic students. These questions will yield important information that will assist examiners in making more valid interpretations of test results.

IN WHICH LANGUAGE(S) SHOULD THE STUDENT BE TESTED?

This question has the examiner involved in asking questions pertaining to language proficiency and language skills of the student. An important aspect of this fact-finding activity is to determine what language the student speaks in different settings and his or her expressive and receptive skills in both English and Spanish. The language in which the student has been taught is also important because it allows the examiner to gain insight into the student's academic language

TABLE 10–3

Questions, procedures, and information which will assist in more valid interpretation of intelligence testing of Hispanic students.

Question	Procedures	Information
In which language(s) should the student be tested?	Administer language dominance/ language proficiency assessment	Predominant language What language is being spoken at home and support for language building Whether the student suffered native language loss
	Select a technically sound standardized instrument	What kind of school support was available for language building Does the student speak standard or nonstandard forms of L1 and L2
	Administer home language use and dynamics	Kind of vocabulary student might have in L1 and L2
What language skills does the student have in L1 and L2?	Examine language loss in family	Examine language base/support within family
	Examine primary language of student	Degree of social academic language and academic language development through schooling in L1 and L2 Kind of vocabulary and language student has
	Examine past educational programs and curricula (Bilingual, ESL, English only, etc.)	Standard and nonstandard L1 and L2
	Determine domain in which each language is used	
	Determine social and academic language	
	Determine code switching, dialect, or nonstandard English patterns	
How do I use language information to interpret test data?	Determine impact of L1 and L2 competence on test performance	Appropriate recommendations for intervention and placement

skills. Low academic language skills will probably interfere with valid results on most test of cognitive ability.

WHAT LANGUAGE SKILLS DOES THE STUDENT HAVE IN L1 AND L2?

The second question examines more closely those aspects that would influence the development or lack of development in L1 and L2. Without addressing this question, the examiner has no sense of whether the language of the test matches the language skills of the student. If the test language is at a higher level than the student's, a low score can be attributed to lower language skills rather than lower cognitive ability. Dialects, code switching, and other linguistic differences can also influence test results.

HOW DO I USE LANGUAGE INFORMATION TO INTERPRET TEST DATA?

A final step is for the examiner to closely analyze the student's language and compare it to the linguistic requirements of the test. If the student has low academic language skills and is administered a test primarily requiring high academic language skills, he or she may be at risk of not being able to fully demonstrate knowledge and skills. Low scores on such tests can indicate a language difference rather than a language deficit.

⅃ᴛ

SUMMARY

Historically, intelligence test scores have not accurately represented the skills of Spanish-speaking students. Low scores on tests of cognitive ability have indicated to school personnel that these students were intellectually deficient. Rather than analyze closely why Hispanic students have scored lower on such tests, a common reaction has been to automatically assume that the scores were true reflections of student abilities and that student skills were in need of remediation. Court cases have demonstrated that testing procedures and intelligence test scores themselves must be scrutinized.

Verbally loaded tests of intelligence have been particularly damaging to Hispanic students from Spanish-speaking backgrounds. Although the problems encountered in the use of such tests have not been totally eliminated, sound decisions can be made when test scores are interpreted properly. This chapter has provided the reader with insights on the most widely used tests of intelligence. This information can be useful in the selection of tests to be used with Hispanic students. Discussions of norms, the nature of tasks on the tests, and the areas that may present particular problems to Hispanic students can be useful to examiners in determining the validity of scores obtained. If intelligence test scores can be viewed as gross indicators of ability rather than definite indicators of potential, better decisions about the abilities of Hispanic students can be made.

⌐⌐

REFERENCES

Altus, G. T. (1953). WISC patterns of a selective sample of bilingual school children. *Journal of Genetic Psychology, 83*, 241–248.

Anastasi, A. (1982). *Psychological testing.* New York: Macmillan.

Berry, G. L., & Lopez, C. A. (1977). Testing programs and the Spanish-speaking child: Assessment guidelines for school counselors. *The School Counselor, 24*(4), 261–269.

Brody, E. B., & Brody, N. (1976). *Intelligence: Nature, determinants, and consequences.* New York: Academic Press.

Brown L., Sherbenou, R. J., & Johnsen, S. K. (1990). *Test of nonverbal intelligence.* Austin, TX: Pro-Ed.

Chandler, J. T., & Plakos, J. (1969). Spanish-speaking pupils classified as educable mentally retarded. *Integrated Education, 7*(69), 28–33.

Cummins, J. (1984). *Bilingualism and special education: Issues in assessment and pedagogy.* San Diego, CA: College-Hill Press.

De León, J. (1990). A model for an advocacy-oriented assessment process in the psycho-educational evaluation of culturally and linguistically different students. The Journal of Educational *Issues of Language Minority Students, 7*, 53–67.

Gould, S. J. (1981). *The mismeasure of man.* Ontario: Penguin Books Canada.

Hamayan, E. V., & Damico, J. S. (1991). *Limiting bias in the assessment of bilingual student.* Austin, TX: Pro-Ed.

Jensen, A. R. (1969). How much can we boost IQ and scholastic achievement?, *Harvard Educational Review, 2,* 1–123.

Kaufman, A. S., & Kaufman, N. L. (1983). *Kaufman Assessment Battery for Children.* Circle Pines, MN: American Guidance Service.

Leiter, R. G., & Arthur, G. (1955). *Leiter International Performance Scale.* Chicago: Stoelting.

Leiter, R. G., & Arthur G. (1979). *Leiter International Performance Scale.* Chicago: Stoelting.

Munford, P. R., & Munoz, A. (1980). A comparison of the WISC and WISC-R on Hispanic children. *Journal of Clinical Psychology, 36*(2), 452–457.

Oller, J. W. (1991). *Language and bilingualism: More tests of tests.* Cranbury, NJ: Associated University Presses.

Oplesch, M., & Genshaft, J. (1981). Comparison of bilingual children on the WISC-R and the Escala de Inteligencia Wechsler Para Niños. *Psychology in the Schools, 18*(2), 159–163.

Raven, J. C., Court, J. H., & Raven, J. (1986). *Manual for Raven's Progressive Matrices and Vocabulary Scales.* London: Lewis.

Thorndike, R. L., Hagen, E. P., & Sattler, J. M. (1986). *Stanford-Binet Intelligence Scale* (4th ed.) Chicago: Riverside.

Wechsler, D. (1982). *Escala de Inteligencia Wechsler para Niños-Revisada.* San Antonio, TX: Psychological Corporation.

Wechsler, D. (1991). *Wechsler Intelligence Scale for Children—III.* San Antonio, TX: Psychological Corporation.

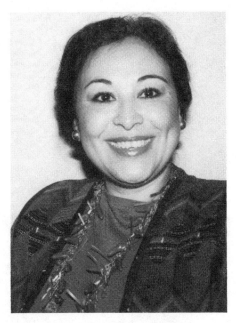

JOZI DE LEÓN, Ph.D.

Dr. De León is an Associate Professor in the Department of Special Education/Communication Disorders at New Mexico State University. She received her bachelor's degree in Early Childhood Education in 1975 from Fayetteville State University in North Carolina, her master's degree in Educational Psychology in 1980 from the University of North Carolina–Chapel Hill, and her doctorate in Bilingual Education/Special Education in 1985 from New Mexico State University. Dr. De León's professional interests have focused on culturally and linguistically diverse exceptional students. She is a certified educational diagnostician concentrating on the assessment of Hispanic bilingual and Spanish-monolingual students. Dr. De León has directed several projects and conducted research in areas of bilingual special education.

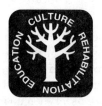

CHAPTER 11

ASSESSMENT OF SPEECH AND LANGUAGE IMPAIRMENTS IN BILINGUAL CHILDREN

HORTENCIA KAYSER, Ph.D.

We just have to rely on the formal tests. It isn't my preference, . . . and it's not my training. (Kayser, 1985, p. 105).

A dart board, I have a dart board it has this much CD (Communication Disorders) and the . . . little wedge is not CD. And then I get about a foot away and throw . . . . it just depends on just what kind of mood I'm in. (Kayser, 1985, p. 113)

If I say in my expert opinion as a language specialist, "this child is communicately disordered in language," somebody will say BS. Your expert opinion is worth nothing; where are your test scores? (Kayser, 1985, p. 105)

ssessing children and adults' speech and language skills is an integral part of our profession as speech-language pathologists.

Test instruments, the tools of our profession, are necessary to determine if a speech and/or language impairment exists, and they are used to describe the performance of an individual on a task. As professionals, our reputations and credibility often depend on the validity and reliability of the test instruments we use. When no instruments are available for the Spanish speaker, or the instruments used are translated from English versions, or the clinician must prepare criterion-referenced instruments, the instruments do not meet the high standards for assessment we provide to English speakers.

Frequently asked questions among clinicians are: Why aren't publishers developing tests? and Why can't we have standardized tests for Spanish speakers? School districts, hospitals, and other agencies have attempted to translate tests and to norm these instruments, hoping to improve services. Often, these measures only increase the number of questions and frustrations. If we can understand why it is impossible to standardize a test in Spanish for bilingual speakers, then maybe clinicians can move on from this test mentality and begin to explore alternative models of assessment of speech and language in Hispanic individuals.

The chapters that discussed speech and language development and bilingualism should provide a foundation for clinicians in understanding the confounding variables that impact test development for Hispanics. What is normal speech and language behavior for developing bilingual children? Should we be looking at other aspects of language development rather than form, content, and use? This chapter will review the procedures recommended for speech-language pathology and special education in assessing communicative impairments in Hispanic children. A discussion follows concerning prereferrals, which includes the case history, questionnaires, and observations. Test instruments and how they can be adapted to fit the needs of students will be discussed briefly. Modified procedures, including a brief discussion of dynamic assessment, will also be presented. Assessment checklists and the interpretation of data will be briefly presented. The chapter concludes with discussion of other important considerations in the assessment process.

占

PREREFERRAL OF HISPANIC CHILDREN

Well I think one of the biggest problems is that the teachers don't really, aren't really tuned in to the kind of problems that these kids are having.

They don't really know what characteristics to make a referral. (Kayser, 1985, p. 95)

We don't go out and seek children and identify them as having problems. And for some reason the teachers are referring primarily Hispanic children for every kind of problem . . . . If the child qualifies, (he) will be placed (Kayser, 1985, p. 96)

REFERRAL CHARACTERISTICS

Boone and Plante (1993) stated that approximately 10% of the population will have a communicative impairment. Olson (1991) states that about 12% of the language minority population in the United States may require special education. But, in many school districts, these students are over- or underpresented in special education because of overzealous referrals, inappropriate referrals, fear of referring and placement, or ignorance.

The reasons for referral of language minority students vary. If the referral is the result of the child's academic failure, the speech-language pathologist will not be the initial recipient of the referral. The child is initially reviewed by a school child study team whose purpose is to help teachers problem solve the difficulties that children have in the classroom. Frequently, child study teams do not serve their designed functions. They should be gatekeepers to special education, but often function more as processors to enter students into special education (Garcia & Ortiz, 1988). Reynolds (1984) reported that 75 to 90% of students who are referred to child study teams are placed into special education.

Kayser (1985) interviewed 20 public school clinicians to determine what descriptors teachers gave on their referrals of Hispanic students for special services. The clinicians gave 14 different descriptions. All of the referral characteristics could be classified into three categories: academics, comprehension, and expression. The most referrals (37.8%) dealt with academic skills, such as reading and writing. Comprehension skills, such as following directions and answering questions about a story, made up 35.5% of the referral descriptions. Only 22.2% of the referral descriptions were related to expressive language skills. These expressive abilities were described in general terms, such as "unintelligible" and "has trouble with English."

Usually seems to be auditory, that they don't follow directions, it's rarely expressive, I don't think. It seems like the ones I've seen it's not like does not express himself well. It's usually does not follow directions, unable . . . you know (to) answer questions about the story, it's usually comprehension type behaviors. (Kayser, 1985, p. 101)

A lot of times they're (teachers) not really specific. They look more at the academics . . . They don't always focus in on language. So I get a lot of information in terms of can't keep up with the rest of the children . . . he's doing very poorly in all his subjects (Kayser,1985, p. 102)

Many of them are second, third grade. That's when they catch them, they're about that time. And I don't know enough about the curriculum off hand to say what it is that teachers are seeing them do or not do in certain areas; that they could pick it up so easily or . . . be so sure that the child is having a problem (Kayser, 1985, p. 102)

Kayser (1985) reported that when a child was referred directly to speech-language pathologists from kindergarten or first grade, the referrals used terms such as "speech unclear." But if the referral came from the second grade or above, academics and comprehension in the classroom were the two primary reasons for referring, not specific oral communication difficulties.

The clinicians also perceived eight demographic characteristics common to the Mexican American children labeled as language impaired and placed in their caseloads. These included: (1) low socioeconomic level; (2) monolingual Spanish-speaking parents; (3) English-only speaking teachers and classrooms; (4) academic difficulties, primarily in reading; (5) comprehension difficulties; (6) referral in the second through fourth grades; (7) poor conversational skills; and (8) bilingual or predominately English speaking. Of interest, when the clinicians' caseloads were examined, 100 of 109 Hispanic students had not received English as a second language classes, and 97 had not received bilingual education. The children were placed directly into speech and language programs without first attempting to assist the student through alternative remedial programs.

These referral characteristics could easily identify any second-language learner as communicatively impaired. There was a salient pattern in the referrals from teachers, and this should alert clinicians of the need of additional information from teachers and parents before testing proceeds. The prereferral process becomes necessary to avoid overreferral to special education and thus the possibility of inappropriate identification of Hispanic children as communicatively impaired.

THE PREREFERRAL

The purpose of preferrals is to reduce the number of inappropriate referrals to speech language services and special education (Ortiz & Maldonado-Colon, 1986). Olson (1991) describes the prereferral as a screening and intervention process that involves identifying the (1) child's problems, (2) source of the problems, and (3) steps to resolve the difficulties within the classroom setting. Garcia and Ortiz (1988) described an eight step prereferal process that will help to reduce inappropriate referrals for second language learners. The basis of these steps is to modify the curriculum and teaching strategies to assist students' learning. The classroom teacher, with assistance from other school staff, explores all other alternatives in assisting students to achieve in the classroom (Olson, 1991). For the speech-language pathologist, the goal of preferral is to assist the special education team in determining the child's language environment (home and school), language use (home and school), and bilingual proficiency.

The Education for All Handicapped Children Act of 1975, Public Law 94-142, requires that children not be placed into special services on the basis of their language, culture, socioeconomic status, or lack of opportunities to learn. The prereferral process protects the rights of children who are acquiring English as a second language.

Three sources of information that assist clinicians in determining the child's language environment, use, and bilingual proficiency are: the case history, questionnaires, and observation of the student.

THE CASE HISTORY

As speech-language pathologists we are aware of the importance of gathering relevant clinical information through the case history. This initial data gathering is essential for the clinician's diagnostic conclusions (Meitus & Weinberg (1983). The case history is especially important for appropriate referrals of second language learners for speech and language intervention. Meitus and Weinberg (1983) suggest taking a detailed case history with 10 categories for investigation: (1) conditions related to the onset and (2) development of the problem, (3) previous diagnostic and (4) rehabilitation results, (5) general developmental status and (6) health status, (7) educational/vocational status,

(8) emotional/social adjustment, (9) pertinent family concerns, and (10) other information volunteered by the respondent.

Appendix B is a Spanish case history form developed over 15 years by two different agencies. The form is detailed. This author's experience with Mexican families indicates that questions should be specific and adequate time must be allowed for the family to think about their responses. Case histories can be sent home with the student, but a personal interview and review of the information with the parent is important to ensure the completeness of the responses to all of the questions.

QUESTIONNAIRES

A number of questionnaires developed for parents and teachers of bilingual students are available. Mattes and Omark (1991) and Langdon and Cheng (1992) provide lists of these instruments. Very few of these questionnaires have determined the validity and reliability of the questions. Kayser (unpublished data) administered the *Bilingual Language Proficiency Questionnaire* (Mattes & Santiago, 1985 Academic Communication Associates) to 10 parents of bilingual students who had been identified as language impaired by two certified bilingual speech-language pathologists. The parents' responses to questions did not indicate any parent concerns or communication or pragmatic difficulty by the students. Further parent questioning indicated that the questions were not specific enough or used terms interpreted differently by the parents. The majority of the questions should have more specific categories (e.g., Does he initiate conversations? to whom, how often, when, are they appropriate, what is the response?) Speech-language pathologists should follow up all questions on a questionnaire with more probing and specific questions to ensure that the parents understand the questions and that correct information is conveyed to the clinician.

Teachers may not have the same difficulty with questionnaires as parents do. If questions are unclear or if the teacher can offer more detailed information, this frequently is offered without further clinician probes.

OBSERVATIONS

A number of language and attention behaviors, listed by Ortiz and Maldonado-Colon (1986), are used by special educators to identify learning disabled students. According to Ortiz and Maldonado-Colon, these same behaviors may also be observed in second language learners. Among the attention behaviors observed both in normal second language learners and learning disabled students are (1) short attention span, (2) distractible, (3) daydreams (4) demands immediate gratification, (5) disorganized, (6) unable to stay on task, and (7) appears confused. The demands of learning English in a classroom may, at times, be overwhelming to a young student and could easily produce the behaviors just listed.

Descriptions of the language behaviors common to both second language learners and learning disabled students (Ortiz & Maldonado-Colon, 1986) include: speaks infrequently, uses gestures, speaks in single words or phrases, refuses to answer questions, does not volunteer information, comments inappropriately, poor recall, poor comprehension, poor vocabulary, difficulty sequencing ideas, difficulty sequencing events, unable to tell or retell stories, confuses similar sounding words, poor pronunciation, and poor syntax.

Now that we know that checklists developed for identification of English speaking learning-disabled students may be misidentifying normal second language learners as language impaired, what do you observe? Table 11–1 is a list of behaviors observed by Mattes and Omark (1991) and Kayser (1990) of bilingual children interacting with peers in the classroom. Both suggest that language-impaired students who are bilingual have difficulty in discourse with peers. Peer relationships are valued among Hispanic students. These observations need further validation, but they are initial attempts to identify behaviors that differentiate impairment from cultural difference.

The prereferral process by speech-language pathologists is necessary so that children are not tested, labeled, and placed into speech-language services inappropriately and unnecessarily. A thorough case history, questionnaires that are clear and specific to the needs of Hispanic families, and observation of behaviors that identify language differences in bilingual children must be part of that process.

ㄌ

SPEECH AND LANGUAGE ASSESSMENT INSTRUMENTS

TEST INSTRUMENTS AND BIAS

The validity and reliability of English tests have been criticized over the years (McCauley & Swisher, 1984; Taylor & Payne, 1983; Vaughn-Cooke; 1983), and the use of these instruments with Hispanic children

TABLE 11–1

Observable communicative behaviors for Spanish- and English-speaking language impaired students.

---

1. Child rarely initiates verbal interactions with peers.
2. Child rarely initiates interactions in peer group activities.
3. Child rarely initiates or organizes play activities with peers.
4. Child does not respond verbally when verbal interactions are initiated by peers.
5. Child's communication has little or no effect on the actions of peers.
6. Child does not engage in dialogue/conversations with peers.
7. Child communicates with limited number of classroom peers.
8. Child generally uses gestures rather than speech to communicate with peers.
9. Facial expressions, eye contact, and other nonverbal aspects of the child's communication are perceived by peers as inappropriate.
10. Facial expressions and/or actions of peers indicate that they may be having difficulty understanding the child's oral and/or nonverbal communications.
11. Peers rarely initiate verbal interactions with the child.

Source: Adapted from *Speech and Language Assessment for the Bilingual Handicapped* (2nd ed.) by L. J. Mattes & D. R. Omark, 1991. Oceanside, CA: Academic Communication Associates; and "Social Communicative Behaviors of Language-disordered Mexican-American Students," by H. Kayser, 1990. *Child Language Teaching Therapy, 6*(3), 255–269.

increases the likelihood of invalid test results. Langdon and Cheng (1992) reviewed 14 articulation and language tests commonly used by bilingual speech-language pathologists. Eight of the tests had no data to support validity or reliability. The other tests had some data on reliability and/or limited review concerning validity. Yet, use of these tests continues to be encouraged and required by state and local educational agencies. Mattes and Omark (1991) and Langdon and Cheng (1992) list the available Spanish tests published in the United States. Table 11–2 summarizes criticisms of the use of standardized tests with Hispanic children.

Vaughn-Cooke (1983) provides an excellent discussion concerning proposed alternatives to traditional testing of minority children. These include the following suggestions.

1. Standardize existing tests on nonmainstream English speakers. Existing tests have been standardized on non-mainstream English speakers (Norris, Juarez, & Perkins, 1989), but Vaughn-Cooke (1983) argues that this results in lower norms and eventually comparisons

TABLE 11–2

Criticisms of tests.

---

1. Lack of validity (does not measure what it is intended to measure). The test does not have
   a. *face validity* (appears sound)
   b. *content validity* (tasks on tests are representative of larger sample of behavior)
   c. *predictive validity* (predicts some later success)
   d. *concurrent validity* (gives results similar to existing tests)
   e. *construct validity* (reflects a valid theory of nature of language and language learning).
2. Lack of reliability (does not consistently give same results). The test does not have:
   a. split-half correlations.
   b. parallel forms.
   c. retesting using the same test.
   d. explicit ratings criteria.
3. Standardization and norms do not include the group to be tested.
4. Development of test construction is limited.
5. Content of test is biased by:
   a. author(s) of test
   b. standardization group
   c. dialect and language group
   d. difficulty of items.
6. Tests are biased due to:
   a. use of middle-class mainstream values and experiences
   b. do not reflect other cultural groups' experiences
7. Test fosters low expectancy for culturally and linguistically diverse children.
8. Test shapes curriculum and does not lead to meaningful instruction.
9. Test evaluates only a segment of child's communicative abilities.
10. Test is viewed as accurate and fixed assessments.
11. Tests is not purely objective.
12. Test lacks linguistic realism and authenticity.

Sources: Adapted from "On Some Dimensions of Language Proficiency by M. Canale, 1983. In J. W. Oller (Ed)., *Issues in Language Testing Research.* Rowley, MA: Newbury House; *Speech and Language Assessment for the Bilingual Handicapped* (2nd ed). by L. J. Mattes & D. R. Omark, 1991. Oceanside, CA: Academic Communication Associates; *Assessing Bilingual exceptional Children: In-service Manual.* by D. R. Omark & D. L. Watson, 1983. San Diego, CA: Los Amigos Research Associates.

between racial groups, which only contributes to lower expectations for minority children.

2. Include a small percentage of minorities in the standardization sample when developing a test. Including a small percentage of minorities in a standardization sample reduces the extent to which the sample represents the average white population. It would be preferable to norm tests to more accurately reflect the population for which they are developed.

3. Modify or revise existing tests in ways that will make them appropriate for nonmainstream speakers. Modifying an existing test does change the original test; therefore, the norms will not be appropriate. Additionally, Vaughn-Cooke warns that clinicians must have a thorough knowledge of nonmainstream dialects before initiating any revisions. This holds true for Spanish-speaking children. This alternative will be discussed further in the next section.

4. Utilize a language sample when assessing the language of nonmainstream speakers. Utilizing a language sample is problematic if the clinician does not have information concerning normal language development for the specific language group being served. This alternative will be presented in Chapter 12 concerning eliciting and analysis of Spanish language samples.

5. Utilize criterion-referenced measures when assessing the language of nonmainstream speakers. Criterion-referenced measures also require information concerning developmental sequences, but this alternative may be more appropriately used for measurement of progress in intervention programs rather than in initial assessment.

6. Refrain from using all standardized tests that have not been corrected for test bias when assessing the language of nonmainstream speakers. There are clinicians who have boycotted the use of standardized tests with Hispanic children and use primarily observations and language samples. But this may not be acceptable in the majority of clinical settings such as schools, children's clinics, and hospitals where third party payments may require objective measures or where state educational agencies define how assessments will be obtained.

7. Develop a new test that can provide a more appropriate assessment of the language of nonmainstream English speakers. This last alternative is an excellent recommendation; unfortunately, test developers have not viewed this as a viable solution. Clinicians will have to request and continue to visit publishers' booths at conventions to convince test developers that there is a critical need and market for Spanish test instruments.

ADAPTING TESTS

Adapting a test instrument means that the tasks and content of the instrument are changed to include culturally appropriate stimuli (Gavillan-Torres, 1984; Kayser, 1989) and are therefore less biased for the Hispanic child. Adapting a test should not be the sole responsibility of an aide, secretary, or even a bilingual professional. Rather, adapting tests should be a concerted effort by a bilingual team. The composition of the team may be different depending on the clinical setting. For example, in a school setting, a group of bilingual specialists may include special and bilingual educators, a reading specialist, and a community member. The teachers may come from different grade levels such as primary and intermediate levels. In a child clinic setting, team members may include an early childhood specialist, a psychologist, nurse, social worker, and a parent. The team should include professionals who are in daily contact with the children.

Kayser (1989) reviewed some of the strategies used by professionals to adapt test instruments. For content revision, the strategies included review of vocabulary to determine appropriateness for the age level of the children, vocabulary substitutions that are more familiar to community members, changing picture stimuli to depict the experiences of the children, and developing story topics that are more familiar for the region. Task revisions included changing formats for appropriate age levels, changing tasks to receptive rather than expressive when necessary, or vice versa, and changing tasks to another modality to assess similar skills.

An understanding of and familiarity with the purpose of testing is necessary for the successful adaptation of test instruments. Discussions among team members will likely lead to frustration because bilingual professionals often have had different experiences with Hispanic children. But the result of these discussions will produce an instrument that will be in the process of development. As the instrument is used with children, specific items can be discussed at a later time and revised or omitted as needed.

MODIFYING PROCEDURES

The test situation is a social communicative event that many Hispanic children have not experienced (Saville-Troike, 1986). Heath (1984) stated that testing has three premises: (a) normal language learners go into a test situation with a known framework for interaction and are expected to use this framework for responses; (b) children are expected to be information givers, interpreters of pictures, and narrators; and (c) children should know how to segment language, so that they know what "words" and "meanings" are, and be able to recognize that there is an agreed-on meaning for a text. Among anthropologists these premises are debated.

A standardized approach to testing limits Hispanic children to a stimulus-response set that is considered to be a western European social communicative event (Taylor & Clark, 1994). Because the purpose of testing is to determine whether a communication impairment exists, modifying procedures may assist clinicians in determining whether an Hispanic student does indeed have a communication difficulty not related to normal second language acquisition. There are three phases for implementing modified procedures; before, during, and after testing. Each of these will be discussed briefly (Erickson & Iglesias, 1986; Kayser, 1989).

BEFORE TESTING

Preliminary precautions should be taken before the testing session begins. These require some time in preparation but are considered to be effective.

1. Reword the instructions so that familiar phrasing, terms, and sentence structure may assist the child to understand what is expected of him.
2. Develop more practice items that will allow the child more examples of the test stimuli.
3. Obtain and use different picture stimuli that may be more representative of the child's culture, or provide a better example of the item.
4. Omit items that you know from your experience are incorrectly identified by Hispanic children.

DURING TESTING

The following modified procedures are presented from the easiest to implement to the most difficult. The more difficult procedures require more practice by the clinician and may take some time to develop.

1. Record all responses, especially if the child changes an answer.

2. Repeat the test stimuli when necessary and more frequently than what is specified or allowed in the test manual.
3. Provide additional time for the child to respond.
4. Watch the child's eye gaze and body movements for referencing when there is no verbal response.
5. Accept culturally appropriate responses as correct.
6. On vocabulary recognition tests, have the child name the picture in addition to pointing to the stimulus item to ascertain the appropriateness of the label for the pictorial representation.
7. Have the child identify the actual object, body part, action, photograph, and so forth, particularly if he or she has limited experience with books, line drawings, or the testing process.
8. Have the child explain why the "incorrect" answer was selected.
9. Continue testing beyond the ceiling.

AFTER TESTING

1. Compare the child's responses to charts on dialect and/or second language acquisition features.
2. Rescore articulation and expressive language samples, giving credit for variation or differences.
3. If the child was uncooperative or unresponsive, complete the testing in several sessions.
4. Consider having a peer, sibling, parent, or trusted adult administer the test items during a second session.

Modifying your procedure is an art and will require clinicians to develop flexibility in their testing protocols. Allowing a student to use a variety of response styles will tap the child's true world knowledge and thereby eliminate inappropriate placement of children into special services.

DYNAMIC ASSESSMENT

The assessment of communicative competency in bilingual children has been described as static (i.e., a measure of a child's ability on one task on one occasion) (Erickson & Iglesias, 1986; Kayser, 1993). Peña and Iglesias (1992) have recommended that dynamic methods of language assessment be used to assess language learning potential in bilingual children. Dynamic assessment focuses on the individual's ability to modify language behavior or ability to learn during the testing process (Erickson & Iglesias, 1986). Thus, the clinician and student interact during the testing session rather than having the child simply respond to test stimuli. The clinician tests, teaches, or mediates, and then retests. Peña and Iglesias (1992) have used this method with preschoolers who were identifed as language impaired and normal. The purpose of their study was to explore home and school demands for labeling versus description and also to demonstrate the efficacy of this approach in differentiating normal from language-impaired children. Peña and Iglesias (1992) reported that the language-impaired children were less responsive to mediation than normals and required more intense effort by the examiner to produce change. Additionally, although the pretest scores for the two groups were similar, the posttest scores after mediation were markedly different. Peña and Iglesias believe that change in the ability to label on a one word expressive test for the normal group helped differentiate them from the language-impaired group.

This method is an experimental and innovative approach to assessing language abilities in Hispanic students. Peña and Iglesias (1992) state that future research directions include comparisions of other language measures, determining whether the mediated skills are transferred to other contexts, and applying learned strategies to new learning situations. There is still much to learn about this method, but it is a promising approach for differentiating language impairments from normal language in developing bilinguals.

INTERPRETING THE DATA

De Leon (1985) reported that team decision making concerning differentiation of children who are language impaired versus normal was more reliable than individual "expert" reviews of the same test data. The teams were from local school districts and were familiar with the community, children, and school expectations for bilingual children. It appears that determining whether a student is speech and language impaired may be improved with the consensus of a team of professionals who routinely provide diagnostic assessments. Speech-language pathologists who review only their own test results may be able to determine normal from deviant, but if the clinician is unsure, discussion of test data with other professionals may bring out information that one person may overlook or not consider.

ᘳ

OTHER CONSIDERATIONS IN ASSESSMENT

TESTING PROCEDURES

A number of practices are used by speech-language pathologists in testing bilingual Hispanic children. When clinicians are unsure of bilingual students' performance, unorthodox procedures may evolve. Table 11-3 summarizes some of the practices that may be used by clinicians who evaluate Spanish-English speaking students (Kayser,

TABLE 11-3
Recommended testing and reporting procedures.

---

1. Use formal and informal measures of language abilities that assess form, content, and use.
2. Administer several test measures that are representative of the population.
3. Use translations of test only if they have been developed by a diagnostic team.
4. Test both languages, but one at a time.
5. Assess bilingual discourse abilities with other bilinguals.
6. Use a minimum of three elicitation procedures to obtain a language sample.
7. Report all adaptations of the test instrument in the evaluation report.
8. Report the nature of the testing procedures, such as the use of an interpreter, language first tested, etc.
9. Report norms only if they are valid for the population tested.

Source: Adapted from "Hispanic Cultures" by H. Kayser, 1993. In D. Battle (Ed.), *Communication Disorders in Multicultural Populations* (pp. 114–157). Boston, MA: Andover Medical Publishers.

1993). Evaluating Hispanic children does require more time and effort than testing an English monolingual student. Using questionable and succinct methods to assess these students will result in invalid assessment results.

THE TRANSLATION OF TESTS

Tests are frequently translated and this process may be considered to be one way of adapting a test instrument. Merely translating the test does not equate to an appropriate adapted assessment instrument (Erickson & Iglesias, 1986; Kayser, 1989). Languages differ in honorifics (formal *Used* versus familiar *tu*), gender markers (*el* and *la*), semantics (*arroz*, tomato based and spicy versus *rice*, white or brown), structural rules (adjective before noun versus adjective after noun), registers (formal educated versus *barrio*), dialectal variations in vocabulary and registers (Cuban versus Mexican), and cultural norms for who speaks what to whom and when. For example, a receptive vocabulary test developed in English for middle-class urban children could be translated. But if two Spanish-speaking children, one reared in Dallas and the other in rural Mexico, were evaluated with this instrument, the test results might indicate that the rural child had an impairment. The urban Spanish-speaking child may have had the experiences of urban life, or at least may have viewed the mainstream culture on television, thereby giving him an edge on this test. The translation of tests is a simplistic attempt to test children, but it neglects complex variables such as culture, language, and children's experiences that allow children to perform at their maximum potential.

THE CLINICIAN'S LANGUAGE PROFICIENCY

There are two issues relative to the assessment of Spanish-speaking children that may have a biasing effect on the child's test performance, the clinician's Spanish or English language proficiency and dialect.

ASHA's (1989) definition for bilingual speech-language pathologists and audiologists states that the clinician must be able to speak his or her primary language and to speak (or sign) at least one other language with native or near-native proficiency in lexicon, semantics, phonology, morphology/syntax, and pragmatics during clinical management. One way of determining bilingual competency is for clinicians to submit to a language proficiency examination administered through language testing agencies. But what if a clinician desires to develop his or her bilingualism? How should his or her proficiency be monitored?

A possible solution would be for the future bilingual clinician is to develop his or her proficiency through a mentoring relationship with another bilingual clinician or other professional. The clinician's proficiency should first be evaluated by the testing agency. A contract could be developed between the two clinicians whereby certain skills would be developed, practiced, and monitored through videotape, tape recording, or live observations. As each of these skills is mastered, the contract is fulfilled. Bilingual clinicians must recognize their own limitations in working in English and/or Spanish. Not all clinicians are able to or interested in working with adults. Similarly, not all bilingual clinicians are capable of working with adults versus children because of fluency and level of language proficiency. The general rule should be, whatever language competency is expected of English-speaking speech-language pathologists, should also be expected of Spanish-speaking clinicians.

DIALECT

Although dialect may have little effect on the comprehension of utterances by adults with other adults, it may have an effect on children who are speech and language impaired. Children do recognize differences in Spanish dialects (Fantini, 1985), but we do not know what effect this may have on the child's testing performance. To illustrate, when a Southerner speaks, it may take a Westerner several minutes to become accustomed to the speech patterns. Spanish-speaking children who use a different dialect from the clinician's dialect may need additional time to become accustomed to and therefore understand the clinician's speech and language. If the child is truly language impaired, the child may have more difficulty than the child with normal language development. Allowing the child to first listen to the clinician's speech patterns during a 10-minute conversational period may improve the child's performance on tests. The same may be true if the child's dialect uses a slower rate of speech than what the clinician uses in her or his dialect. The clinician's language proficiency and dialect should be considered and monitored for potential biasing effects on children's test performance.

THE CLINICIAN-CHILD INTERACTION

A significant and yet little explored variable is the cultural difference in verbal and nonverbal communication behaviors between the clinician and the child during the speech-language assessment event. Taylor (1986) has suggested that clinicians should recognize that the different modes, channels, and functions of communication events in which individuals are expected to participate in a clinical setting may result in differing levels of linguistic or communicative performance.

It is assumed that clinicians who are from the same ethnic and cultural background as the client may have the cultural sensitivity to recognize clinical practices that might affect the performance of the client. Kayser (1994) described the verbal and nonverbal communicative behaviors of two clinicians during a speech and language screening event with monolingual English- and monolingual Spanish-speaking Hispanic preschoolers. One clinician was a native monolingual English speaker and the other was a bilingual Mexican American whose first language was Spanish when she entered the public schools. They each screened 10 Hispanic children.

The two clinicians differed in four nonverbal areas of interaction: (1) touching for behavior control, (2) head nodding or shaking, (3) facial expression, and (4) eye gaze. Touching was not observed for the English-speaking clinician (EC), but was a behavior consistently used by the Spanish-speaking clinician (SC). Touching was used to control the child's behavior or to get his or her attention on the immediate task. SC touched the child's hands, fingers, and back. SC also used head nods and shakes to affirm, agree, and disagree with the child. These nonverbal acts were frequently the only communicative acts used by SC. Although EC frequently smiled and was friendly, SC's facial affect had much more variation. She would show facial grimaces that expressed confusion if the child's utterances were unclear, dissatisfaction if the child did not behaviorally comply, and interest in the child's background and knowledge. Of particular interest was the increased use of eye gaze by the Hispanic clinician to control the child's behavior. A stern look at the child was frequently all that was necessary to regain attention for a task.

The sequence of interactions used by these two clinicians as they administered a test stimulus was also different. After EC administered a test stimulus, she looked down at her protocol and then looked up at the child. The Hispanic child would respond either verbally or nonverbally. If the child responded nonverbally, EC would miss the nonverbal responses such as eye gaze for referencing or the slight movement of the child's body to indicate the answer (e.g., child lifts shoulder to show his or her "shoulder"). The Hispanic clinician's nonverbal interactions were different from EC's because she continued to observe the child after giving the stimulus. If the child responded nonverbally, SC accepted or rejected the response and then proceeded to mark her protocol.

Three differences were observed in the clinicians' linguistic behaviors. These included the use of (1) directives, (2) clarifications, and (3) explanations. The Hispanic clinician was direct in her requests of the child's behavior and performance on the screening test. Her directives were performatives such as *di* (say) or *haz* (do). In contrast, EC was indirect in her requests of the child's behavior and performance on the test. Her directives were in the form of hints (e.g., "Did you have milk or orange juice?" after asking "Can you tell me what a glass is used for?"), questions (e.g., "Can you point to your nose?"), permission statements (e.g., "Can we finish this?"), and statements of need (e.g., "I want you to do some things for me"). The overall communicative style of the Hispanic clinician was direct, whereas the Anglo clinician's style was polite and indirect.

The second linguistic difference between the two clinicians was in the use of clarifications during communication breakdown. SC used repetition as the means for clarifying with the children. Repetitions ranged from one to four times for the same test stimulus, without a change in the form. EC used rephrasing as the means for clarifying information for the children. If the child did not respond to the clinician's statement, the clinician immediately rephrased the test stimulus.

The third linguistic difference between the two clinicians was in the use of explanations by EC to introduce each subtest. The clinician would give an explanation and then ask if the child understood and was ready to begin the testing. The Hispanic clinician did not provide explanations but instead was directive and told the child what to do next. The Hispanic clinician's interaction lacked explanations and used no transition into the next subtest.

In summary, the verbal and nonverbal communication behaviors of the two clinicians as they interacted with the children were distinctly different in style, form, and use. Of course, more study is necessary to better understand cultural and linguistic differences in communication by Hispanic and Anglo clinicians. But the more we learn about differences in clinical interactions, the more better we will be able to serve Hispanic children in the assessment "event."

⊔⌐

SUMMARY

The purpose of this chapter was to review recommended procedures for speech and language assessment of Spanish-English-speaking students. Prereferral procedures, which include the case history, questionnaires, and observations will assist clinicians in determining whether further testing is warranted. Tests and their criticism, adaptations, and use through modified procedures were discussed. Other considerations for assessment such as translation of tests, dialect and language proficiency of the clinician, and child-clinician interactions were reviewed. Diagnostic assessment of bilingual children is not an easy or simple task. Individuals who continue to find simple, fast, and expedient methods for assessments may not understand the complexity of the issues involved in testing children who are learning a second language or educational systems that fail to consider the effects of English-only instruction and the use of standardized tests with bilingual students.

⊔⌐

REFERENCES

American Speech-Language-Hearing Association. (1989). Bilingual speech-language pathologists and audiologists. *Asha, 31*(3), 93.

Boone, D., & Plante, E. (1993). *Human communication and its disorders.* Englewood Cliffs, NJ: Prentice-Hall.

Canale, M. (1983). On some dimensions of language proficiency. In J. W. Oller (Ed.), *Issues in language testing research* (pp. 331–342). Rowley, MA: Newbury House.

DeLeon, J. (1985). *An investigation into the development and validation of an assessment procedure for identifying language disorders in Spanish-English bilingual children.* Unpublished doctoral dissertation, New Mexico State University. Las Cruces.

Education of All Handicapped Children Act of 1975. 20 U.S.C.A. 1411-1420: P.L. 94-142 (1975).

Erickson, J. G., & Iglesias, A. (1986). Assessment of communication disorders in nonEnglish proficient children. In O. Taylor (Ed.), *Nature of communication disorders in culturally and linguistically diverse populations.* (pp. 181–218). San Diego, CA: College-Hill Press.

Fantini, A. E. (1985). *Language acquisition of a bilingual child*. San Diego, CA: College-Hill Press.

Garcia, S., & Ortiz, A. (1988). Preventing inappropriate referrals of language minority students to special education. The National Clearinghouse for Bilingual Education. *Occasional Papers in Bilingual Education, 5*.

Gavillan-Torres, E. (1984). Issues of assessment of limited-English-proficient students and of truly disabled in the United States. In N. Miller (Ed.), *Bilingualism and language disability: Assessment and remediation* (pp. 131–153). San Diego, CA: College-Hill Press.

Heath, S. B. (1984, November). *Cross cultural acquisition of language*. Paper presented at the annual convention of the American Speech-Language-Hearing Association. San Francisco, CA.

Kayser, H. (1985). *A study of speech-language pathologists and their Mexican-American language disordered caseloads*. Unpublished doctoral dissertation, New Mexico State University, Las Cruces.

Kayser, H. (1989). Speech and language assessment of Spanish-English speaking children. *Language, Speech, and Hearing Services in Schools. 20*, 226–244.

Kayser, H. (1990). Social communicative behaviors of language-disordered Mexican-American students. *Child Language Teaching Therapy. 6(3)*, 255–269.

Kayser, H. (1993). Hispanic cultures. In D. Battle (Ed.) *Communication disorders in multicultural populations* (pp. 114–157). Boston, MA: Andover Medical Publishers.

Kayser, H. (1994). Intervention with children from linguistically and culturally different backgrounds. In M. E. Fey, J. Windsor, & S. F. Warren (Eds.), *Language intervention: Preschool through the elementary years* (pp. 315–331). Baltimore, MD: Paul H. Brookes.

Langdon, H., & Cheng, L. (1992). *Hispanic children and adults with communication disorders*. Gaithersburg, MD: Aspen.

Mattes, L. J., & Omark, D. R. (1991). *Speech and language assessment for the bilingual handicapped (2nd ed.)* Oceanside, CA: Academic Communication Associates.

Mattes, L. J., & Santiago, X. X. (1985). *Bilingual Language Proficiency Questionnaire*. Oceanside, CA: Academic Communication Associates..

McCauley, R., & Swisher, L. (1984). Psychometric review of language and articulation tests for preschool children. *Journal of Speech and Hearing Disorders, 49(1)*, 34–42.

Meitus, I. J., & Weinburg, B. (1983). *Diagnosis in speech-language pathology*. Baltimore, MD: University Park Press.

Norris, M. K., Juarez, M. J., & Perkins, M. N. (1989). Adaptation of a screening test for bilingual and bidialectal populations. *Language, Speech, and Hearing Services, 20(4)*, 381–389.

Olson, P. (1991). Referring language minority students to special education. ERIC Clearinghouse on Languages and Linguistics. Washington, DC: Center for Applied Linguistics.

Omark, D. R., & Watson, D. L. (1983). *Assessing bilingual exceptional children: In-service manual*. San Diego, CA: Los Amigos Research Associates.

Ortiz, A., & Maldonado-Colon, E. (1986). Reducing inappropriate referrals of language minority students in special education. In A. C. Willig & H. F. Greenberg (Eds.), *Bilingualism and learning disabilities* (pp. 37–52). New York: American Library.

Peña, E., & Iglesias, A. (1992). The application of dynamic methods to language assessment: A nonbiased procedure. *The Journal of Special Education. 26*(3), 269–280.

Reynolds, M. (1984). Classification of students with handicaps. In E. W. Gordon (Ed.), *Review of research in education* (pp. 63–92). Washington, DC: American Educational Research Association.

Saville-Troike, M. (1986). Anthropological considerations in the study of communication. In O. Taylor (Ed.), *Nature of communication disorders in culturally and linguistically diverse populations* (pp. 47–72). San Diego, CA: College-Hill Press.

Taylor, O. (1986). Historical perspectives and conceptual framework. In O. Taylor (Ed.), *Nature of communication disorders in culturally and linguistically diverse populations* (pp. 1–18). San Diego, CA: College-Hill Press.

Taylor, O. L., & Clark, M. (1994). Culture and communication disorders: A theoretical framework. *Seminars in Speech and Language, 15*(2), 103–114.

Taylor, O. L., & Payne, K. T. (1983). Culturally valid testing: A proactive approach. *Topics in Language Disorders. 3*, 1–7.

Vaughn-Cooke, F. B. (1983). Improving language assessment in minority children. *Asha, 25*(9), 29–34.

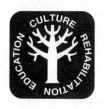

CHAPTER 12

LANGUAGE SAMPLES: ELICITATION AND ANALYSIS

HORTENCIA KAYSER, Ph.D.
MARÍA ADELAIDA RESTREPO, M.A.

If the child has been real verbal, then I usually feel pretty comfortable with the work. If I've had a very hard time eliciting any kind of verbalizations, then I feel real uncomfortable in terms of how adequate that language sample is. (Kayser, 1985, p. 112)

Eliciting a language sample is an art. Clinicians develop this skill over years of experience. They recognize that the materials, tasks, and interactions of the clinician will determine the representativeness of the language sample obtained from the child or adult. Eliciting the language sample becomes more difficult when the child or adult is from another culture. We know that Hispanic children have unequal roles and status from adults (Heath, 1986). This unequal status then contributes to the child's perceptions of what can be said, to whom, and when. This difference for Hispanic children and adults affects the interaction when a stranger, such as a speech-language pathologist, attempts to elicit language utterances (Kayser, 1989).

How the language sample is analyzed depends on the clinician's language framework. A number of analysis procedures are available, most are time-consuming, but all are valuable in determining the strengths and weaknesses of children and adults who speak English and Spanish. Analyzing the Spanish language sample is problematic because limited developmental data are available to make a definitive determination as to whether a language impairment does indeed exist. This chapter will discuss the elicitation procedures commonly used by clinicians and the importance of the child's culture in defining appropriate roles and tasks. The second section will provide suggestions for initial interactions with preschoolers, school-age children, and adolescents. A brief discussion and examples of standard procedures for eliciting language samples that are recommended for use by speech-language pathologists and researchers in second language acquisition and bilingual education will be provided. Finally, analysis procedures for form, content, and use that can be applied to Spanish language samples will be discussed in detail.

ᒡ

HOW DO WE ELICIT LANGUAGE SAMPLES?

Kayser (1985) conducted open-ended interviews with 20 speech-language pathologists concerning the elicitation procedures they used with Hispanic children. These clinicians recognized that test scores were more valued than language samples by psychologists and educational diagnosticians, but they also stated that many of the language tests they used were not reliable measures of the children's language abilities. Several of the clinicians stated that they used only the language sample to qualify children as language impaired.

All 20 clinicians depended heavily on the language sample in determining whether a child was language impaired. The child's comprehension of language could be evaluated with formal tests, but to evaluate the child's expressive language, both formal tests and language samples were utilized. Specific areas that were evaluated in the language sample included: syntactic structures; conversational skills such as topic maintenance, turn-taking, and clarification ability; questions; detailed descriptions; coherence in explanations; and the ability to express opinions. During the language sample elicitation, the child's behavior and auditory processing abilities were observed. These cognitive skills included attending to the task, auditory memory and sequencing, response time, and auditory discrimination. The linguistic background that each clinician brought to the evaluation determined what was elicited and how a language sample was analyzed (Kayser, 1985).

How the speech-language pathologists elicited the language sample determined the child's language performance. The technique most often used by the clinicians was to have a conversation with the child. Other techniques included narratives, with or without books, descriptions of objects or pictures, explanations of activities, information gathering, and questioning. Conversational skills were considered important, not only for developing rapport before formal testing, but also for further elicitation of language after testing. Conversations were elicited during play by talking about cartoons, the children's family, a popular television program, or whatever the clinician believed would be interesting to the child. Each clinician based the topic of the conversation on his or her past experience as to what had worked for other Hispanic children.

The narrative was elicited by providing the child with a book, a sequence of pictures, or asking the child to retell a story that the clinician first told. The narratives were then analyzed for content, sequence, and story structure. Some clinicians believed that the narrative gave more information concerning children's organizational abilities than conversations because some children never learned to retell a story, even after months of therapy. Other clinicians stated that the conversational sample was more valuable than narratives because the children gave a variety of grammatical structures that were not seen in the narratives. Some clinicians used both procedures. There were clinicians who based the language impairment decision only on the narrative; others used only the conversational analysis. All of the clinicians reported that the language sample was the most representative sample of the child's expressive language abilities. The language sample could be elicited several weeks later and the only difference would be the quantity of language, but not the quality. Narratives provided a good means for assessing a child's cognitive and organizational abilities with language, whereas conversational skills more accurately assessed a child's grammatical and interactional social abilities (Kayser, 1985).

CULTURE AND THE CLINICIAN'S PROCEDURES

Eliciting a language sample from an Hispanic child, teenager, or adult may be biased by the procedures used by clinicians. Two variables must be considered when attempting to elicit the sample. The first is the clinician-child or -adult interaction; the second involves the tasks of using conversation and narrative. Both procedures are culturally bound (i.e., different cultures define the rules differently for conversations and the presentation of narratives).

ROLES AND STATUS

Heath (1986) has described the Mexican American child as having unequal conversational status with adults. This means that having a conversation with a stranger such as a speech-language pathologist may be an awkward event for the child. By giving the child a role of having equal status, where the child must inform, explain, describe, direct, and so on, the clinician is breaking a cultural rule, that adults have more status and children do not assume equality to an adult. This may explain why many Hispanic children are reticent to speak to clinicians.

CONVERSATIONS AND NARRATIVES

The second variable is the use of conversation and narratives to elicit the language samples. We know that Hispanic children do have conversations, but primarily with peers, siblings, and intimate family members (Heath, 1986; Kayser, 1990). Conversations then must be viewed as culturally bound (i.e., who should speak what to whom is culturally determined). Narratives, as explained by Gutierrez-Clellan in Chapter 5, are also culture-bound. Children learn the narrative style of their families and culture (Heath, 1986). Therefore, for many Hispanic children, using a book is an unfamiliar interaction between an adult and child and an unfamiliar style of telling stories. For Mexican Americans, narratives are oral. There is retelling of the family history and travels. These stories may have a moral or explain appropriate behavior as a purpose. The type of narrative and the style that is produced by Hispanic children would have to be familiar to the clinician.

CONSIDERATIONS IN ELICITING LANGUAGE SAMPLES

There are three age groups of children from whom clinicians attempt to elicit languages samples, preschool, school-age (kindergarten through 6th grade), and adolescents (7th through 12th grades). There are specific cultural norms that each age group will respond to, which facilitate eliciting the language sample.

PRESCHOOL-AGE CHILDREN

Many Hispanic preschool children have strong attachments to their mothers. Their unwillingness to accompany the clinician to a room to "play" is often displayed through tears, lack of responsiveness, or gestures. Two suggestions may help clinicians obtain a representative language sample. The first is to elicit the sample in the preschool classroom with classmates; the second is to elicit the sample with the mother in the therapy room.

Taking a language sample of a child in the classroom is not difficult. A wireless microphone can be attached to the child's clothing, and the tape recorder with receiver can be stored near the clinician or teacher's desk. The clinician can observe the child's interactions and chart the child's initiations and responses to other children's initiations for conversations. The clinician also can observe the other children's responses to the child's communication attempts. The clinician can then begin interaction with the target child with other children near to contribute to the conversations. This allows the target child to become comfortable with the adult. A language sample can be obtained in 30 minutes if the clinician chooses scheduled classroom events that are conducive to talking.

A child who will not separate from a mother or caregiver may require more time to elicit the language sample. One technique I have used with these young children is to allow the mother and child to play with toys in the room and record their interactions using a video camera. The language sample is first elicited through a mother-child interaction. The clinician's instructions to the mother should reflect the need for a language sample. Using the phrase "play with your child" may not be appropriate for the Hispanic mother, because play is appropriate for children, but not for adult-child interactions. Instructions to the mother can include: "Teach your child how to use this . . . ." "Show the child what this is used for." "See if the child will imitate your phrases."

Once the child appears to feel comfortable, the clinician enters the room. The clinician talks to the mother, either about the family or the child. The clinician slowly approaches the child and begins to play with both mother and child. The clinician may touch the child's head, which is culturally appropriate for Mexican and Mexican American mothers and children (Maestas & Erickson, 1992). For the parent, touching the child may relieve some anxiety, because there are beliefs a curse is placed on a child (*Mal ojo* or evil eye) when an adult admires the child and does not touch his or her head or face. The clinician begins to play primarily with the child, occasionally touching the child's hands. The child will eventually recognize that the mother is comfortable and allows the clinician to play and thus join the interaction. A third alternative would be to allow a sibling to "play" with the preschooler to elicit a sibling- or peer-child interaction.

The use of all three types of interactions will provide the clinician with different contexts and interactors for analysis and comparisons.

SCHOOL-AGE STUDENTS

Younger school-age children (5 to 9 years) may still be using the cultural norm that children do not have conversations with adults. This depends on the acculturation and assimilation of the student. Hispanic children who have recognized that it is acceptable to talk to adults in school may not have the refined conversational skills that are seen in English-speaking children. Eliciting language samples from these primary and intermediate grade students will require a second context other than the clinician-child interaction. The second context may be a peer-child interaction with familiar and/or unfamiliar students. Peer-peer interactions tend to be more directive than when the child is speaking to an adult (Fantini, 1985). This context will provide the clinician with a means of determining whether the child does use differing social registers.

ADOLESCENTS

Three types of adolescents are referred for evaluations: the Spanish monolingual, the English speaker who has lost Spanish proficiency, and the Spanish speaker who was educated in this country and has some English abilities but has not become proficient in English.

The elicitation of the language sample for each type of student requires an understanding of how much education the child has received in this country and his or her experiences with mainstream English speakers. If the students are interacting primarily with Spanish-speaking individuals in the classroom and the community, they may still adhere to cultural rules of adult-child interactions. Additionally, the type of task used to elicit the sample will depend on their literacy skills (English or Spanish), exposure to English narratives, and the number of years of education in Latin America. Conversational interactions may be awkward for the student; therefore, an interview format may be more appropriate with this age level. Students at this age level are more than willing to answer questions and provide information if it is known to them. A conversation with an adult stranger concerning personal or unusual topics may be more difficult and uncomfortable for them.

MORE SUGGESTIONS FOR ELICITING LANGUAGE SAMPLES

Cornejo, Weinstein, and Najar (1983) described a number of techniques that are used by researchers in second language acquisition and bilingual education. These elicitation procedures are summarized in Table 12-1. The techniques were designed to encourage children to spontaneously express themselves with minimal probing from an adult. All of the techniques were field-tested and refined to maximize their effectiveness. Langdon (1992) also provides a number of techniques that can be used with Hispanic students. Selecting a culturally appropriate technique may require time to determine if certain tasks are unnatural or offensive. This can only be determined by asking the student, parent, or caregiver.

Eliciting a language sample is an art. It takes practice and often years of experience to develop an ability to elicit specific forms, use,

TABLE 12-1
Elicitation techniques.

Technique	Description	Application	Examples	Age Level
Probe	Student responds to open or closed-ended questions	Elicits yes/no or short response	Why did he do this? Does he cook at home?	Children/Adults
Description	Describes an object	Use variety of stimuli Children use toys Adults use pictures	Tell me about the picture.	Children/Adults
Narration	Describes a sequence of events	Can talk about play event, retell cartoons just seen, wordless picture books, comic books, or folktale.	What's he doing?	Children/Adults
Interpretation	Provides meanings of stimuli	Child interprets motives of characters, artist's intended meaning, music's message	Why would the monster want to?	Adolescents/ Adults
Expression	Reacts personally to a stimulus	Present several toys and ask why chose that toy, ask for story where there is conflict, relate a meaningful incident.	Tell me about the time you were embarrassed in class.	Children/Adults
Explication	Provides information about a process or procedure	Verbal directions to get to neighborhood, street map and ask how to get from one point to next. Building a house, toy, make foods.	Tell me step by step.	Children/Adults

TABLE 12–1 (continued)

Technique	Description	Application	Examples	Age Level
Elaboration	Must expand on topic	Ask for elaboration on topic already introduced in interaction	Tell me more.	Children/Adults
Role-playing	Must use language appropriate for situation.	Suggest an imaginary situation: parent/teacher caught you fighting, arguing with brother, asking for a date, clearing up a misunderstanding, apologizing to friend, forgetting a meeting.	Excuse me. May I help you?	Children/Adults
Games/problem solving	Must verbalize answer to problems	Counting games, identifying errors or inconsistencies, guessing games, how a toy/machine works.	What's wrong with it?	Children/Adults
Sustained production	Produces a stream of uninterrupted language	Recites as many words as possible without stopping or length of words or topics	I want you to say as many words in English as you can.	Children/Adults
Paraphrase	Asked to express an idea another way.	Express an idea differently without changing the meaning	Say this differently.	Adolescents/ Adults

Source: Adapted from *Eliciting Spontaneous Speech in Bilingual Students: Method and Techniques,* by R. J. Cornejo, A. C. Weinstein, and C. Najar, (1983). Educational Resources Information Center (ERIC), Clearinghouse on Rural Education and Small Schools (CRESS). Las Cruces: New Mexico State University.

and content from children. Limiting the elicitation process to a narrative or a conversation limits the representativeness of the language sample for Hispanic children. A variety of samples is required, and hopefully, the different contexts with different interactors will provide the clinician with a rich language sample that is representative of the Hispanic student's capabilities.

ꓶ

LANGUAGE ANALYSIS

When assessing a child through language sample analyses, the main purposes of the analyses are (1) to determine the presence or absence of a language impairment and (2) to describe a child's language and language goals for intervention. These two purposes require clinicians to have developmental information to determine whether the child's language is age-appropriate. Although normative data for Spanish development are limited, Anderson (see Chapter 3) provides a summary of developmental data to assist clinicians in differentiating normal from deviant language development in Spanish-speaking children. More research is needed in both normal and impaired populations to increase our ability to identify language impairments in Spanish-speaking children more efficiently and effectively. However, with Anderson's information and the clinician's comparison of a child's language sample to those of children from the local community, a clinician may be able to determine whether a child has a language impairment.

When a clinician obtains a language sample, the main areas of analyses are form, content, and use (Swisher, 1994). If the purpose of the analysis is to determine whether a child has a specific language impairment, the most efficient approach is to analyze form. However, if the purpose of the analysis is to describe the language of a child with a different diagnosis or to determine whether a child has a language deficit secondary to a primary disorder, analyses of language content and use also should be completed. For example, if a child has a possible diagnosis of autism, semantic and pragmatic abilities would be important skills to analyze to determine the child's language goals. If a child has suffered meningitis and is reentering school, the clinician should analyze the child's form, content, and use at the discourse level in addition to the test battery to determine whether the child has a language/cognitive deficit. In addition, older school-age children with language impairment develop semantic and pragmatic deficits that significantly affect their academic and communicative skills. Therefore, thorough language analyses with this age group are essential for establishing language goals.

ANALYSIS OF LANGUAGE FORM

The most common clinical analyses of form are morphology, syntax, and discourse structure.

MORPHOSYNTAX

Syntactic complexity can be analyzed by mean length of response (MLR) per utterance in words. Mean length of utterance (MLU) in morphemes is not indicative of sentence complexity in Spanish (Barrera & Barrera, 1989, cited in Schnell de Acedo, 1994) given that ellipsis are quite frequent forms. Kvaal, Shipstead-Cox, Nevitt, Hodson, and Launer (1988) found that MLU in preschool-age children increased with age in Spanish-speaking children; however, other authors disagree with the use of this procedure in Spanish. The use of mean length of response is recommended for highly inflected languages such as Spanish (Schnell de Acedo, 1994).

To obtain (MLR) scores, the clinician first transcribes the sample and then determines the utterances. The criteria for an utterance in Spanish are the same as the criteria for English. An utterance is marked by a rising or falling intonation contour and a terminal pause (Miller, 1981). Once the utterances are identified, the number of words per utterance are counted and averaged across the total number of utterances.

Mean length of response in utterances should be used with younger children; however, for older children, like English, sentence complexity should be analyzed with Terminal Units (T-units) (Hunt, 1965). Utterances become difficult to segment with older children and thus there may be over inflation of the MLR score (Siguan, Colomina, & Vila, 1990). Gutierrez-Clellen and Hofstetter (1994) found that mean length of T-unit increased with age in Spanish-speaking children in the United States. They also analyzed sentence complexity utilizing a subordination index which also increased with age.

T-units are defined as any clause and its subordinate clauses. For example, the simple sentence, *El perro esta dormido*, is a T-unit. An example of a sentence with a subordinate clause is: *El perro esta tan cansado que no lo podemos despertar*. Similarly to MLR, once a transcript is divided into T-units, the number of words per T-units is counted and averaged. The index of subordination is obtained by adding the number of clauses per T-unit, and then averaging. Thus, the first sentence would have a subordination score of 1, and the second sentence would have a subordination score of 2. Because there is greater use of elliptical sentences in Spanish, some authors (e.g., Gutierrez-Clellen & Hofstetter, 1994) do not count elliptical sentences (unlike English scoring) as part of a T-unit. This prevents an overinflation of the mean length of the T-unit score. However, the use of elliptical utterances should not be ignored because they are cohesion discourse strategies.

Another syntactic analysis in Spanish is the *Developmental Assessment of Spanish Grammar* (DASG) (Toronto, 1976). This analysis is not commonly used clinically because it is time-consuming. Research using this analysis is also limited and does not always result in positive results. For example, Linares-Orama and Sanders (1974) found that this analysis differentiated children by age and presence of impairment. However, McKaig (1988) found that it did not differentiate Spanish-speaking children with normal language from those with language impairment. The difference in results may be related to problems in the subject selection criteria in the McKaig study. Other variables may also exist, but more research is necessary to determine the reliability and validity of this procedure.

The DASG is an adaptation of the *Developmental Sentence Scoring* (Lee, 1974) and was locally normed in Chicago. Clinician's who use this procedure may want to obtain new norms and obtain discriminant validity, or use it for descriptive purposes (research is underway to determine whether the DASG is valid for purposes of identifying language impairment in Spanish-speaking children). DASG is limited in its range of analyses, but does provide a general indication of syntactic development as children get older.

The DASG requires that the clinician segment the transcript into sentences, which according to Toronto's (1976) description, appear to be the equivalent of T-units (i.e., a clause and its subordinate clauses), except when there are two coordinated clauses. These are to be counted as one sentence to allow the clinician to count the use of the conjunction. The grammatical categories analyzed include: (a) indefinite pronouns and modifiers, (b) personal pronouns, (c) primary verbs, (d) secondary verbs, (e) conjunctions, and (f) interrogatives. In addition to these specific categories, the children's use of negation and number is analyzed. However, negation is limited to some pronouns and negative sentences are not necessarily scored as more complex structures. Similarly, formulation of yes/no questions is not included in the analysis. The clinician is referred to the original article for a detailed description of the analysis procedures.

AGREEMENT OF NOUN AND VERB PHRASES

In morphosyntactic analyses, the clinician should first segment the sample into utterances or T-units, depending on the child's language level. Segmenting the transcript into utterances or T-units facilitates analysis at the morphosyntactic level.

Once segmentation is completed, the clinician can analyze the use of different morphosyntactic aspects within sentences. Because Spanish is a highly inflected language, it is important to analyze agreement of both verbs and noun phrases. Verbs need to agree in person (i.e., the subject and the verb conjugation should match). For instance, the verb phrase, *El se fue corriendo,* agrees in person with third person singular; however, if the subject was first person plural *nosotros,* the verb would not agree and therefore would be marked as incorrect. In addition to person agreement, verbs need to agree across sentences on person, mood, aspect, and tense.

Noun phrases should agree in number and gender (i.e., articles, adjectives, and nouns should match in number, as singular or plural, and in gender, as masculine or feminine). For instance, the article and adjective in the phrase, *la cosa rosada,* agree both in number, singular, and in gender, feminine, with the noun. However, the phrase *la casa blanco* fails to agree in gender. Lastly, the phrase *los tres carro* fails to agree in number with the noun. The noun or pronoun determines both gender and number for the phrase.

Agreement analyses for the verb and noun systems help in determining the nature of the language difficulties the child is having (i.e., whether there are specific problems with the verb, the noun phrase, or both). The problem may lie in the use of pronouns, tense or aspect, gender agreement, plurals, number agreement, or person agreement. Once a frequency count of the different types of agreement errors is established in a 50-utterance sample, the clinician can determine whether the sample is deviant or normal.

ARTICLES

Articles have different uses in Spanish and English. The use of English articles may present problems for second language learners.

For example, monolingual Spanish speakers use the definite article to describe body parts, weights and measures, titles, and days of the week; it also precedes infinitives, generic nouns, clothing, and abstract nouns. In addition, Spanish speakers tend to use the definite article with exophoric reference more frequently than English (Restrepo, 1992). Indefinite articles, on the other hand, are used less frequently in Spanish than in English. They are used to differentiate definiteness and indefiniteness and they precede qualified abstract nouns. Thus, when a clinician analyzes whether a child uses articles appropriately in spontaneous speech, if the clinician uses English as the basis, he or she may think that the child is overusing the definite article. However, a clinician should keep in mind that a child learning to speak both languages may use a combination of English and Spanish rules.

Difficulties with article use may include omissions of the article or substitution of the article because of number or gender agreement errors. In addition, the article may be used incorrectly by providing the wrong definite or indefinite form, and in turn confusing whether a referent has been presented or not. Thus, the clinician needs to indicate what type of difficulty the child has and whether article use is influenced by the second language. For example, a child with specific language impairment may omit unstressed articles such as *un*. A child who speaks both languages may use the possessive pronoun with body parts instead of the definite pronoun (i.e., *me voy a lavar mis manos/las manos*; I am going to wash my hands/the hands). A school-age child may use the definite article to introduce new information, thus making a reference error.

Schnell de Acedo (1994) reported that, although articles appear to be well developed by age 3 in Spanish monolinguals, investigators using bilingual children as subjects have noted article errors well beyond this age. She explains that these errors may occur in part because the bilingual children had been exposed to English and Spanish early in their development. In addition, Lopez-Ornat (1988) believes that the problem may exist because the analyses do not differentiate between article-noun agreement and article-adjective-noun agreement. Thus, structure of the language and the languages the child speaks should always be considered when analyzing language samples and determining whether a child has a language deficit.

PREPOSITIONS

In addition to number and gender agreement, it is important to look at the child's use of prepositions. Unlike English, Spanish does not emphasize location as frequently as English. In Spanish, direction and location are expressed with verbs of direction and a general locative. In English, direction and location are explicitly expressed with prepositions (Slobin & Bocaz, 1988). Thus, to expect a Spanish-speaking child to express whether an object is in a specific location is not appropriate. For example, if a child is asked where the ball is, a response such as *en la caja* (in/on the box) would be correct if the ball is on the box. It would be inappropriate to expect the child to say *sobre la caja* (on the box). However, a child who speaks both English and Spanish may use both forms of coding location or path. For example, in the Southwest it is not uncommon to see the expression *se subio arriba* (went up up). In this expression, the child expresses direction with the verb and the preposition, which is not common in monolingual Spanish-speaking populations.

Spanish-speaking children with language impairment omit or substitute prepositions. One commonly omitted preposition is *a* (to); however, when transcribing a language sample, the clinician should attend to the possible prolongation of the vowel before the *a*, which would indicate that the child is using that form. For example, a child may say *se vaa ir* (subject is going to leave). This would indicate that the child is prolonging the *a* to mark the preposition *a* (to). Other children demonstrate difficulty with other prepositions such as *detras* (behind) and *abajo/debajo* (below). However, the difficulty is more semantic. That is, they do not understand the relational concept, and therefore use more substitutions. Thus, clinicians should categorize prepositional errors based on which preposition the error occurred on and the type of error to determine whether the difficulty is based on semantics or form. For example, a child may demonstrate substitution of prepositions such as *con* to indicate *en* (in/on). Thus, the child should work on the differences in meaning between the two concepts. In summary, omissions may occur when the preposition is unstressed, and substitutions may occur when there is uncertainty with the prepositional concept.

PRONOUNS

The correct use of pronouns is a difficult skill for children to acquire, especially at the discourse level. It has been reported that pronouns are well established in early preschool years; however, language analyses of normal school-age bilingual children indicate that they may still have difficulties at the discourse level, especially with gender agreement. Masculine forms appear to develop early and are used more frequently before the child can use all of the pronouns correctly.

To analyze pronouns, the clinician should count all of the obligatory contexts in which the pronoun should occur or the pronouns that are present in the language corpus. The clinician should then count the correct usage of the pronoun to determine a ratio of number of correct to number of total possibilities. Please note that elliptical phrases should not be considered obligatory contexts. The clinician then can establish the number and type of missing pronouns and the number and type of substituted pronouns.

STORY STRUCTURE

Several writers have described analyses of story structure (e.g., Stein & Glenn, 1979; Westby, 1992). Some analyses of story structure can be quite complex; however, there are some major components that a clinician can analyze that are not too complex and time-consuming. To complete this analysis, the clinician should attempt to obtain a story narrative. Procedures used to elicit story narratives vary. Therefore, the information included in the narratives varies according to the elicitation procedure, channel in which the story is presented, channel in which the child narrates, and context in which the narrative is being presented (Scott, 1988).

When analyzing narratives, the clinician should keep in mind that the child's cultural background influences the type of information in the narrative. For example, Slobin and Bocaz (1988) found that Spanish-speaking children tend to describe the result and imply the action. English-speaking children tend to describe the action and imply the results. Thus, Spanish-speaking children allow the listener to assume how events occur, and English-speaking children allow the listener to assume the end result. Spanish-speaking children also devote more attention to establishing the static locations of objects and participants in scenes. English-speaking children, in contrast, devote less attention to static descriptions and attend more to the elaboration of trajectories, leaving much of the arrangement to be inferred.

Westby 1992) adapted Stein and Glenn's (1979) story structure. To analyze story structure in a narrative, the clinician first needs to segment the story into T-units, as described above. The clinician can then categorize the T-units into the following categories:

Setting: sets the conditions for the events in the story.

Initiating event: initiates a reaction or response.

Reaction: characters react to the initiating event with overt reactions or attempts.

Consequence: the result of the characters' reaction.

Resolution: the characters thoughts of the consequence.

Ending or result: the child terminates the story.

Given the components of a story narrative, we may expect to find more information in the setting and result of Spanish-speaking children's narratives, whereas we may see more information in the action in the English-speaking child. Note that this information is not based on data, but on inferences from data, and thus further research is needed in this area.

The clinician also needs to understand the developmental aspects of children's narratives when analyzing story narratives. For example, preschool-age children develop narratives initially with an adult providing all of the contextual support. They then proceed to being independent and providing their own support (Eisenberger, 1988). In addition, children initially provide poor relations between sentences even if they use conjunctions, which initially serve to connect unrelated sentences and later develop to establish semantic relations. Children's early story narratives provide little background information to orient the listener. Thus, children's narrative story structures follow a developmental course.

ANALYSIS OF CONTENT

Language content is the objects, actions, and relations people talk about. All people learn to talk about objects, actions, and relations. Languages and cultures may differ in the vocabulary or the topics people use, but the content of what they say is the same across ages, languages, and cultures (Lahey, 1988). Thus, the description of language content in this section does not differ among languages because it is universal.

Lahey described three language content categories: (a) objects, (b) object relations, and (c) event relations. Objects refer to specific objects (i.e., dog, cookie, Martin are specific objects) and to classes of objects (i.e., dogs, cookies, people, virtues). Type/token ratios (TTRs) have been used to describe the diversity of a child's vocabulary; however, in several English studies, TTRs have been highly unreliable depending on the topic, length of the sample, context in which the sample is elicited, manner in which the sample is elicited, and knowledge of the listener (Hess, Haug, & Landry, 1989; Richards, 1987). Thus, the use of TTRs is not recommended as a vocabulary measure in Spanish either. Across cultures and languages, children do differ on the use of labels that are given to objects.

Object relations are relations of the object with itself, such as existence (*esta es una casa*/this is a house); in comparison to other objects, such as attribution (*la casa verde*/the green house); and in relation to other objects, such as in location (*la bola esta debajo de la mesa*/the ball is under the table). The reader is referred to Lahey (1988) for further detail on this topic.

Developmental data on content categories in Spanish, are not, to the authors' knowledge, available. The clinician is referred to Lahey (1988) for an overview of the development of the categories. However, the expression of these categories may be dependent on the complexity of the language required to express it. Therefore, the developmental hierarchy of categories in English may differ from Spanish.

COHESION

Cohesion analysis is often used to describe how well a person can maintain relationships between clauses. *Cohesion* is the process of establishing nonstructural semantic relations that exist within the text. Cohesion occurs when the interpretation of one element in discourse is dependent on another (Halliday & Hassan, 1976).

Cohesion ties are the elements in the text that establish cohesion. Ties link items below or above the clause whether they are related structurally or not. Halliday and Hassan (1976) in a seminal work described English cohesion. This type of analysis can be adapted to Spanish, although it is not exact because certain forms like determiners work differently in the two languages. There are five types of cohesion ties: reference, conjunction, causal, lexical, and ellipsis. The most clinically useful types of cohesion are referential and conjunction. In Spanish, elliptical cohesion is also important because it is maintained through agreement and is used more frequently than in English. Thus, the issues described above for agreement should be considered across sentences. **Referential cohesion** can be divided into three types:

Personal reference, which includes
personal pronouns: *yo, tu, el, nosotros, ustedes, ellos*
possessive determiners: *mi, su, tu*
possessive pronouns: *mio, suyo, tu*

Demonstrative reference, which includes demonstrative adjectives: *este, ese, aquel, en ese entonces*, etc.

Comparative reference, which includes *mas que, igualmente, menos que, mismo*, etc.

Conjunction cohesion ties the meaning of a previous sentence to the content that follows. There are four main types of conjunctions:

Additive conjunctions establish a relation of added information, similarity of meaning, and alternative meaning: *y, e, o, ni, que, ya, ademas, de la misma manera*

Adversative conjunctions establish a relation that is contrary to the expected: *sin embargo, mas, pero, aunque, sino, siquiera, con todo*

Causal conjunctions establish a relation that is a result, reason, or purpose: *que, porque, pues, pues que, puesto que, a causa de que*

Temporal conjunctions establish a relation that specifies time: *entonces, despues, eventualmente, finalmente*

Clinically, cohesion analysis helps clinicians determine how well a child determines and maintains semantic relations across sentences. When a clinician is doing cohesion analysis, he or she should analyze one type of cohesion at a time. For example, referential cohesion at the same time. The clinician should categorize all the ties, establish all the obligatory contexts in which ties should occur, and divide by the number of correct responses in those contexts. The number obtained indicates the percentage of successful cohesion ties. For example, if a 12-year-old child is successful in making referential ties in three out of nine attempts (33% of the time), the child demonstrates significant cohesion problems. The same procedure should be followed for each category. This allows the clinician to determine which aspects of cohesion is difficult for the child.

⊔

SUMMARY

The purpose of this chapter was to discuss elicitation and analyses procedures that may be used with Spanish-speaking individuals. A study of the elicitation practices used by speech-language pathologists revealed that conversations and a variety of narrative tasks were the primary procedures used to elicit language samples. The influence of culture on the use of narratives was discussed. The cultural roles of adults and children during conversation also has an effect on the language performance of children with clinicians. Suggestions for interacting with and eliciting language samples from preschool, school-age, and adolescents were recommended so that language samples are not based only on clinician-child conversations and narratives. Finally, Spanish language analyses for form, content, and use were discussed with the purpose of providing clinicians with analysis procedures that have been used in research and clinical practice.

Analysis of language samples is time-consuming, but the information that is gained in terms of developmental data and intervention goals outweigh the time and effort spent in completing these procedures. Because few Spanish tests are available, children and adults will benefit from the thorough analysis of their expressive language abilities.

⊔

REFERENCES

Cornejo, R. J., Weinstein, A. C., & Najar, C. (1983). *Eliciting spontaneous speech in bilingual students: Methods and techniques.* Las Cruces, NM: Educational Resources Information Center, Clearinghouse on Rural Education and Small Schools New Mexico State University.

Eisenberger, A. R. (1988). Learning to describe past experiences in conversation. *Discourse Processes, 8,* 177–204.

Fantini, M. (1985). *Language acquisition of a bilingual child.* San Diego, CA: College-Hill Press.

Gutierrez-Clellen, V. F., & Hofstetter, R. (1994). Syntactic complexity in Spanish narrative: A developmental study. *Journal of Speech and Hearing Research, 37*, 645–654.

Halliday, M. A. K., & Hassan, R. (1976). *Cohesion in English*. London, UK: Longman.

Heath, S. B. (1986). Social cultural contexts of language development. In *Beyond language: Social and cultural factors in schooling language minority students* (pp. 143–186). Los Angeles: California State Department of Education: Bilingual Education Office. Evaluation, Dissemination and Assessment Center.

Hess, C. W., Haug, H. T., & Landry, R. G. (1989). The reliability of type-token ratios for the oral language of school age children. *Journal of Speech and Hearing Research, 32*, 536–540.

Hunt, K. (1965). *Grammatical structures written at three grade levels* (Research Report No. 3). Champaign, IL: National Council of Teachers of English.

Kayser, H. (1985). *A study of speech language pathologists and their Mexican American language disordered caseloads*. Unpublished doctoral dissertation, New Mexico State University, Las Cruces.

Kayser, H. (1989). Speech and language assessment of Spanish-English speaking children. *Language,Speech,Hearing, Services in Schools, 20*, 226–244.

Kayser, H. (1990). Social communicative behaviors of language-disordered Mexican-American students. *Child Language Teaching Therapy, 6*(3), 255–269.

Kvaal, J. T., Fitzgerald, M. (1985). The relation between grammatical development and acquisition of 10 Spanish morphemes by Spanish-speaking children. *Language, Speech, Hearing Services in the Schools, 19*, 384–394.

Kvaal, J. T., Shipstead-Cox, S. G., Nevitt, S. G., Hodson, B. W., & Launer, P. B. (1988). The acquisition of 10 Spanish morphemes by Spanish-speaking children. *Language, Speech, and Hearing Services in Schools, 19*, 384–394.

Lahey, M. (1988). *Language disorders and language development*. New York: Macmillan.

Langdon, H. W. (1992). Speech and language assessment of LEP/bilingual Hispanic students. In H. W. Langdon & L. Cheng (Eds.), *Hispanic children and adults with communication disorders: Assessment and intervention* (pp. 201–271). Gaithersburg, MD: Aspen.

Lee, L. L. (1974). *Developmental Sentence Analysis*. Evanston, IL: Northwestern University Press.

Linares-Orama, N., & Sanders, L. J. (1974). Evaluation of syntax in three-year-old Spanish-speaking Puerto Rican children. *Journal of Speech and Hearing Research, 20*, 350–357.

Lopez-Ornat, S. (1988). On data sources on the acquisition of Spanish as a first language. *Journal of Child Language, 15*, 679–686.

Maestas, A. G., & Erickson, J. G. (1992). Mexican immigrant mothers' beliefs about disabilities. *American Journal of Speech-Language Pathology, 1*(4), 5–10.

McKaig, M. (1988). *Language skills of normal and language impaired kindergarten and first grade English-Spanish bilingual children.* Unpublished doctoral dissertation. The University of Oklahoma, Norman.

Miller, J. (1981). *Assessing language production in children.* Baltimore, MD: University Park Press.

Restrepo, M. A. (1992). Spanish and English cohesion: A contrastive analysis of the definite article in both languages. Unpublished manuscript.

Richards, B. (1987). Type/token ratios: What do they really tell us? *Journal of Child Language, 14,* 201–209.

Schnell de Acedo, B. (1994). Early morphological development: The acquisition of articles in Spanish. In J. L. Sokolov & C. Snow (Eds.), *Handbook of research in language development using CHILDES* (pp. 210–253). Hillsdale, NJ: Lawrence Erlbaum.

Scott, C. (1988). A perspective on the evaluation of school children's narratives. *Language, Speech, and Hearing Services in the Schools, 19,* 67–82,

Siguan, M., Colomina, R., & Vila, I. (1990). *Metodologia para el Estudio del Lenguaje Infantil.* España: Abril Editorial.

Slobin, D. A., & Bocaz, A. (1988). Learning to talk about movement through time and space: The development of narrative abilities in Spanish and English. *Lenguas Modernas, 15,* 5–24.

Stein, N., & Glenn, C. (1979). An analysis of story comprehension in school children. In R. Freedle (Ed.), *New directions in discourse processes* (Vol. 2, pp. 53–120). Norwood, NJ: Ablex.

Swisher, L. (1994). Language disorders in children. In F. D. Minifie (Ed.), *Introduction to communication sciences and disorders* (pp. 243–280). San Diego, CA: Singular Publishing Group.

Toronto, A. S. (1976). Developmental assessment of Spanish grammar. *Journal of Speech and Hearing Disorders, 41,* 150–171.

Westby, C. (1992). Narrative analysis. In W. Secord (Ed). *Better Practices in School Speech Pathology: Descriptive Nonstandardized Language Assessment Manual* (pp. 53–63). San Antonio, TX: The Psychological Corporation.

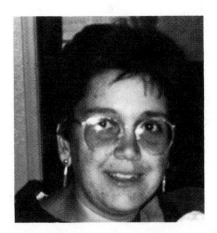

MARÍA ADELAIDA RESTREPO, M.A., CCC-SLP

Ms. Restrepo, who received her master's degree in 1986 from the University of Massachusetts, is a doctoral candidate in the Department of Speech and Hearing Sciences at The University of Arizona. Her primary interest is on the identification of language disorders in Hispanic children. She is currently involved in finding methods that accurately identify language impairment in Spanish-speaking children between the ages of 5 to 7. Her previous employment includes Bilingual speech-language pathologist at Holyoke Hospital in Holyoke, Massachusetts and in a private practice in Springfield, Massachusetts. In both positions, she served Spanish-speaking children and adults with speech and language problems. She has also worked at Carondelet Health Services in Tucson, Arizona, serving both children and adults, and has served as a consultant for their bilingual speech-language pathologists. She occasionally reviews materials with a multicultural focus for Communication Skill Builders.

PART III

CONCLUSIONS

The final chapter is a discussion of the importance for practicing bilingual and monolingual clinicians to become clinical researchers. The importance of reducing research bias with Hispanic populations and the necessity of researchers becoming culturally sensitive to the populations they study is discussed. Suggestions also are given on how clinicians may develop their own research abilities.

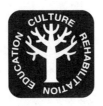

CHAPTER 13

RESEARCH NEEDS AND CONCLUSIONS

HORTENCIA KAYSER, Ph.D.

Culture should reside at the core of our understanding of research in virtually all aspects of deafness and other communication disorders. All communication, normal and pathological, is reflective of culture, and culture plays a significant role in how cultural groups define pathology, the priorities they place on various pathologies, the precursors of pathology for a particular group and appropriate strategies for culturally valid assessment and management. (Orlando Taylor, 1992, p. 2)

The research needed for working with children and adults from linguistically and culturally diverse populations with communication impairments is of a magnitude that is beyond description. Each of the authors of this textbook shared a segment of his or her research interests and activities, but much still needs to be investigated. In his review of over 200 articles in journals of speech, language, and hearing sciences published in the last 2 years, Glattke (1994) reported that none addressed the communication disorders of children and adults from culturally and linguistically diverse populations. The need for research quickly becomes evident to practicing clinicians when they attempt to provide assessment and intervention for these populations.

Research in communication disorders and sciences with multicultural populations is still in its formative stage primarily because of three factors. First, we do not have a cadre of minority researchers. Second, the research paradigms currently used by mainstream researchers in our profession are not compatible with the differences and needs of a culturally and linguistically diverse population. The third reason relates to the competency of existing researchers and their understanding of culturally and linguistically different populations. Some mainstream researchers have an interest, but they lack an understanding of biasing effects in their hypotheses, tasks, and interpretation of results. Competencies in addition to statistics and standard research methods are needed if research with Hispanics or any other group is to present a valid and an accurate representation of Hispanics. Each of these factors can be viewed as barriers to research (Cole, 1992) in communication disorders in multicultural populations, but each can also be viewed as needs for improvement in research training institutions.

This chapter will discuss issues concerning the need for new researchers and how clinicians can develop their abilities in clinical research. How established researchers must examine their research questions and designs for cultural biases will also be considered. Culturally competent researchers and their characteristics will be discussed. The final sections of the chapter will review research questions and needs that were discussed at a 1992 working conference on the Research and Training Needs of Minority Individuals sponsored by the National Institute on Deafness and other Communication Disorders. The participants in this working conference emphasized the need to train new and competent minority researchers and the need to educate existing and practicing researchers of the need for change in their own perceptions of research with culturally and linguistically diverse populations.

WANTED: RESEARCHERS

In speech-language pathology and audiology, the master's degree is considered the clinical degree and the doctoral degree is regarded as the research credential. Cole (1992) reported that approximately 3,000 members of the American Speech-Language-Hearing Association have doctorates in speech-language pathology and audiology. Only 188 of the ASHA members with doctorates are minorities. Only 356 members with doctorates describe themselves as full-time researchers. In this group, a total of 20 (0 American Indian, 2 Hispanic, 6 African American, and 12 Asian) minorities are full-time researchers in communication sciences and disorders. An additional 56 minority members with doctorates consider research as a secondary activity. Therefore, there are 76 minority researchers in the United States who may or may not be actively completing research with culturally and linguistically diverse populations. Of these 76, approximately 10 are Hispanic. Unquestionably, there is a paucity of minority researchers who can serve as role models and mentors. The American Speech-Language-Hearing Association has recognized this problem and recommended an assertive effort to recruit minorities into the professions as well into doctoral programs. Until doctoral programs can recruit, retain, and graduate Hispanic researchers in communication sciences and disorders, maybe our efforts to increase our knowledge about Hispanic populations should be toward retooling practicing clinicians' competencies in research.

A goal could be to retool clinicians who are actively providing services to Hispanic children and adults for research. The first objective for these clinicians would be to join forces with others in their work settings who have an interest in research. Hispanic and mainstream clinicians could be paired and mentored by researchers who have an interest in this area. Local universities may have faculty who would agree to be mentors for clinicians who are interested in developing and implementing research designs. These universities may also have programs to assist field researchers in their analysis and writing of projects.

If no local university or researcher is interested in collaborating in research, networking within the various ASHA groups such as the Minority Concern's Collective and the Hispanic Caucus are alternative resources for research mentors. Finding the right mentor will take time and may require that the clinician examine the potential mentor's background, research interests, and understanding of first and second authorship of manuscripts. Knowing a potential mentor's interests and strengths will increase the clinician's success and likelihood of finding a suitable mentor.

Other options for learning and mentoring relationships for clinicians include joining an ongoing research project or seeking out researchers in other disciplines such as second language acquisition, literacy, Spanish, bilingual, early childhood, and regular education. Their methodologies may be different from those used by speech-language pathology or audiology researchers, but the experience is invaluable.

In a hospital or clinic setting, there are pediatricians, neurologists, psychologists, neuropsychologists, and other medical professionals who may have an interest in research. Investigations could include a retrospective study of files or a case study of an individual child or adult. There are a number of possibilities, but the clinician must take the initiative in developing collaborative and mentoring relationships for research projects within his or her own clinical population and setting.

⊔

RESEARCH AND A PARADIGM SHIFT

Researchers in the field of communication sciences and disorders have traditionally used English-speaking middle-class individuals as control subjects in research designs. These subjects serve as the control group that are compared to the disordered group. This type of comparison has been extended to culturally and linguistically different groups who have now become the "new disordered" population (Cole, 1986). This experimental model has been used as the paradigm for research whereby comparisons are made between the middle-class English speaking "normal" and the minority group. Perspectives concerning subject selection, research design, and researcher competencies must shift if progress is to be made in our understanding of communication impairments in culturally and linguistically diverse populations.

SUBJECTS AS VICTIMS

Cole (1986) stated that it is all too acceptable for behavioral researchers to compare low socioeconomic level minorities with middle- and upper-class whites. The results of such research are predictable. The minority group is always lower, less able, and fails in comparison to the "normal" group. The hypothesis of "there is a difference" becomes a euphemism for "they are inferior" (p. 93). Cole (1986) has described this type of research as "victim analysis." This perspective in research perpetuates negative stereotypes, reduces behavioral expectations, and contributes to a self-fulfilling prophecy. That is, minority children will do poorly whatever the measure, task, or skill. Research with Hispanic populations has reflected this philosophy in cross-cultural comparisons, and this type of research continues to be offered as attempts to understand other cultures and languages. The argument is that there must be a norm or a standard to study variation. However, a counter-argument can be made that this type of design was not used for understanding English-speaking children and adults.

Cole (1986) has stated that it is the social responsibility of the researcher to ask him- or herself the following questions when conducting research and interpreting the findings:

1. Does the research question address a need among minorities?
2. Is the performance variable based on white middle-class expectations?
3. How can the hypothesis be examined without a victim analysis paradigm?
4. Are the findings interpreted in terms of a deficit theory?
5. Could the findings be misinterpreted to the detriment of minority individuals?

This self-examination of research questions and procedures is necessary so that the professions are not innundated with information that may be biased and invalid and increase the misunderstanding of persons from culturally and linguistically different backgrounds.

A RESEARCH PARADIGM SHIFT

Taylor (1992) and Saville-Troike (1986) have recommended that the study of culturally and linguistically diverse groups include an understanding of the culture. The research methodology that encourages the use of the culture's perspective in the research question is called ethnography. *Ethnography*, a branch of anthropology, is the science of describing a group and its culture through observation, interviews, notes in a diary, or a multitude of other data collection techniques (Lutz, 1980). This research methodology is inductive in that few explicit assumptions are made about relationships. In the experimental model, the researcher pursues a deductive research approach based on a priori assumptions about relationships (Taylor,

1992). Ethnographic research has no set assumptions, and the results and conclusions are interpreted from the perspective of the population under study. This research paradigm has been termed the ethnography of communication (Hymes, 1962).

Although this methodology may be viewed as subjective by experimental researchers, the study of culturally and linguistically different populations must include the perspective of the individuals who are studied. An experimental design must take into consideration the culture and its possible influence on the subjects. Adding the culture's perspective provides the framework from which to develop designs, tasks, and procedures that can measure the target behaviors that are of interest to the researcher and of importance to the community. Understanding the cultural impact on a variety of variables requires the researcher to become culturally competent.

⌐

THE CULTURALLY COMPETENT RESEARCHER

An interest in a culturally and linguistically diverse population is an important asset for a researcher, but it is only one of many characteristics necessary to become a culturally competent researcher. Taylor (1992) suggests eight attributes. The researcher knows that:

1. Truth is determined by the preceptor's culture. That is, each culture views what is true from its own experiences and beliefs.
2. Culture and cultural diversity should be part of every segment of research in communication sciences and disorders. This should include developmental, cognitive, epidemiological, normative, assessment procedures, and treatment efficacy research.
3. Research topics and what is researchable are culturally determined. What has been researched and may seem appropriate for English-speaking subjects may be inappropriate and offensive for the minority population of interest.
4. Research results are never generalized from one subgroup of minority subjects to a larger group of minorities or to the majority culture. These overgeneralizations are ethnocentric and do not consider variation within a culture.
5. The interpretation of the results by the researcher is culture-bound. Therefore, errors are inevitable without sensitivity and

knowledge of differences within and between culturally and linguistically diverse populations.

6. Issues, research designs, and instruments to measure independent variables are culturally driven. A task and its measurement may be appropriate for one group but insignificant for another group.
7. Culture must be taken into consideration when framing research questions, methodologies, and analyses.
8. Cross-cultural comparisons that examine cultural differences should be completed without contamination from variables such as socioeconomic status, gender, education, and geography.

There may be other characteristics and definitely skills that must be developed to become a culturally competent researcher. The researchers who have contributed to this textbook have all been trained with a sensitivity to culture and its effects on the investigation. The Latino researchers have also brought their innate sensitivity of what is appropriate, necessary, and important for research with Hispanic populations. We are still learning and, hopefully, taking notice of unacceptable assumptions that have slowly entered into our research designs from our past mentors and colleagues.

RESEARCH ISSUES

The National Institute of Deafness and Other Communication Disorders, one of the National Institutes of Health, invited researchers and research trainers to discuss research needs and training issues for minority populations. Individuals involved in training and research with minority subjects were asked to develop papers that addressed the most pressing needs in research in the major disorder areas, such as voice, language, fluency, and hearing. Each participant was asked to address two questions: What do we know? and What do we need to know? The following are summaries of the participants' responses to "What do we need to know?" The discussions concerning fluency, voice, and neurogenics will be briefly reviewed and other considerations for Hispanic populations will be provided.

WHAT DO WE NEED TO KNOW?

LANGUAGE

Kayser (1992) reported that there are methodological issues that must be taken into consideration before research questions can be successfully answered and later reported on issues that need to be addressed in children who are learning two languages. Studies reported in the last 20 years concerning Hispanic bilingual students and language impairments have had flaws in design, and therefore, their conclusions may be suspect.

McLaughlin (1984) has made suggestions concerning methodological issues in the study of normal bilingual populations. The same recommendations should be considered in the design of studies with Hispanic children and adults with speech and language impairments. He stated that the researcher should:

1. Look for bias in any form in the design of the study.
2. Critique the study's hypothesis for conflict with previous research. This is accomplished successfully only after careful study of the literature in childhood and adult second language acquisition.
3. Subject selection should include rigorous controls for any investigation with bilingual populations. The number, gender, and ages of subjects should be stated and kept to homogeneous groupings. Social roles are different for males and females in many Hispanic cultures; therefore, this variable should be monitored.
4. The socioeconomic status of subjects.
5. The educational background of the family and subjects should also be factors in the subject selection. Families with greater literacy and experental backgrounds may have different interactional styles and funds of knowledge that would influence language learning in the subjects.
6. Intelligence levels are important in language learning; therefore, the subjects should be described and controlled for intelligence levels. This requires nonbiased assessment of intelligence and possibly nonverbal measures.
7. He suggests that a detailed description of the bilingualism in the subjects be offered by the researcher. This should include information concerning the subjects' length of residency and the type of exposure to English.

8. The researcher may also include the proficiency levels of the subjects in each language.
9. If measures are used to describe the proficiency levels, a description of the test instruments, including reliability and validity is warranted.
10. Descriptions of language mixing and code-switching events should be noted and should also be important to the research.
11. An interesting area that McLaughlin believes should also be controlled within the study, is the attitude of the subjects and family toward bilingualism. A positive attitude toward the majority language may be a motivator for language learning and therefore would affect the dependent variable in any investigation.

Once these subject variables are controlled, there are three broad areas that should be research priorities (Kayser, 1992). The first area is the description of the various types of speech and language disorders in the bilingual child. The second is the assessment process itself, including alternative, innovative, and nonstandardized methods and models, and the third is the intervention and management of speech and language impairments in bilingual children.

DESCRIPTIONS

Minority language children who are monolingual Spanish-speaking and bilingual children should be described and studied within a communicative competency framework. The grammatical, sociolinguistic, discourse, and strategic competencies of these children must be studied in-depth and through collaboration with family and community members. These descriptions may follow the same broad age groups used in infant bilingual studies: simultaneous bilinguals, children under the age of three learning two languages in the home; preschool successive bilinguals, children who learn English after the age of 3 years; and school-age successive bilinguals children who learn English after the age of 5. The school-age population may be further subdivided into age groups that relate to the changes in classroom demands and curriculum. The age at which a second language is introduced does have an effect on the bilingualism of the normal child. We can only assume that age of acquisition of a second language will also affect the child with a language impairment. There must be systematic studies of child language disorders in bilingual populations in the same groups that traditionally have been used in the infant bilingual studies.

There are phenomena in language learning that occur only in bilingual communities. These phenomena can and do confound the study of bilingualism and do affect the diagnosis of a language impairment in the bilingual individual. These phenomena include interference or transference, language mixing, language loss, and code-switching.

Interference between the two languages has been studied in normal bilingual children and we know that the influence of one language on another may be a series of strategies that the child is using to acquire the second language. We do not know to what extent interference or transference of features of one language on the other has on both languages in bilingual children with language impairments.

Closely related to interference is the phenomenon of language mixing in young children. We know that normal populations do mix the languages but progressively separate the two language systems. How does mixing differ for the language-impaired child who is bilingual in form, content, and use, from the normal bilingual child? Does mixing continue for shorter or longer time periods for the language-impaired child? How can a retrival disorder be differentiated in discourse when the child is language mixing?

Code switching, the alternating use of two languages, has been observed in normal bilingual children and found to progress through a hierarchy of functions depending on the child's proficiency in the two languages and his or her age. The rules for code switching may not be salient for the language-impaired child. We know that bilingual individuals can identify appropriate code switching, but how do bilingual children with language impairments perceive and negotiate this sociolinguistic phenomenon within their community?

Language loss, the loss of the home language after exposure to a second language, is known to occur in normal bilingual children. Too often, if the child is losing one language and learning a second language, the child appears to lack proficiency in both languages. This area of study is problematic because children are often identified as language disordered during this stage of second language acquisition. How can language loss be differentiated in the child who is language impaired and the child who is simply in a stage of second language acquisition? Does the language-impaired child retain the first language longer than the normal bilingual child or does he or she lose the first language more readily?

ASSESSMENT

A greater understanding of child language impairments in bilingual populations would help in the assessment of bilingual children. It would be too simple to state that we need to develop appropriate and better test instruments for the infant-toddler, preschool, primary, and secondary school-age populations. What is needed is to look at the whole evaluation process to determine if a different model would better meet the needs of minority language children. In addition to tests, the literature suggests that we should also be determining the language status of the child, observing children in natural contexts, administering questionnaires to parents and teachers, and of course eliciting a number of language samples from the target child. All of these suggestions appear to be appropriate, but we do not have research that validates the use of any of these procedures. For example, we have not studied the effects of a variety of language sampling procedures with any bilingual children who are speech and language impaired. Questionnaires have been developed by many school systems, but it is not known if any have undergone item analysis and/or validity studies. There is much to learn about assessing bilingual children for language disorders.

INTERVENTION AND MANAGEMENT

A variety of treatment and management programs are popular in the profession. The frameworks used for these programs were developed for the monolingual English-speaking child. One approach to remediation that has received considerable attention is the whole language approach to language intervention. This philosophy of language learning has been studied in regular and bilingual classrooms and found to be successful with Hispanic populations and other groups. Will this approach be effective with bilingual populations who have language impairments? Will traditional therapy be more effective than a collaborative approach with bilingual populations? Because there are so few bilingual speech-language pathologists, what is the effect of providing therapy only in English to bilingual language-impaired populations? Would teaching English using English developmental norms be more effective in language learning than teaching English concepts that are already known in the child's first language? Would teaching language learning strategies to bilingual language-impaired children be more effective in language development than teaching English using traditional English as a second language methods? Second language teaching by clinicians to language-impaired children is practiced daily in this country, but we have no understanding of the effectiveness of these approaches.

Family and caregiver roles and their effects on interactions with language-impaired children is another area needing study. What is appropriate and acceptable counseling for these families, when a child is in a bilingual environment and the parent only speaks the minority language? How do we help the family facilitate language development in the developmentally delayed child? Intervention and management of language impairments in children who speak more than one language needs a tremendous amount of study.

Kayser (1992) presented primarily macro issues in assessment and intervention, but a number of micro issues also need to be studied, including conversational analysis; phonological, syntactical, semantic, and narrative development; and parent- and teacher-child interactions. The disorder areas of speech and language still must be defined for Hispanic populations.

FLUENCY

Conrad (1992) gave five recommendations for research among multicultural populations. She stated that we must: (1) determine what is normal fluency for each major cultural group; (2) identify what factors of normal fluency vary with cultural difference; (3) understand how fluency interacts with language learning (whether first or second language) and with attitudes and perceptions about individuals; (4) understand how the language of the culture facilitates or impedes treatment of that disorder as well as (5) which treatment procedures are more successful with subjects from a specific culture.

In addition to these areas, other basic information needed regarding Hispanic populations and fluency includes incidence information, including sex ratio; comparisons of stuttering in the first and second languages; fluency development in bilingual/bicultural children; stuttering predictors in bilingual/bicultural children; paralinguistic and linguistic influences on treatment targets; relationship between sociocultural variables and stuttering; and the client-clinician relationship and interaction (Watson, 1991; Watson & Kayser, 1994).

VOICE

Agin (1992) reviewed 50 years of literature concerning voice disorders and found that very few reported research with subjects from culturally and linguistically diverse populations. She stated what is assumed to be a disorder among Caucasians should not be assumed to be a disorder in another culture. Therefore, it is possible that some clinical methods and procedures traditionally used with dysphonic Caucasians may not apply to persons from culturally and linguistically different groups. Specific cross-cultural and cross-racial investigations of acoustic parameters, discourse variables, anatomical and physiological bases for diversity, incidence and variability of disorders, and assessment and intervention methods are research areas needed with diverse populations.

The few studies that have been completed with Puerto Rican and Mexican students indicate that there is a higher incidence of vocal nodules and hoarseness. Why this is a problem among Hispanic youth is unknown. Laryngeal cancer is known to have a higher incidence among African Americans after age 60. Because Hispanics generally have been counted as white in many studies, it is not known whether Hispanic adults have a higher incidence of laryngeal cancer than white populations.

HEARING

Scott (1992) gave seven recommendations for research: (1) epidemiological studies of auditory disorders across all racial groups; (2) studies in the change in hearing sensitivity as a function of age across all racial groups, including pure tone thresholds, speech thresholds, speech recognition skills, central auditory processing skills, and psychoacoustic abilities; (3) investigations on the effects of industrial and nonindustrial noise exposure on auditory thresholds on all racial groups; (4) examination of the role of the eustachian tube in the development of otitis media and other middle ear diseases; (5) studies on peripheral sensorineural hearing loss, including studies on the effects of sickle cell anemia; (6) service delivery issues among culturally and linguistically different groups; and (7) studies on the deaf cultures and sign language among different multicultural populations.

Hearing loss among young Hispanic children is a concern, because many of these children may not have access to medical assistance or may not be identified as having a hearing loss until the child is past the critical age for language learning (Hodgson & Montgomery, 1994). Issues such as cochlear implants, language barriers in assessment and management, as well as appropriate amplification are concerns for speech-language pathologists and audiologists.

NEUROGENICS

Wallace (1992) gave three recommendations to the working group concerning neurogenics. She stated that (1) formal investigations are needed to explore the occurrence and causes of communication disorders resulting from neurological impairment within minority groups; (2) investigations are needed to explore factors associated with prognosis and recovery for these populations; and (3) data are needed on the specific rehabilitation needs of culturally and linguistically diverse populations.

The assessment and intervention of Hispanic patients with neurogenic disorders have the same variables that will affect any bilingual community. Therefore, understanding the premorbid condition of the patient's language use, bilingualism, literacy, educational status, and so on (McLaughlin, 1984) are all important factors in the success and effectiveness of the assessment and intervention process.

⊔

SUMMARY

The purpose of this chapter was review the needs in research with Hispanic populations. The most important of these issues is the development of researchers among practicing clinicians. Clinicians can develop their abilities in research design with mentoring, coursework, and active participation with experienced researchers. Culturally competent researchers who understand that culture is at the basis of valid research designs, procedures, and subject selection are needed in all areas of communication sciences and disorders. Their questions should reflect what is important and necessary to know about the Hispanic cultures being studied rather than a comparison of their performance with white populations (i.e., victim analysis). Finally, current research needs extend from early intervention to adult neurogenics in all areas of speech and language impairments. The few researchers who are beginning the trek to understanding the speech and language of children and adults from Hispanic populations are recognizing that more researchers are needed to answer the many questions related to development, disorders, and assessment and intervention programs.

CONCLUSIONS

This book presentated ideas, experiences, and initial investigations by a few of the researchers interested in the communicative impairments of Spanish-English speaking children and adults. Their Hispanic focus included not only their research populations, but, for many of the contributors, their own Hispanic backgrounds, which helped to bring perspectives that may not be seen by mainstream investigators. Research generally generates more questions than it answers. Hopefully, the research presented here will see fruition in many journals in the near future. Also, we can hope that the many concepts that have been presented will serve as seeds for further investigation among clinical researchers in clinics, hospitals, and school settings.

REFERENCES

Agin, R. (1992, April). *Voice disorders in diverse cultural populations.* Paper presented to the Working Group: Research and Research Training Needs of Minority Persons and Minority Health Issues, National Institute on Deafness and Other Communication Disorders, National Institutes of Health. Bethesda, MD.

Cole, L. (1986). The social responsibility of the researcher. *ASHA Reports, 16,* 93–100.

Cole, L. (1992, April). *Cultural and institutional barriers to research careers in deafness and other communication disorders.* Paper presented to the Working Group: Research and Research Training Needs of Minority Persons and Minority Health Issues, National Institute on Deafness and Other Communication Disorders, National Institutes of Health. Bethesda, MD.

Conrad, C. (1992, April). *Fluency disorders in culturally diverse populations.* Paper presented to the Working Group: Research & Research Training Needs of Minority Persons and Minority Health Issues, National Institute on Deafness and Other Communication Disorders, National Institutes of Health. Bethesda, MD.

Glattke, T. (1994, April). *Culturally sensitive and appropriate research designs.* Paper presented at Challenges in the Expansion of Cultural Diversity in

Communication Sciences and Disorders conference of the American Speech-Language-Hearing Association, Sea Island, GA.

Hodgson, W. R., & Montgomery, P. (1994, May). Hearing impairment and bilingual children: Considerations in assessment and intervention. *Seminars in Speech and Language, 15*(2), 174–181.

Hymes, D. (1962). The ethnography of speaking. In T. Gladwin & W. C. Sturtevant (Eds.), *Anthropology and human behavior* (pp. 13–53). Washington, DC: Anthropological Society of Washington.

Kayser, H. (1992, April). *Child language disorders in bilingual populations.* Paper presented to the Working Group: Research and Research Training Needs of Minority Persons and Minority Health Issues, National Institute on Deafness and Other Communication Disorders, National Institutes of Health. Bethesda, MD.

Lutz, F. (1980). Ethnography—The holistic approach to understanding schooling. In Green, J. & Wallet, C. (Eds.), *Ethnography and language in educational settings* (pp. 5—63). Norwood, NJ: Ablex.

McLaughlin, B. (1984). Early bilingualism: Methodological and theoretical issues. In M. Paradis (Ed.), *Early bilingualism and child development* (pp. 19–45). Amsterdam: Swets and Zeitlinger.

Saville-Troike, M. (1986). Anthropological considerations in the study of communication. In O. Taylor (Ed.), *Nature of communication disorders in culturally and linguistically diverse populations* (pp. 47–72). San Diego: College-Hill Press.

Scott, D. (1992, April). *Hearing science and cultural diversity: What we know, what we need to know, and recommendations for NIDCD.* Paper presented to the Working Group: Research and Research Training Needs of Minority Persons and Minority Health Issues, National Institute of Deafness and Other Communication Disorders, National Institutes of Health. Bethesda, MD.

Taylor, O. (1992, April). *Research designs and methodologies that NIDCD should encourage and support for intramural and extramural research on people of color.* Paper presented to the Working Group: Research and Research Training Needs of Minority Persons and Minority Health Issues, National Institute on Deafness and Other Communication Disorders, National Institutes of Health. Bethesda, MD.

Wallace, G. L. (1992, April). *Adult neurogenic disorders.* Paper presented to the Working Group: Research and Research Training Needs of Minority Persons and Minority Health Issues, National Institute on Deafness and Other Communication Disorders, National Institutes of Health. Bethesda, MD.

Watson, J. B. (1991). Graduate seminar in stuttering. Texas Christian University. Fort Worth.

Watson, J. B., & Kayser, H. (1994). Assessment of bilingual/bicultural children and adults who stutter. *Seminars in Speech and Language, 15*(2), 149–164.

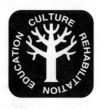

APPENDIX A

ENGLISH AND SPANISH PROFESSIONAL TERMINOLOGY

Terminology	Terminologia
academic achievement	aprovechamiento escolar
adaptations	adaptaciones
adaptive techniques	técnicas adaptativas
adaptive behavior	conductas adaptativas
adaptive tools	herramientas (de adaptación)
articulation	articulación
assessment	evaluación
assistive technology	tecnología de apoyo
at-risk children	niños en riesgo
audiogram	audiograma
audiological evaluation	evaluacion audiológica
audiology	audiología
auditory discrimination	discriminación auditiva
behavior management plan	plan de control de manejo de conducta
borderline	limítrofe (area fronteriza)
brain lesion	lesión cerebral
CEC=Council for Exceptional Children (U.S.)	Consejo para Niños Excepcionales
certification	certificación
child-find and screening	ubicación e identificación de niños
cleft palate	paladar hendido
cognitive development	desarrollo cognitivo
cognitive skills	habilidades cognitivas
Communication development	desarrollo de la comunicación
concrete experiences	experiencias concretas
consonants	consonantes
continuum	continuo
critical thinking	pensamiento crítico
deaf	sordo
delays	retrasos
developmentally appropriate	prácticas apropiadas para el desarrollo
practices	practicas

Terminology	Terminologia
diagnosis	diagnostico
dysphagia	disfagia
ear infection	infección del oido
ear (middle, inner, outer)	oido (medio, interno, externo)
early childhood	infancia
early intervention	intervención temprana
empower	aumentar potencial
enable	facilitar
enhance	acentuar/aumentar
excessive nasality	exceso de nasalidad
fetal alcohol syndrome	sindrome de alcoholismo fetal
fine and gross motor	motor fino y grueso
frenum	frenillo
gestures and signs	gestos y señas
goals and objectives	metas y objetivos
hearing impairment	impedimento auditivo
hearing loss	pérdida de audición
higher order thinking skills	procesos ejecutivos—variables de alto orden
hoarseness	ronquera
I.Q.	cociente intelectual
individual education plan	plan educativo individual
infant/toddler	infante
knowledge	conocimiento
language impairment	on alteración de lenguaje
larynx	laringe
learning problems	problemas de aprendizaje
learning disabilities	incapacidad de aprendizaje
lesson plans	planes de clase
life skills	habilidades para la vida
literacy development	desarrollo de la lectoescritura
literacy	lectoescritura
mentally retarded	retrasado mental

Terminology	Terminologia
modality	modalidades
moderate delay	retraso moderado
movement	movimiento
multi-handicapped	con discapacidades múltiples
multicultural	multicultural
muscular dystrophy	distrofia muscular
NABE=National Association of Bilingual Education (U.S.)	Asociación Nacional para la Educación Bilingue
neurological evaluation	evaluación neurológica
occlusions	oclusivas
omission (to omit a sound)	omisión (dejar de pronunciar un sonido)
otologist	otólogo (especialista del oido)
paralysis	parálisis
paraplegic	parapléjico
paraprofessionals	paraprofesionales
phonological disorder	desorden fonológico
phonological processes	procesos fonológicos
physical development	desarrollo físico
preschool	preescolar
problem-solving	procesos de resolución de problemas
procedures	procedimientos
psychological evaluation	evaluación psicológica
psychosocial	psicosocial
rationale	justificación
reading/writing development	desarrollo de la lecto estritura
resource-room	cuarto de apoyo pedagógico
screening	prueba de selección
screening process	proceso de detección
self-contained	auto contenido
service sites	clínicas de servicio
severe	severo
social skills	habilidades sociales

Terminology	Terminologia
socio/emotional development	desarrollo social y emocional
special education placement	ubicación en el programa de educación especial
speech/language delay	retraso de habla y lenguaje
speech/language pathology	patología del habla y lenguaje
speech/language evaluation	evaluación del habla y lenguaje
speech mechanism	mecanismo del habla
standardized tests	pruebas estandarizadas
strategies	estrategias
stutterer	tartamudo (a)
stuttering	tartamudear
substitution (to replace 1 sound for another)	sustitución (reemplazar un sonido por otro)
team	equipo
techniques	técnicas
tonsils	amigdalas
training	entrenamiento
treatment	tratamiento
transition	transición
visual discrimination	discriminación visual
visual impairment	impedimento visual
visual-motor	viso-motriz
velum	velo del paladar
vocal cords	cuerdas vocales
vocal exercises	ejercicios vocales
vocal intensity	intensidad de voz
vocal quality	calidad de voz
voice	voz
voice (harsh, strident, rough)	voz (aspera, estridente, ronco)
vowels	vocales
whole language	lenguaje integral

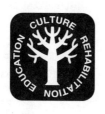

APPENDIX B

SPANISH CASE HISTORY FORM

HISTORIA DE HABLA Y LENGUAJE

IDENTIFICACION:

Nombre:_____ Fecha de nacimiento:_____

Domicilio_____

        calle   ciudad   estado   z.p.

Numero de telefono_____ Sexo_____ Edad_____

Referido por_____ Medico_____

DESCRIPCION DEL PROBLEMA:

Describa el problema del habla o lenguaje del niño (a)_____

_____

_____

_____

_____

_____

En su conocimiento, cuándo se dio Ud. Cuenta del problema?_____

_____

_____

_____

_____

HISTORIA DE LA FAMILIA:

	Nombres	Edad	Ocupacion	Educacion
Madre:				
Padre:				
Niños:				

_____

_____

_____

Otras personas:

_____

_____

_____

Que idioma(s) se habla en el hogar?_____

DURANTE EL EMBARAZO DE ESTE NIÑO (A) HUBO:

toxemia (envenenamiento de la sangre)_____

Diferencia entre los tipos de sangre_____

Diabetes_____

Sarampion Aleman_____

Enfermedades (mencione especificamente)_____

_____

_____

Golpes o heridas (mencione especificamente)

_____

_____

Medicación_____

radiografias (rayos X)_____

Hemorragias_____

Anemia_____

Otros_____

_____

_____

Fue este nino (a) prematuro?

Favor de indicar como fue este parto:

Normal_____

De operacion cesarea_____

Venía de pies_____

Otros_____

_____

Sufrio complicaciones en el embarazo?_____

_____

_____

Durante el primer mes su nino (a) tuvo . . . ?

Falta de oxígeno_____

piel amarilla_____

que pasar tiempo en la incubadora_____

    Por cuanto tiempo?_____

Problema al mamar or al comer_____

_____

Babeaba demasiado_____

DESARROLLO:
Escriba el edad cuando su nino/(a) . . :

se sentó solo_____

gateó_____

se paró solo_____

caminó solo_____

tuvo control del orin_____

Hubo algo en el desarrollo de su nino (a) que le preocupo durante los primeros 18 meses?

HISTORIAL MEDICO:
Enfermedades previas. (Favor de indicar la fecha y la edad del niño (a) cuando tuvo estas enfermedades, se es que las padecio).

Sarampión_____

Encefalitis_____

Meningitis_____

Viruela loca (varicela)_____

Paperas_____

Fracturas en los brazos o en las piernas_____

Fracturas en el craneo (descalabradas)_____

Contuciones (golpes)_____

Ingestión de veneno (tomo veneno)_____

Infecciones continuas en los oidos_____

Infeccion respiratoria_____

Pulmonía_____

Alergias_____

Otros_____

Describa las veces que fue hospitalizado, incluyendo las visitas a la sala de emergencia. Cual fue la razon de las visitas y la fecha?_____

_____

_____

_____

Describa la salud de su niño (a)._____

_____

_____

Tiene su nino?:

Defecto visual_____   Usa lentes?_____

Defecto del oido?_____   Usa aparato para oir?_____

Abertura en el paladar?_____

Defecto en la lengua, quijada, dientes, labios?_____

_____

Problemas emocionales o del comportamiento?_____

_____

Defecto físico?_____

HABLA Y LENGUAJE:

Hizo su niño (a) sonidos durante los primeros seis meses?_____

Que edad tenia cuando hablo su primera palabra?_____
Que edad tenia cuando empezo a usar dos o tres palabras combinadas?

_____

Por lo regular, cuantas palabras usa en frase hoy?_____

COMPRENSION: Indique si o no

    Entiende solamente movimientos expresivos_____

    Responde a mandatos simples o sencillos_____

    Responde a mandatos verbales complicados_____

EXPRESION:

    Se comunica principalmente por medio de acciones_____

    Conversa con frases simples_____

    Habla con palabras limitadas o frases sencillas_____

    Conversa a un nivel normal o avanzado_____

HABLA:

    Se da a entender solamente con los padres o familiares_____

    Se da a entender con otras personas_____

FLUIDEZ:

    Normal_____

    Repite palabras_____

    Repite sílabas_____

    Repite sonidos_____

    Prolonga sonidos_____

    tensión en la cara_____

Comprende (reconoce) su niño (a) que tiene problemas con el habla?
Si la respuesta es afirmativa, Cuando se dio cuenta?_____

_____

_____

Ha tratado de corregirse a si mismo?_____

Como lo ha hecho?_____

_____

Presenta este niño (a) algun problema de comportamiento?

    en casa_____

    en el barrio o vecinidad_____

    en la escuela_____

HISTORIA EDUCATIVA:
Escriba el nombre de las escuelas a las que haya asistido, incluyendo
las escuelas pre-escolares.

Escuela	Ciudad	Fecha	grado o ano

RESUMEN:
Si ud. fuera la persona que evaluara los factores que podrian estar
relacionados con los problemas de habla y lenguaje de su niño (a), que
mas agregaria?
Marque los factores que Ud. Cree que existan.

Problemas del oido_____   Problemas al tomar alimento_____

Problemas emocionales_____   Falta de amigos con quien jugar___

Parálisis cerebral_____   Falta de estímulo adecuado_____

Epilepsia_____   Problemas de comportamiento___

Disturbio visual_____   Retardo mental_____

Celos hacia los hermanos_____   Problemas del ambiente_____

Caprichudo (terco)_____

_____
Nombre de la persona quien lleno esta
forma

_____   _____
       Fecha   Cual es su relacion familiar con el
                                 niño (a)

Source: St. Mary's Hospital & Health Center, Tucson, Arizona, Texas Christian University, Fort Worth, Texas. Adapted by H. Kayser, 1994.

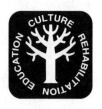

APPENDIX C

ENGLISH AND SPANISH PARENT LETTER

⊔

THE BILINGUAL CHILD

Becoming bilingual in English and Spanish is an ideal that many of us would like to have but do not always achieve. We constantly hear of the importance of knowing two languages for education, international trade, the military, and local businesses. With many of our Hispanic children, becoming bilingual is a natural occurrence within our school. Unfortunately, many of our children lose the ability to speak and eventually understand Spanish. As a parent who uses Spanish only in the home, or is bilingual, you may have concerns about speaking Spanish, learning English, school achievement, and what you can do to help your children during this time of learning two languages. This newsletter will provide some information that will help you understand bilingualism and how you, as a parent, can help your child to become bilingual.

PARENTS' ATTITUDES TOWARD SPANISH

For the Spanish-speaking parent, there are several attitudes about using Spanish. Some parents believe that only Spanish should be used in the home; others tell their children not to speak Spanish at all, to only use English. Some bilingual parents may use Spanish only when they want to keep a secret from the children; other bilingual parents actively use the two languages and expect the children to answer in the appropriate language. The rules parents make for using Spanish in the home will tell the child how important and valuable the language is to the family. The parent's attitude toward Spanish and the speakers of Spanish is one of the most important factors in whether the child will continue to use and learn Spanish as an adult. When the parents and the teachers tell the child with their actions and words that Spanish is not important, the child will probably do what comes naturally, use English, the language of education and the general community.

The child's loss of Spanish not only affects the child's communication with the family, but also his or her feelings about himself. The child not only loses Spanish, but he also loses ties with parents, grandparents, uncles, aunts, and his identify as an Hispanic. In many cases, children become anxious because they do not know which culture they belong to or which language they should use. With some children, losing the language causes emotional problems because of the loss of communication with the parents. Once the child loses his or her ability to communicate in spanish, the parents, extended family, and the Spanish- and English-speaking communities condemn the child for not keeping the language. Adults who lose their ability to speak Spanish, feel remorse at the loss of the language and often are alienated from the family and community. More and more parents are now realizing that bilingualism is beneficial and necessary for the family. The following are suggestions taken from studies on bilingualism, bilingual education, and language development in bilingual children.

HOW TO PROMOTE BILINGUALISM IN YOUR CHILD

1. Support a positive attitude toward the home language and the dominant language. This attitude comes from pride in your heritage and language and should carry over to the school and community. Make sure that the school promotes and encourages expression in English and Spanish.

2. Encourage cultural activities and events in the home, community, and the school. Part of bilingualism is becoming bicultural. These cultural events provide opportunity to talk about the culture, the traditions, history, and values of the people.

3. Encourage bilingual education in your schools. If your child receives only English for instruction, he or she may not be learning all that he or she can because of lack of understanding. If your child is not understanding in school, get help through bilingual education, tutoring through older siblings, or the schools.

4. Help the child learn about the community. Allow the child to visit the public library, recreation centers, churches, and other group organizations. This is where the child will learn English and all of its uses outside of the school.

5. Speak Spanish in the home. We know that when children learn Spanish in the home and are encouraged in Spanish to read, write, have discussions, ask questions, and are taught the correct use of Spanish grammar and vocabulary, they learn and have a good command of English. What is learned in the home transfers to English once the child has learned to speak English. What is being taught in Spanish is not just a language, but thinking skills and learning language through the use of that language. Children who are not encouraged to speak Spanish in the home do not learn English at a level that will help them to achieve in the schools.

Learning two languages is difficult even for children. Helping your child to become an active bilingual adult depends on the parents' attitudes and willingness to use and expose the child to both languages in many situations. If you have any questions or concerns about your child's speech and language development, see a speech-language pathologist near you. The speech-language pathologist in your child's school can offer more suggestions concerning activities on how to develop language in your child.

Hortencia Kayser, Ph.D.

⊔

EL NIÑO BILINGUE

Hacerse bilingue en inglés y español es un ideal que muchos de nosotros quisiéramos tener pero no siempre conseguimos. Constantemente oímos hablar de la importancia de saber dos lenguas para la educación, el comercio internacional, la milicia, y negocios locales. Con muchos de nuestros niños Hispanos, hacerse bilingue es una cosa natural dentro de nuestras escuelas. Desafortunadamente, muchos de nuestros ninos pierden la habilidad de hablar y con el tiempo pierdan la habilidad de entender español. Como un padre de familia que usa el espanol solamente en casa, o es bilingue, usted debe preocuparse de que su hijo hable español, aprenda inglés, salga bien en la escuela, y todo lo que usted pueda hacer para ayudar a su hijo durante este tiempo de aprendizaje de dos idiomas. Este boletin de noticias proveera algo de información que le ayudara a entender lo que es ser bilingue y cómo usted como padre de familia puede ayudar a su hijo a hacerse bilingue.

ACTITUDES DE LOS PADRES HACIA EL ESPAÑOL

Para el padre de familia que habla español, hay varias actitudes acerca de usar el español. Algunos piensan que el espanol debe de usarse solamente en el hogar, mientras que otros les dicen a sus hijos que no hablen español para nada, que usen ingles solamente. Los padres bilingues pueden usar español únicamente cuando quieren ocultar algun secreto de sus hijos, mientras que otros padres bilingues usualmente se valen de las dos lenguas y esperan que los hijos contesten en la lengua apropiada. Las reglas para usar el español en casa le diran al niño qué tan importante y valioso es el idioma para la familia. La actitud del padre hacia el español y los hispanoparlantes es uno de los factores más importantes si el niño va a continuar usando y aprendiendo español como adulto. Cuando los padres y maestros les dicen a los niños con sus acciones y palabras que el español no es importante, el niño probablemente hara lo que le viene mas natural, usar inglés, la lengua de la educación y de la comunidad en general.

La pérdida del español para el niño no solo afecta la comunicación del niño con la familia, pero también sus sentimientos hacia si mismo. El niño no solo pierde el español, sino que tambien pierde los lazos con los padres, abuelos, tios, tias, y su identidad como hispano. En muchos casos, los niños se ponen ansiosos porque no saben a qué cultura pertenecen o cual lengua deben usar. Con algunos niños, la pérdida de la lengua causa problemas emocionales debido a la pérdida de la comunicación con los padres. Una vez que el niño pierde la habilidad para comunicase en español, los padres, la familia extendida, las comunidades de habla hispana, e inglés condenan al niño por no mantener la lengua. Los adultos que pierden su habilidad para hablar español, sienten remordimiento por la perdida de la lengua y a menudo se separan de la familia y de la comunidad. Más y más padres se estan dando cuenta ahora que el bilingualismo es beneficioso y necesario para la familia. Las siquientes son sugerencias tomadas de estudios sobre bilingualismo, educación bilingue y el desarrollo de la lengua en niños bilingues.

COMO PROMOVER BILINGUALISMO EN SU HIJO

1. Apoye una actitude positiva hacia la lengua de la casa y la lengua dominate. Esta actitud viene del orgullo en su herencia y en su lengua y debe de continuar hacia la escuela y la comunidad. Asegúrese de que la escuela promueva y anime la expresión en inglés y en español.

2. Anime las actividades culturales y eventos en la casa, la comunidad, y en la escuela. Parte del bilingualismo esta en hacerse bicultural. Estos eventos culturales proveen la opportunidad de hablar acerca de la cultura, las tradiciones, la historia, y los valores de la gente.

3. Apoye la educación bilingue en sus escuelas. Si su hijo recibe solamente ingles en su instrucción, el o ella puede que no este aprendiendo todo lo que el o ella puede aprender debido a la falta de entendimiento. Si su hijo no esta entendiendo en la escuela, obtenga ayuda por medio de educacion bilingue, tutoría de sus hermanos mayores o de la escuela.

4. Ayude al niño a aprender acerca de la comunidad. Permita al niño que visite la biblioteca publica, centros de recreación, iglesias, y otras organizaciones de grupo. Aquí es donde el niño va a aprender inglés y todos sus usos fuera de la escuela.

5. Hable español en la casa. Nosotros sabemos que cuando los ninos apreden español en casa y son apoyados en español para leer, escribir, tener discusiones, hacer preguntas, y se les enseña el uso correcto de la gramatica y vocabulario españoles, ellos aprenden y tienen buen dominio del inglés. Lo que se aprende en casa se transfiere al inglés una vez que el niño ha aprendido a hablar inglés. Lo que se enseña en español, no es unicamente una lengua, sino habilidad para pensar y aprender la lengua por medio del uso de esa lengua. Los niños que no son animados a hablar español en casa, no aprenden inglés a un nivel que les ayude a desarrollarse en la escuela.

Aprender dos idiomas es dificil aún para los niños. Ayudar a su hijo a hacerse un adulto bilingue activo depende de las actitudes y la voluntad de los padres para usar y exponer al niño a las dos lenguas en distintas situaciones. Si usted tiene preguntas o inquietudes acerca del habla de su niño y del desarrollo de su lengua, consulte a un patólogo de habla y lenguaje cerca suyo. El patólogo de habla y lenguaje en la escuela de su niño puede ofreces mas sugerencias concernientes a actividades sobre como desarrollar la lengua de su niño.

Hortencia Kayser, Ph.D.
Traducido por Gilberto Hinojosa
          Tarrant County Junior College
          Claudio Milstein
          University of Arizona

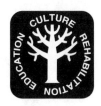

INDEX

A

American Speech-Language-Hearing
    Association (ASHA)
  bilingual speech-language pathology
    position statements, 1–13, 258
  Code of Ethics, 5
  Hispanic Caucus, 4, 293
  Minority Concern's Collective, 293
  minority membership in, 76
  Multicultural Issues Board, 4
  support personnel policies,
    209–211
Assessment of speech and language
    impairments, 243–265
  adapting tests, 253
  bias in, 249–252
  case history, 247–248
  clinician-child interaction, 260–261
  clinician's language proficiency
    and, 258–259
  data interpretation, 256–257

  dialect and, 259
  dynamic assessment, 255–256
  instruments for, 249–257 (*see also*
    Tests)
  observation, 248–249
  prereferrals, 244–245, 247–249
  procedure modifications, 253–255
  questionnaires, 248
  referral characteristics, 245–246
  research needs, 301
  testing procedures, 257–258
  translating tests, 258

B

Babbling, 23
Biculturalism, 7–9
Bilingual Language Proficiency
    Questionnaire, 248
Bilingual speech-language
    pathology, 1–13

Bilingual speech-language
   pathology *(continued)*
  academic competencies required,
   11–12
  ASHA position statements, 3–6, 258
  certification of, 6–7
  classroom role of, 141–146
  clinical practicum for, 9–10
  competencies required of, 6–11, 258
  defined, 4, 10
  development of, 10
  language competencies required,
   6–11, 258
Bilingualism, 160–167
  bilingual family types, 190–191
  code switching, 163–167
  definitions and descriptions, 161–163
  language impairments and, 192–202
  myths about, 185–192
  parent letter for prompting, 321–327

C

Case history form, Spanish, 313–319
Classroom intervention processes,
  129–146
Clausal word order, 52
Clinical practicum, 9–10
Code switching, 163–167, 170
  language impairment versus,
   165–167, 170
  research needs, 300
  vocabulary or word finding problem, 191–192
Complex sentences, 54–55
Consonants, 19–23
Conversation instruction, 139–141
Cultural speech patterns, 82–83
Cultural values, 78–82, 87
  interactional, 173–174
  language sampling and analysis
   and, 268–269
  locus of control, 172–173

relational patterns, 175–176
research needs, 291–306
time concepts, 173–174

D

Dialects, 20–21, 35, 43
  language assessment and, 259

E

Early intervention, 75–95
  case studies, 88–90
  cultural speech patterns, 82–83
  cultural values and, 78–82
  early language socialization, 78–82
  goals of, 86–88
  minority statistical problems,
   75–76
  program philosophy, 83–85
  service delivery, 85–86
English as a second language (ESL),
  130 (*see also* Language assessment
  and instructional programming,
  129–152)
Ethnography, 295–296

F

Fluency, 302

H

Hearing, 303
Hispanic demographics, 153–160
  age, 154–155
  cardiovascular disease, 157–158
  diabetes, 158
  education, 155
  family ties, 175
  geographic distribution, 154
  health care, 156–157
  income, 156
  infectious disease, 159–160
  trauma, 158–159

I

Inflection, 43–51, 58–61
Intelligence testing, 223–241
  Binet's scale and, 223–224
  court cases affecting, 225
  factors affecting performance,
    226–235
  heredity and, 224–225
  *Kaufman Assessment Battery for
    Children* (K-ABC), 232–233, 234
  language choice for testing, 236–238
  language proficiency and, 236–238
  nonverbal tests, 233–235
  *Stanford-Binet Intelligence Scale,
    Fourth Edition*, 226–227
  *Wechsler Intelligence Scale for Children,
    Third Edition* (WISC-III), 227–232
Interpreters, 207–222
  ASHA support personnel policies,
    209–211
  assessment and, 216–217
  conferences and, 217–218
  defined, 208
  intervention and, 218–219
  qualifications, 211–213
  training, 213–216
  translator, 208
  utilization of, 219

L

Language assessment and instruc-
    tional programming, 129–152
    (*see also* Assessment of speech
    and language impairments)
  case studies, 135–136
  classroom based, 137–141
  code switching, 165–167, 170
  mediated learning experience
    (MLE), 143–146
Language impairments, 192–202
  case studies, 195–202
  defined, 192–193
  diagnosis of, 200–202

  expressive language statistics, 195
  identification of, 192–195
  linguistic competency, 201–202
  research needs, 301–302
Language research needs, 298–302
Language sampling and analysis,
    265–286
  adolescents, 271
  articles, 277–278
  cohesion, 282–284
  content analysis, 281–284
  cultural factors, 268–269
  elicitation procedures, 266–274
  language analysis, 274–284
  morphosyntax, 275–280
  noun and verb phrases, 277
  prepositions, 278–279
  preschoolers, 269–270
  pronouns, 279–280
  school-age children, 269–270
  story structure, 280–281
Language socialization, 78–82
Limited English proficient (LEP)
    students, 129 (*see also* Language
    assessment and instructional
    programming, 129–152)

M

Mediated learning experience (MLE),
    143–146
Morphosyntactic development,
    41–74
  basic characteristics, 43–55
  case studies, 64–68
  grammatical development, 55–64
  inflectional morphology, 43–51
  syntactical development, 62–64
  syntactic structure, 52–55, 62–64

N

Narrative development and disorders,
    97–127

Narrative development and disorders
    (continued)
  age-appropriate interventions,
    116–118
  assessment, 103–104
  case histories, 119–123
  differences versus disorders, 115–116
  early narrative development,
    100–109
  family mediation, 104–109
  preschool narratives, 109–115
  school-age children, 118–123
National Institute of Deafness and
    Other Communication
    Disorders, 295
Negative sentence formation, 53
Neurogenic disorders, 153–182
  assessment and treatment, 167–171
  bilingualism and, 160–167
  case history taking, 168–169
  code switching and, 163–167, 170
  cultural factors, 171–176
  language choice for therapy,
    169–171
  research needs, 302
Non-English proficient (NEP) stu-
    dents, 129 (see also Language
    assessment and instructional
    programming, 129–152)
Noun phrase
  inflection, 60–61
  morphology, 50–51
  word order, 53

P

Parent letter, English and Spanish,
    321–327
Phonological development, 17–40
  assessment and treatment, 30
  babbling, 23
  case studies, 29–34
  consonant and vowel system, 18–21
  dialects, 20–21

normative data, 21–29
  preschoolers, disordered, 25–27
  preschoolers, normal, 25
  school-age children, disordered,
    28–29
  school-age children, normal, 27–28
  "standard" Spanish, 19–20
  two-year-olds, 24
  vowels, 23–24
Pronouns
  case, 47–50
  personal, 61–62
Public Law 99–457, 75

Q

Question formation, 54

R

Recitation instruction, 137–139
Research, 291–306
  culture competence, 296–297
  ethnography, 295–296
  fluency, 302
  hearing, 303
  language, 298–302
  minority research statistics, 293
  neurogenics, 304
  "victim analysis," 294–295
  voice, 302–303
Resource specialist (RSP), 130

S

Speech-language pathology. See
    Bilingual speech-language
    pathology
Syntax. See Morphosyntactic
    development

T

Terminology, professional, English
    and Spanish, 307–311

Tests
  adapting, 253
  Austin Spanish Articulation Test, 30
  *Assessment of Phonological
    Disabilities—Spanish* (APD-S),
    26, 30, 31, 33, 34, 35
  *Assessment of Phonological Processes—
    Spanish* (APP-S), 26, 28, 30, 65
  bias in, 249–253
  *Clinical Evaluation of Language
    Function*, 200
  *Development Assessment of Spanish
    Grammar*, 276
  *Escala Wechsler de Inteligencia para
    Niños-Revisada*, 227
  *Expressive One-Word Picture
    Vocabulary Test*, 81
  *Fundación MacArthur: Inventario del
    Desarrollo de las Habilidades
    Comunicativas* (IDHC), 104
  *Kaufman Assessment Battery for
    Children* (K-ABC), 232–233, 234
  *Leiter International Performance
    Scale*, 235
  procedures for, 257–258
  Raven's Progressive Matrices, 235
  *Sequenced Inventory of Communication
    Development*, 80, 81
  Southwest Spanish Articulation Test, 30

  *Spanish Structured Photographic
    Expressive Language Test—
    Preschool*, 65
  *Stanford-Binet Intelligence Scale,
    Fourth Edition*, 226–227
  *Test for Auditory Comprehension of
    Language*, 194
  Test of Early Language Development,
    200
  Test of Language Development, 200
  Test of Nonverbal Intelligence
    (TONI), 235
  Token Test for Children, 200
  translation of, 258
  *Wechsler Intelligence Scale for
    Children, Third Edition*
    (WISC-III), 227–232
  *Wechsler Intelligence Scale for
    Children Revised—Mexican Adap-
    tation* (WISC-RM), 130

Verbs
  conjugation, 73
  morphology, 43–47, 58–60
Voice, 302–303
Vowels, 23–24